T0200225

Postoperative Care Handbook of the Massachusetts General Hospital

A Lippincott Williams & Wilkins

Handbook

HB

Postoperative Care Handbook of the Massachusetts General Hospital

Sheri Berg, MD
Medical Director of the Post-Anesthesia Care Units
Staff Anesthesiologist and Intensivist
Department of Anesthesia, Critical Care, and Pain Medicine
Massachusetts General Hospital
Boston, Massachusetts

Edward A. Bittner, MD, PhD
Associate Professor of Anesthesia
Department of Anesthesia, Critical Care, and Pain Medicine
Massachusetts General Hospital
Boston, Massachusetts

Wolters Kluwer

Philadelphia • Baltimore • New York • London
Buenos Aires • Hong Kong • Sydney • Tokyo

Acquisitions Editor: Keith Donnellan
Editorial Coordinator: Lauren Pecarich
Production Project Manager: Bridgett Dougherty
Design Coordinator: Teresa Mallon
Manufacturing Coordinator: Beth Welsh
Marketing Manager: Dan Dressler
Prepress Vendor: S4Carlisle Publishing Services

Copyright © 2018 Wolters Kluwer.

All rights reserved. This book is protected by copyright. No part of this book may be reproduced or transmitted in any form or by any means, including as photocopies or scanned-in or other electronic copies, or utilized by any information storage and retrieval system without written permission from the copyright owner, except for brief quotations embodied in critical articles and reviews. Materials appearing in this book prepared by individuals as part of their official duties as U.S. government employees are not covered by the above-mentioned copyright. To request permission, please contact Wolters Kluwer at Two Commerce Square, 2001 Market Street, Philadelphia, PA 19103, via email at permissions@lww.com, or via our website at lww.com (products and services).

9 8 7 6 5 4 3 2 1

Printed in China

Library of Congress Cataloging-in-Publication Data

ISBN-13: 978-1-4963-0104-8
ISBN-10: 1-4963-0104-8

Cataloging-in-Publication data available on request from the Publisher.

This work is provided "as is," and the publisher disclaims any and all warranties, express or implied, including any warranties as to accuracy, comprehensiveness, or currency of the content of this work.

This work is no substitute for individual patient assessment based upon healthcare professionals' examination of each patient and consideration of, among other things, age, weight, gender, current or prior medical conditions, medication history, laboratory data and other factors unique to the patient. The publisher does not provide medical advice or guidance and this work is merely a reference tool. Healthcare professionals, and not the publisher, are solely responsible for the use of this work including all medical judgments and for any resulting diagnosis and treatments.

Given continuous, rapid advances in medical science and health information, independent professional verification of medical diagnoses, indications, appropriate pharmaceutical selections and dosages, and treatment options should be made and healthcare professionals should consult a variety of sources. When prescribing medication, healthcare professionals are advised to consult the product information sheet (the manufacturer's package insert) accompanying each drug to verify, among other things, conditions of use, warnings and side effects and identify any changes in dosage schedule or contraindications, particularly if the medication to be administered is new, infrequently used or has a narrow therapeutic range. To the maximum extent permitted under applicable law, no responsibility is assumed by the publisher for any injury and/or damage to persons or property, as a matter of products liability, negligence law or otherwise, or from any reference to or use by any person of this work.

LWW.com

RRS1708

William (Jay) Gerald Austen, MD
Associate Professor of Surgery
Massachusetts General Hospital
Boston, Massachusetts

Elisabeth M. Baker, NP
Massachusetts General Hospital
Boston, Massachusetts

Joanne E. Baker, MS, CNP
Nurse Practitioner
Department of Critical Care
Massachusetts General Hospital
Boston, Massachusetts

William Benedetto, MD
Assistant Anesthetist
Department of Anesthesia, Critical Care, and Pain Medicine
Harvard Medical School
Assistant Professor of Anesthesia
Department of Anesthesia, Critical Care, and Pain Medicine
Massachusetts General Hospital
Boston, Massachusetts

Sheri Berg, MD
Medical Director of the Post-Anesthesia Care Units
Staff Anesthesiologist and Intensivist
Department of Anesthesia, Critical Care, and Pain Medicine
Massachusetts General Hospital
Boston, Massachusetts

Alana B. Birner, RN
Massachusetts General Hospital
Boston, Massachusetts

Edward A. Bittner, MD, PhD
Associate Professor of Anesthesia
Department of Anesthesia, Critical Care, and Pain Medicine
Massachusetts General Hospital
Boston, Massachusetts

Kevin Blackney, MD
Department of Anesthesia, Critical Care, and Pain Medicine
Massachusetts General Hospital
Boston, Massachusetts

Katherine Boudreault, MD
Clinical Fellow in Neuro-Ophthalmology
Department of Ophthalmology
Massachusetts Eye and Ear Infirmary
Boston, Massachusetts

Yuriy Bronshteyn, MD
Assistant Professor of Anesthesiology
Duke University School of Medicine
Durham, North Carolina

Kathryn L. Butler, MD
Instructor in Surgery and Associate Director of the Surgical Clerkship
Harvard Medical School
Assistant in Surgery
Division of Trauma, Emergency Surgery, and Surgical Critical Care
Massachusetts General Hospital
Boston, Massachusetts

Dean Cestari, MD
Department of Ophthalmology
Massachusetts Eye and Ear Infirmary
Boston, Massachusetts

Jonathan Charnin, MD
Senior Associate Consultant
Department of Anesthesiology and Perioperative Medicine
Mayo Clinic
Rochester, Minnesota

Yufei Chen, MBBS
Clinical Fellow in Surgery
Department of Surgery
Massachusetts General Hospital
Boston, Massachusetts

Martha DiMilla, MS, RN, APRN, ACNP-BC
Department of Anesthesia, Critical Care, & Pain Management
Massachusetts General Hospital
Boston, Massachusetts

Carlos Fernandez-Robles, MD
Assistant Professor of Psychiatry
Massachusetts General Hospital
Boston, Massachusetts

Edward George, MD, PhD
Assistant Professor of Anesthesia
Massachusetts General Hospital
Boston, Massachusetts

Jeremy Goverman, MD, FACS
Assistant Professor in Surgery
Harvard Medical School
MGH Trustee's Fellow in Burns
Massachusetts General Hospital
Boston, Massachusetts

Rebecca L. Grammer, MD, DMD
Department of Oral and Maxillofacial Surgery
Massachusetts General Hospital
Boston, Massachusetts

Michael Hermann, MD
Department of Anesthesia, Critical Care, and Pain Medicine
Massachusetts General Hospital
Boston, Massachusetts

Mark Hoeft, MD
Larner College of Medicine
University of Vermont
Burlington, Vermont

Benjamin Hollingsworth, NP
Department of Orthopedics
Massachusetts General Hospital
Boston, Massachusetts

Ashlee Holman, MD
Assistant Professor
Department of Pediatric Anesthesiology
University of Michigan Health System
C. S. Mott Children's Hospital
Ann Arbor, Michigan

Ryan J. Horvath, MD, PhD
Instructor and Critical Care Fellow
Department of Anesthesia, Critical Care, and Pain Medicine
Massachusetts General Hospital
Boston, Massachusetts

Caroline B. G. Hunter, MD
Department of Anesthesia, Critical Care, and Pain Medicine
Massachusetts General Hospital
Boston, Massachusetts

Craig S. Jabaley, MD
Assistant Professor
Department of Anesthesiology
Associate Medical Director
Emory University Hospital
Emory University
Atlanta, Georgia

Christina Anne Jelly, MD
Department of Anesthesia, Critical Care, and Pain Medicine
Massachusetts General Hospital
Boston, Massachusetts

Haytham M. A. Kaafarani, MD, MPH, FACS
Assistant Professor of Surgery,
Harvard Medical School
Director, Patient Safety & Quality
Director, Clinical Research
Co-Director, Trauma Injury Prevention & Outreach Program
Division of Trauma, Emergency Surgery, and Surgical Critical Care
Massachusetts General Hospital
Boston, Massachusetts

Rebecca I. Kalman, MD
Department of Anesthesia, Critical Care, and Pain Medicine
Massachusetts General Hospital
Boston, Massachusetts

Tara Kelly, MD
Department of Anesthesia, Critical Care, and Pain Medicine
Massachusetts General Hospital
Boston, Massachusetts

Jean Kwo, MD
Assistant Professor
Department of Anesthesia
Harvard Medical School
Staff Anesthesiologist
Department of Anesthesia, Critical Care, and Pain Medicine
Massachusetts General Hospital
Boston, Massachusetts

Jarone Lee, MD, MPH
Medical Director
Blake 12 Surgical ICU
Surgery and Emergency Medicine
Massachusetts General Hospital
Harvard Medical School
Boston, Massachusetts

Erin J. Levering, NP
Multidisciplinary Intensive Care
Massachusetts General Hospital
Boston, Massachusetts

Mazen Maktabi, MB, BCh
Department of Anesthesia, Critical Care, and Pain Medicine
Massachusetts General Hospital
Boston, Massachusetts

John J. A. Marota, MD, PhD
Assistant Professor
Department of Anesthesia, Critical Care, and Pain Medicine
Massachusetts General Hospital
Boston, Massachusetts

Meredith Miller, MD
Department of Anesthesia, Critical Care, and Pain Medicine
Beth Israel Deaconess Medical Center
Boston, Massachusetts

Christopher R. Morse, MD
Assistant Professor
Department of Surgery
Massachusetts General Hospital
Harvard Medical School
Boston, Massachusetts

Yasuko Nagasaka, MD, PhD
Department of Anesthesia, Critical Care, and Pain Medicine
Massachusetts General Hospital
Boston, Massachusetts

Ala Nozari, MD, PhD, DEAA
Associate Professor
Department of Anesthesia
Harvard Medical School
Chief, Orthopedic Anesthesia
Department of Anesthesia, Critical Care, and Pain Medicine
Massachusetts General Hospital
Boston, Massachusetts

Roy Phitayakorn, MD
Assistant Professor
Department of Surgery
Massachusetts General Hospital
Boston, Massachusetts

Richard M. Pino, MD, PhD, FCCM
Associate Professor
Division Chief, Critical Care; Vice Chair for Regulatory Affairs
Anesthesia
Harvard Medical School
Department of Anesthesia, Critical Care, and Pain Medicine
Massachusetts General Hospital
Boston, Massachusetts

Elie P. Ramly, MD
Department of Surgery
Massachusetts General Hospital
Boston, Massachusetts

Nailyn Rasoul, MD
Clinical Fellow in Neuro-Ophthalmology
Department of Ophthalmology
Massachusetts Eye and Ear Infirmary
Boston, Massachusetts

Heather Renzi, NP
Massachusetts General Hospital
Boston, Massachusetts

Uma M. Sachdeva, MD, PhD
Department of Surgery
Massachusetts General Hospital
Boston, Massachusetts

Adeola Sadik, MD
Department of Anesthesia, Critical Care, and Pain Medicine
Massachusetts General Hospital
Boston, Massachusetts

Naveen F. Sangji, MD, MPH
Clinical Fellow
General Surgery
Massachusetts General Hospital
Boston, Massachusetts

William Schoenfeld, MD
Department of Anesthesia, Critical Care, and Pain Medicine
Massachusetts General Hospital
Boston, Massachusetts

Joseph Schwab, MD
Associate Professor
Orthopedic Surgery
Massachusetts General Hospital
Harvard Medical School
Boston, Massachusetts

Erik Shank, MD
Assistant Professor
Department of Anesthesiology
Harvard Medical School
Division Chief
Pediatric Anesthesia
Massachusetts General Hospital
Boston, Massachusetts

Milad Sharifpour, MD
Department of Anesthesia, Critical Care, and Pain Medicine
Massachusetts General Hospital
Boston, Massachusetts

Kenneth Shelton, MD
Department of Anesthesia, Critical Care, and Pain Medicine
Massachusetts General Hospital
Boston, Massachusetts

Tao Shen, MD
Clinical Fellow
Department of Anesthesia, Critical Care, and Pain Medicine
Massachusetts General Hospital
Boston, Massachusetts

Matthew Sigakis, MD
Clinical Lecturer
Anesthesia, Division of Critical Care
University of Michigan Medical School
Ann Arbor, Michigan

Bryan Simmons, MD
Department of Anesthesia, Critical Care, and Pain Medicine
Massachusetts General Hospital
Boston, Massachusetts

Matthew Tichauer, MD
Director, Division of Emergency Critical Care
Assistant Professor of Critical Care and Emergency Medicine
Department of Emergency Medicine, Traumatology & Critical Care
Hartford Hospital & Hospital of Central Connecticut
University of Connecticut School of Medicine
Hartford, Connecticut

Maria J. Troulis, DDS
Associate Professor
Director, Residency Program, Oral and Maxillofacial Surgery
Department of Oral and Maxillofacial Surgery
Massachusetts General Hospital
Harvard Medical School
Boston, Massachusetts

Elizabeth Turner, MD
Clinical Fellow in Acute Care Surgery/Surgical Critical Care
Division of Trauma, Emergency Surgery, and Surgical Critical Care
Massachusetts General Hospital
Harvard Medical School
Boston, Massachusetts

Andrew Vardanian, MD
Health Sciences Assistant Clinical Professor
Division of Plastic Surgery
University of California Los Angeles Medical Center
David Geffen School of Medicine at UCLA
Los Angeles, California

Connie Wang, MD
Department of Anesthesia, Critical Care, and Pain Medicine
Massachusetts General Hospital
Boston, Massachusetts

Daniel Dante Yeh, MD
Associate Professor of Surgery
DeWitt Daughtry Family Department of Surgery
University of Miami Miller School of Medicine
Trauma Surgeon
Ryder Trauma Center
Miami, Florida

Kevin H. Zhao, MD
Anesthesiologist and Intensivist
Anesthesiology Associates of Ann Arbor
Ann Arbor, Michigan

CONTENTS

Patient Care

SECTION I

Patient Care

Head and Neck Surgical Patient

Rebecca L. Grammer and Maria J. Troulis

I. INTRODUCTION

A. Demographics of OMFS and ENT Patients

Patients undergoing oral and maxillofacial surgery (OMFS) and ENT procedures vary in age from infants to elderly. Most procedures are scheduled and not emergent; thus, patients may be optimized from a medical perspective preoperatively. Acute life-threatening conditions that compromise the airway include infections or bleeding. Patients with acute infections have the potential for serious complications, particularly because many head and neck infections may affect airway patency. This is also true of intraoral bleeding or bilateral mandibular fractures. In these patients, often awake, fiberoptic intubation is a necessity, and patients may require prolonged intubation for airway protection and/or admission to the Surgical Intensive Care Unit for airway monitoring.

B. Disposition from the Operating Room

Postoperatively, most oral and maxillofacial surgery patients are extubated in the operating room and transferred to the postanesthesia care unit. Patients undergoing major maxillofacial operations such as orthognathic surgery or reconstruction after maxillofacial trauma are often admitted overnight for observation. Patients undergoing minor procedures, such as sinus surgery or dentoalveolar surgery, may be discharged home after recovery from anesthesia. Patients with intraoral incisions, who have had a bone graft, are maintained on a clear liquid diet for 48 hours postoperatively. Those patients undergoing maxillary or mandibular surgery requiring osteotomies or open reduction and internal fixation of fractures are maintained on a blended, "no chew" diet for 6 weeks postoperatively.

OMFS and ENT patients may require an ICU stay with or without intubation. Such cases include those with concern for severe airway edema, patients with prolonged intubation for long cases, extensive maxillofacial trauma, tongue lacerations, or obstructive sleep apnea. Rarely, patient may be placed in maxillomandibular fixation for immobilization.

II. COMMON POSTOPERATIVE PROBLEMS

A. Pain

Postoperative pain is expected after any surgical procedure, including maxillofacial surgery. The degree of pain depends on the type and extent of operation, individual pain tolerance, preoperative pain including severity, duration, and etiology (such as myofascial pain, headaches, temporomandibular joint [TMJ] pain, or trauma), and preoperative narcotic requirement. As well, systemic diseases such as fibromyalgia, connective tissue or autoimmune disorders, vascular disease, and diabetes may affect postoperative pain. Patients undergoing TMJ surgery, orthognathic surgery, surgical repair of facial fractures, or incision and drainage of extensive maxillofacial infections may have high levels of postoperative pain. Traumatic fractures are often less painful once the fractures have been immobilized. Postoperatively, pain is often well controlled initially with intraoperative local anesthesia, but as this wears off, intravenous and oral pain medications must be titrated for effect. Narcotic pain medications are often required in the postoperative period.

B. **Nausea/Vomiting**

Postoperative nausea is the most common postoperative complication of maxillofacial surgery, occurring in as many as 40% of patients and often resulting in vomiting. Risk factors include female gender, history of motion sickness, vertigo, migraines, and prior postoperative nausea and vomiting (PONV). TMJ and ear surgery can cause postoperative vertigo, which may contribute to nausea. Medications that may contribute include volatile anesthetic, narcotics, and antibiotics. Nasal intubation, maxillary osteotomies, turbinectomies, nasoseptoplasty, and sinus surgery cause postoperative bleeding with nasal and pharyngeal drainage. Some of this bloody drainage is swallowed, which causes significant irritation to the gastrointestinal tract, resulting in nausea. Postoperative placement of orogastric or nasogastric tube to suction the stomach before extubation may reduce postoperative nausea. Adverse consequences of nausea/vomiting may include wound dehiscence, bleeding, hematoma, dehydration, and aspiration. Anesthesia literature suggests multimodal approach to prevention and management of PONV.

C. **Swelling**

Postoperative swelling of the tissues is expected following maxillofacial surgery. Procedures involving the mandible, particularly those with extensive dissection on the lingual aspect, may cause swelling of the floor of mouth or oropharynx and, in rare cases, concern for airway compromise. Contributing factors may include length of operation, extent of dissection, surgical trauma, and patient factors, such as anticoagulation. Swelling usually peaks at 24 to 48 hours postoperatively. It begins to improve over 3 to 4 weeks, but may take longer in certain cases, such as orthognathic surgery. In cases where severe airway edema is expected, extubation may be delayed until the edema subsides. Depending on the procedure, methods to minimize postoperative edema may include applying ice to the face for the first 48 hours, keeping the head of bed elevated for 1 week, and administration of perioperative steroids.

D. **Ecchymosis**

Postoperative skin discoloration is common after surgery, particularly in maxillofacial surgery. This is a result of extravasation of blood subcutaneously. Ecchymosis will evolve from purple to green to yellow, similar to a bruise, will resolve in 2 to 4 weeks, and moves inferiorly with gravity.

E. **Hematoma/Hemorrhage**

Life-threatening bleeding is rare after most oral and maxillofacial surgery. Incidence has been reported between 1% and 12.5%. Severe hypertension in the postoperative period for patients on therapeutic anticoagulation may contribute to postoperative bleeding. Most hematomas are minor; however, floor of mouth hematoma may cause airway obstruction. Postoperative bleeding can usually be controlled with compression or occlusive suturing. Rarely, vessel ligation or embolization is needed.

F. **Nasal Airway Obstruction**

After maxillofacial surgery, it is common for patients to experience postoperative nasal obstruction, particularly after maxillary/LeFort osteotomy, turbinectomy, nasoseptoplasty, sinus surgery, rhinoplasty, or nasotracheal intubation. Airway obstruction is caused by postoperative edema, nasal secretions, postoperative nasal/sinus bleeding, and anatomic variation. Secretions can be suctioned from the nose postoperatively, and in some cases nasal trumpet may be needed. Postoperatively, patients can be monitored with pulse oximetry to evaluate oxygenation. As well, adjunctive measures that help with nasal airway obstruction include keeping head of bed elevated, and humidified oxygen by face tent to keep the mucous membranes moist. Nasal sprays, including saline, phenylephrine, or oxymetazoline, decrease nasal mucosal swelling and minimize secretions in the immediate postoperative period. Systemic antihistamines or pseudoephedrine may also decrease nasal secretions. Manual irrigation and debridement of the nose postoperatively to clean crust and secretions will assist with nasal obstruction.

G. Nasal Bleeding

Postsurgical bloody nasal discharge is anticipated after maxillofacial surgery involving the nose, maxillary sinuses, or maxilla. Examples of operations may include maxillary surgery including LeFort osteotomies, turbinectomies, and other sinus or nasal surgeries. The sinuses are often filled with blood after the procedure, and this is a natural process for clearing the blood from the sinuses. Patients can be treated with a decongestant, such as pseudoephedrine, and saline nasal spray. This usually occurs primarily in the immediate postoperative period and resolves by 12 to 24 hours postoperatively. Some blood-tinged drainage may last for 10 to 14 days postoperatively. In rare cases, more severe bleeding can occur. Anterior and posterior nasal packing should be placed to control the bleeding. Rarely, treatment may require embolization or vessel ligation.

H. Infection

Postoperative infections may develop in any surgical patient. As in all surgical patients, this is usually a later complication in the days following the procedure. Owing to the highly vascular anatomy of the head and neck, postoperative infections are less common than in other surgical sites. However, because of this anatomy, these infections are concerning because of risk of spread through local tissue planes or retrograde through valveless facial and angular veins. Early signs may include tachycardia, fever, edema, erythema, leukocytosis, and later purulent drainage from the incision. The initial management includes perioperative antibiotics and then, if needed, surgical intervention for incision and drainage.

Upper facial infections result from infections of the upper face structures including parotid duct, periorbital region, maxillary sinus, orbits, maxillary teeth, and parotid gland. For periorbital infections, one must evaluate for preseptal versus postseptal infection. Ophthalmology should be involved as needed. Lower facial infections are considered those localized to the buccal space or from the parotid duct, mandibular teeth, submandibular or sublingual salivary glands, lymph nodes, and floor of the mouth structures. These patients suffer from pain, swelling, and trismus. Maxillofacial infections are commonly caused by penicillin-sensitive organisms. In patients who do not respond to penicillin, the most common organism cultured is a resistant *Staphylococcus aureus*.

I. Sensory Nerve Injury

After maxillofacial surgery, branches of the trigeminal nerve may have been traumatized, resulting in temporarily diminished sensation or altered sensation. Affected structures depend on location of the operation, but may include lips, teeth, tongue, gingiva, nose, chin, or cheeks. In less extensive operations, diminished sensation may be because of local anesthesia and may recover within hours of the procedure. In more extensive operations, it may take up to 1 year for functional recovery, and in rare cases there may be permanent sensory deficit including anesthesia, dysesthesia, or paresthesia. Nerves most at risk include the lingual nerve, inferior alveolar nerve in cases of mandibular osteotomy, mental nerve in genioplasty, and, less frequently, infraorbital nerve in maxillary osteotomy. The hypoglossal nerve may also be affected, depending on the procedure, such as resection.

J. **Motor Nerve Injury**

Branches of the facial nerve may be injured during maxillofacial surgery, particularly during TMJ surgery and all operations via extraoral approach, particularly those using a submandibular incision. Injury to the facial nerve may result in weakness of the muscles of facial expression, appearing as facial droop. Up to 50% are related to nerve stretching, and injury is often temporary, but may be permanent.

III. **CONSIDERATIONS IN ENT AND OMFS PATIENTS**

A. Postoperatively, maxillofacial surgery patients are occasionally kept in maxillomandibular fixation (MMF) with wire or elastics. In some cases, a splint is secured to the upper or lower jaw postoperatively. Particularly for patients in MMF, heavy scissors or wire cutters must be at the bedside postoperatively. In the event of an airway emergency or aspiration event, the wire or elastics can be cut.

B. Because many maxillofacial surgery patients are numb, from anesthetic or nerve injury during the operation, they may have difficulty managing their secretions in the early postoperative period. Maxillofacial surgery patients should have a yankauer or soft suction at the bedside and head of bed elevated to 30 degrees or higher, at all times.

C. Owing to difficulty breathing through the nose, patients should have humidified face tent, both for supplemental oxygen and to keep the oral and nasal mucosa moist.

D. Patients having undergone maxillary or sinus surgery should be on strict sinus precautions. Sinus precautions include the following: avoid blowing the nose, only wipe nasal secretions; avoid sneezing or sneeze with mouth open; avoid drinking from a straw; avoid smoking; avoid heavy lifting; avoid bending over; keep head of bed elevated at all times.

E. Owing to numbness and swelling, patients have difficulty drinking from a cup. When patients are awake enough to tolerate an oral diet, clear liquid diet should be administered via a syringe connected to a long tube such as a rubber catheter or "sippy cup." Fluids can then be administered to the posterior oropharynx slowly in small volumes. Patients can be taught to feed themselves with this instrument or a spoon.

F. Nasal intubation is commonly used in maxillofacial surgery. Nasal intubation is best for all cases requiring checking occlusion, such as mandible or maxillary fractures, or orthognathic surgery. Oral intubation is usually indicated for maxillary and nasal surgeries. Other types of intubation used less frequently include tracheostomy or submental intubation, which may be indicated in panfacial trauma or patients requiring prolonged airway protection.

G. For patients on therapeutic anticoagulation, coagulation factors should be checked preoperatively, when applicable. As well, these patients are at high risk of bleeding intraoperatively and postoperatively. Local measures should be taken intraoperatively to prevent postoperative bleeding. As well, nasal intubation should be avoided if possible, because of the risk of nasal bleeding.

H. Pediatric ENT and maxillofacial surgery patients with congenital deformities and acquired maxillofacial deformities are often difficult to ventilate by mask and difficult to intubate. Face mask should be chosen for a careful fit, particularly in the setting of maxillofacial deformities. Anesthesia providers should be prepared for a difficult airway. Adjuncts include oral airway, nasal trumpet, and laryngeal mask airway. Consider awake or awake sedated fiberoptic intubation.

l. Controlled hypotensive anesthesia is often employed in maxillofacial surgery to reduce perioperative blood loss and operative time. Deliberate hypotension is described as a 30% decrease in mean arterial pressure, with systolic pressures in the 80 to 90 mm Hg range.

Suggested Readings

Alcantara CEP, Falci SGM, Oliveira-Ferreira F, et al. Pre-emptive effect of dexamethasone and methylprednisolone on pain, swelling, and trismus after third molar surgery: a split-mouth randomized triple-blind clinical trial. *Int J Oral Maxillofac Surg* 2014;43(1):93–98.

Brookes CD, Berry J, Rich J, et al. Multimodal protocol reduces postoperative nausea and vomiting in patients undergoing Le Fort I osteotomy. *J Oral Maxillofac Surg* 2015;73:324–332.

Dan AEB, Thygesen TH, Pinholt EM. Corticosteroid administration in oral and orthognathic surgery: a systematic review of the literature and meta-analysis. *J Oral Maxillofac Surg* 2010;68:2207–2220.

Geha H, Nimeskern N, Beziat JL. Patient-controlled analgesia in orthognathic surgery: evaluation of the relationship to anxiety and anxiolytics. *Oral Surg Oral Med Oral Pathol Oral Radiol Endod* 2009;108:e33–e36.

Jahromi HE, Gholami M, Rezaei F. A randomized double-blinded placebo controlled study of four interventions for the prevention of postoperative nausea and vomiting in maxillofacial trauma surgery. *J Craniofac Surg* 2013;24(6):e623–e627.

Phillips C, Brookes CD, Rich J, et al. Postoperative nausea and vomiting following orthognathic surgery. *Int J Oral Maxillofac Surg* 2015;44(6):745–751. doi:10.1016/j.ijom.2015.01.006.

Robl MT, Farrell BB, Tucker MR. Complications in orthognathic surgery: a report of 1000 cases. *Oral Maxillofac Surg Clin North Am* 2014;26:599–609.

van der Vlis M, Dentino KM, Vervloet B, et al. Postoperative swelling after orthognathic surgery: a prospective volumetric analysis. *J Oral Maxillofac Surg* 2014;72:2241–2247.

Wolford LM, Rodrigues DB, Limoeiro E. Orthognathic and TMJ surgery: postsurgical patient management. *J Oral Maxillofac Surg* 2011;69:2893–2903.

2 Ophthalmologic Surgical Patient

Elizabeth Turner, Nailyn Rasoul,
Katherine Boudreault,
and Dean Cestari

I. INTRODUCTION

The ophthalmic surgical patient can undergo either intraocular or extraocular surgery. Depending on the type of surgery that has been performed, different complications can result. In addition, different modes of anesthesia, including topical, regional, or general anesthesia, can be used. Topical and regional blocks have unique complications that are important to be aware of when managing the postoperative ophthalmic patient. The most common ophthalmic procedures and their operative and associated anesthetic complications will be discussed in the sections below.

II. OPHTHALMIC SURGERY

Ophthalmic procedures can generally be divided into intraocular and extraocular surgery. Intraocular procedures can include surgeries for cataract, corneal diseases, glaucoma, retinal repairs, and ruptured globe repairs. Extraocular procedures include strabismus and oculoplastic surgeries. Ophthalmic procedures are typically performed on an outpatient basis, and the patient is often discharged home from the postanesthesia care unit the same day. Depending on the type of procedure, different types of anesthesia may be required. General anesthesia is mandatory in cases of ocular perforation and intraorbital procedures.

A. Intraocular Surgery May Result in Pain and Discomfort if an Abrasion Exists

1. **Cataract surgery**

   a. Cataract surgery is performed when the natural intraocular lens becomes cloudy. In most uncomplicated cases, it is performed using only topical and intracameral (within the anterior chamber) anesthesia. The surgeon makes two small incisions through the cornea and uses phacoemulsification (powerful ultrasound) to remove the lens and place a synthetic lens in the eye. Wound closure often does not require a suture, but with complicated cases or with larger incisions, a small suture may be necessary. Patients are discharged from the hospital the same day with postoperative follow-up the following morning.

   b. Most complications of cataract surgery occur during the procedure itself (e.g., rupture of the posterior capsule occurs in approximately 1.9% of cases) and managed acutely by the surgeon.

   c. Early postoperative complications include:

      1. Corneal edema presenting as a decrease in vision and may result in pain and discomfort if an abrasion exists.

      2. Intraocular pressure spikes resulting in pain and nausea. This is uncommon, but can be seen if the viscoelastic substance used intraoperatively is not completely removed at the time of surgery. Additionally, low intraocular pressure can occur secondarily to a leaking wound, resulting in visual disturbances, often without pain.

      3. Uveitis (inflammation) typically presents with blurred vision, conjunctival erythema, discomfort and photophobia.

4. Endophthalmitis is an intraocular bacterial or fungal infection and is a severe and sight-threatening major postoperative complication. Fortunately, it occurs rarely in approximately 0.05% to 0.33% of cases, and usually presents 3 to 7 days after surgery. This is an absolute emergency and needs to be addressed urgently.

2. **Corneal surgery**
   a. Corneal surgeries include corneal transplants and refractive surgery. Performing a penetrating keratoplasty (corneal transplant) implies that the eye will be open to the air for a few minutes during the surgery, with risk of expulsion of the intraocular contents. Retrobulbar blocks are mandatory and sedation is often necessary. During an endothelial keratoplasty, only the deeper part of the cornea is replaced.
   b. Postoperative complications include:
      1. Weak sutures with or without leakage of aqueous humor resulting in hypotonia.
      2. Suture infections and endophthalmitis resulting in pain, photophobia, and visual impairment.
      3. Corneal erosions, graft rejection, and uveitis presenting with pain, photophobia, and decreased vision.

3. **Glaucoma**
   a. Glaucoma surgery is performed to decrease uncontrolled intraocular pressure that fails to respond to medical management. There are generally two types of glaucoma: open-angle glaucoma and closed-angle glaucoma. "Open angle" means that the angle where the iris meets the cornea is as wide and open as it should be. Glaucoma can result when the trabecular meshwork (the eye's drainage system) has become blocked, thereby increasing the intraocular pressure in the eye. When the angle is closed, it is the narrowness of the angle that blocks the trabecular meshwork from draining the aqueous humor, thereby increasing the intraocular pressure.
      In general, the purpose of glaucoma filtering surgery is to create a new drainage canal that allows external filtration of aqueous into the subconjunctival space. The aqueous can be drained via the conjunctiva (bleb) or through a device (tube shunt) and may be reabsorbed through the ophthalmic veins.
   b. Postoperatively, patients can experience temporary mild to moderate ocular discomfort and are discharged home the same day.
   c. Major early postoperative complications (i.e., those occurring in less than 3 months) include low intraocular pressure (from leakage of the conjunctiva, from excessive filtration, or associated with choroidal effusion), high intraocular pressure (from malignant glaucoma, pupillary block, or subchoroidal hemorrhages), infection (blebitis/endophthalmitis), hyphema (blood in the anterior chamber), or uveitis (inflammation in the eye).

4. **Trauma**
   a. Globe perforations need to be repaired under general anesthesia and the patient is typically admitted overnight. The mechanism of trauma itself as well as duration of the surgical repair may increase the risk of infection. Pre- and postoperative antibiotics are usually provided, as well as intravitreal injection of antibiotics, if there is a possibility that the vitreous may have been contaminated.
   b. Postoperative complications include those associated with intraocular surgery, such as corneal erosion, exposed or infected sutures, wound leakage with or without hypotony, elevated

intraocular pressure, and infections (endophthalmitis). Postseptal cellulitis is a rare complication.

5. **Retina**

   a. Retinal detachment, macular holes, complicated cataract surgeries with rupture of the posterior capsule and trauma are examples of indications for posterior segment surgeries. Retrobulbar anesthesia is performed in these cases to ensure complete akinesia of the eye, with analgesia of the intra- and extraocular contents. Patients are typically discharged the same day.

   b. The two main types of ocular surgery for retinal detachment repair are scleral buckle and vitrectomy.

      1. A scleral buckle is a piece of silicone, rubber, or semihard plastic placed on the sclera. The material is sewn to the eye to relieve vitreal traction on the retina. This allows the retinal tear to settle against the wall of the eye. Retrobulbar anesthesia usually precludes the development of the oculocardiac reflex (OCR) when the muscles are stretched or pulled. Patients may experience moderate pain postoperatively and may require pain medicine in most cases. Postoperative complications include double vision (usually resolving without treatment), infection (postseptal cellulitis), or failed retinal apposition.

      2. Pars plana vitrectomy is an intraocular surgery that involves removal of vitreous from the eye using three surgical ports through the sclera. In many cases, gas will be injected into the eye at the end of the procedure. Patients need to keep a specific head down position in order to keep the gas within the eye in the proper position. Postoperative complications include increased intraocular pressure, low intraocular pressure, infection (endophthalmitis), failure to reattach the retina, and inflammation (uveitis).

B. **Extraocular Surgery**

   1. **Strabismus**

      a. Strabismus surgery is used to correct misaligned eyes. Most surgeons operate under general anesthesia for the patient's comfort. The muscles, in one or both eyes, are detached from the globe, then either resected (strengthened) or recessed (weakened) to enable both eyes to orient in the same direction and maximize motility. It is a fairly well-tolerated surgery, and patients are discharged home the same day.

      b. One frequent intraoperative complication encountered by the surgeon and anesthesiologist is bradycardia associated with pulling or stretching of the extraocular muscles. Use of adjustable sutures has become a popular method of strabismus correction, and patients may experience significant vasovagal responses during the adjustment period, but this is not an issue once the patient is discharged home.

      c. Postoperatively, complications can include slippage of the reattached extraocular muscle. This often results in significant diplopia and limitation of eye movement, in the direction of action of the slipped extraocular muscle. This is often the result of a broken suture and the patient should be evaluated by his or her strabismus surgeon immediately. Infections such as intraorbital cellulitis or the development of abscesses are rare complications and tend to occur later in the postoperative course. A conjunctival granuloma can be seen as part of the chronic healing process as a result of a local reaction to the suture material and usually responds to topical corticosteroid drops.

2. Oculoplastic surgery

a. Eyelid procedures are typically performed under local anesthesia, whereas orbital procedures are performed under general and peribulbar anesthesia. Peribulbar anesthesia is also used to decrease bleeding by vasoconstriction. The development of a retrobulbar hematoma leading to visual impairment (by causing a compressive optic neuropathy) is a rare, but serious complication that can be associated with elective blepharoplasty and presents in the early postoperative period with proptosis, chemosis, and decreased vision. This is an ophthalmic emergency requiring urgent recognition and treatment with canthotomy and cantholysis. (I feel urgent CT would actually be a mistake here and fail to decompress the optic nerve STAT to restore vision).

b. Other major complications include infections, such as preseptal or postseptal cellulitis, or the development of abscesses.

III. PITFALLS OF COMMON OPHTHALMIC SURGICAL PROCEDURES

A. Extraocular Surgery

1. Oculocardiac reflex

a. Presentation/Signs

The OCR often presents with sinus bradycardia, but other arrhythmias have also been identified, including atrioventricular block, junctional rhythms, ectopic beats, ventricular tachycardia, and asystole.

b. Etiology

1. The OCR may result from traction or pressure on the globe, orbital contents, or extraocular muscles, and has been associated with cardiac arrests during ocular surgery.

2. The afferent stimulus begins at the ophthalmic division of the trigeminal nerve that synapses in the main trigeminal sensory nucleus. The second-order neuron then synapses with the visceral motor vagal nucleus. The third-order neuron, innervates the sinoatrial node resulting in bradycardia.

3. It is thought that retrobulbar blocks may prevent OCR by inhibiting first-order neural transmission.

c. Management

If the OCR is suspected perioperatively or postoperatively, the anesthesiologist should notify the surgeon to stop orbital stimulation, and optimize oxygenation and ventilation. Atropine may be considered in more severe cases.

2. Retrobulbar hemorrhage

Retrobulbar hemorrhage will be discussed in anesthetic complications.

3. Postseptal cellulitis

a. Presentation

Postseptal cellulitis may present as pain, red eye, blurred vision, double vision, eyelid swelling, infra- and/or supraorbital pain or hypoesthesia.

b. Signs

Signs of postseptal cellulitis include conjunctival chemosis and injection, eyelid chemosis and erythema, proptosis and restricted ocular motility with pain on attempted eye movement, and signs of optic neuropathy, such as decreased vision, afferent pupillary defect, and decreased color vision.

c. Management

1. Consult ophthalmology and infectious disease urgently.

2. Request imaging of the orbit (CT scan with contrast) to rule out the presence of an intraorbital abscess.

3. Start intravenous empiric antibiotics.

B. **Intraocular Surgery**
  1. **Endophthalmitis**
     a. Presentation
        Endophthalmitis presents with sudden onset of decreased vision and increasing eye pain 3 to 7 days after an intraocular surgery.
     b. Signs
        The signs begin with decreased visual acuity, inflammatory cells and fibrin in the anterior chamber which aggregate (hypopyon), decreased red reflex, corneal edema, intense conjunctival injection, and eyelid edema.
     c. Management
        1. Ophthalmology should be consulted urgently.
        2. The patient usually requires intraocular injection of antibiotics and, might need a vitrectomy.
  2. **Corneal erosion**
     a. Presentation
        The patient may present with a foreign body sensation, tearing, discomfort with blinking, sharp pain, or photophobia as soon as they wake up from the surgery or when the local anesthesia wears off. Infection at the site of erosion is unlikely in the early postoperative phase, but can occur if a corneal erosion is not managed well at the time of presentation.
     b. Signs
        Corneal erosion may cause moderate conjunctival injection and the cornea may be slightly hazy with mild eyelid chemosis.
     c. Management
        1. Obtain an ophthalmology consult.
        2. Never patch an eye with corneal erosion.
        3. Prescribe antibiotic ointment (e.g., erythromycin, bacitracin, or polysporin q4h) during the day and at bedtime, until the patient is seen by ophthalmology, or for a minimum of 2 to 5 days with resolution of the pain and improvement of vision.
  3. **Elevated intraocular pressure**
     a. Presentation
        1. High intraocular pressure may be secondary to pupillary block, retained viscoelastic material or lens particles, hyphema, pigment dispersion, and generalized inflammation after an intraocular surgery. The angle may be open or closed. The most common cause of elevated intraocular pressure postoperatively is undiagnosed preoperative open- or closed-angle glaucoma.
        2. Can present with decreased vision, constant ocular pain, colored halos around lights, frontal headache, nausea, and vomiting.
     b. Signs
        Signs of elevated intraocular pressure include moderate conjunctival injection, slightly hazy cornea, and fixed and mid-dilated pupil.
     c. Management
        1. Obtain an ophthalmology consult.
        2. The management will depend on the cause of the increased pressure.

IV. **COMMON ANESTHETIC-RELATED PITFALLS IN OPHTHALMIC SURGERY**
  A. **Topical Anesthesia**
     Topical anesthesia is the most common type of anesthesia used in ophthalmic procedures. For office procedures, ester agents, such as proparacaine hydrochloride 0.5% and tetracaine hydrochloride 1%, are often used. Subconjunctival lidocaine (xylocaine) (1% to 2%) (with

and without epinephrine) may be used to anesthetize a focal area of the ocular surface and for cataract surgery.

Complications of the use of topical anesthesia include:

1. **Hypersensitivity reactions**
   a. Patients treated with topical proparacaine or tetracaine during a procedure can rarely develop a hypersensitivity (or toxic) reaction, presenting as softening and erosion of the corneal epithelium, conjunctival congestion, and occasionally subconjunctival hemorrhage.
   b. Clinically, patients present with pain, photosensitivity, discomfort, and conjunctival injection.
   c. Further topical anesthesia should be avoided and lubricating agents may be used for treatment.
   d. Allergic reactions to topical anesthetics are rare, but have been reported mostly with the ester class of analgesics such as proparacaine and tetracaine. Patients will report itching, conjunctival injection, chemosis, and eyelid swelling. The practitioner should use the amide class of analgesics thereafter (such as lidocaine and bupivacaine), although corneal toxicity increases with this class of medications and, unfortunately, these are not available in topical solution.

2. **Cardiac conduction depression**
   a. Rarely, a toxic amount of lidocaine injected subconjunctivally can result in cardiac conduction depression.
   b. Practitioners should monitor for light-headedness, hypotension, and an irregular heart rate.
   c. Patients should be placed in a unit with cardiorespiratory monitoring and support if necessary.

3. **Central nervous system**
   a. Rarely, a toxic amount of lidocaine injected subconjunctivally can result in central nervous system (CNS) depression.
   b. Patients tend to present with drowsiness, weakness, and fatigue.
   c. Patients should be placed on a monitored unit to ensure cardiorespiratory and neurologic stability.

B. **Regional Anesthesia: Sub-Tenon's, Peribulbar, and Retrobulbar Blocks**

   In many ophthalmic surgical cases, topical anesthetics are not sufficient to provide the level of anesthesia necessary to perform the procedures. There are three types of regional blocks used in ophthalmic procedures: sub-Tenon's, peribulbar, and retrobulbar. All three blocks provide ocular anesthesia; however, the retrobulbar block also prevents movement (akinesia) and sight from the eye. Amide local anesthetics (such as lidocaine [xylocaine] and bupivacaine [Marcaine]) are preferred to ester agents for retrobulbar blocks because the amides have a longer duration of action and less systemic toxicity.

   A peribulbar implies the anesthetic mixture injected around the eye, but not within the muscle cone; therefore, the risk for intraocular injection, intraconal hemorrhage, and optic nerve damage is greatly decreased. Patients also maintain some level of vision during the surgery. Retrobulbar blocks, in contrast, temporarily extinguish vision because of placement of anesthesia within the muscle cone, resulting in impairment of neural conduction along the optic nerve.

   1. **Sub-Tenon's block**
      a. The sub-Tenon's block is performed using surgical scissors to create a small hole in the conjunctiva and the underlying Tenon's capsule. A cannula is inserted beneath the Tenon's capsule to infiltrate anesthetic solution. Sub-Tenon's blocks have lower complication rates in comparison to other regional anesthetic modalities.

  b. Complications from sub-Tenon's blocks include:
   1. Pain upon injection, chemosis, and subconjunctival hemorrhage, which occurs due to anterior spread of the local anesthetic agent and damage to minor blood vessels with the needle tip. These complications often resolve spontaneously without treatment.
   2. Very rare complications include globe perforation perioperatively, retrobulbar hemorrhage, myotoxicity, CNS depression from anesthetic spread, and chronic dilatation of the pupil.
2. **Peribulbar block**
   A peribulbar block is the infiltration of anesthetic mixture around the eye, but not within the muscle cone. It is completed with a shorter needle and produces anesthesia of the eye but not akinesia. The risk of accidental intraocular injection, intraconal hemorrhage, and optic nerve damage is far less than with retrobulbar blocks. Peribulbar blocks tend to present with more conjunctival edema, erythema, and subconjunctival hemorrhage because of the larger volume of anesthetic agent necessary and spread of the anesthetic agent more readily in a peribulbar block in comparison to a retrobulbar block.
3. **Retrobulbar block**
   A retrobulbar block is the injection of anesthetic within the muscle cone producing not only anesthesia, but also akinesia. There is also temporary loss of vision secondary to impairment of neural conduction along the optic nerve. Some complications for peribulbar and retrobulbar blocks are similar (Fig. 2.1).
   a. Retrobulbar hemorrhage
    1. This serious complication can occur following both intraconal and extraconal regional anesthetic blocks (as well as orbital surgeries), and results from bleeding (venous or arterial) posterior to the globe within the orbit. When comparing extraconal (peribulbar) versus intraconal (retrobulbar) injection techniques, a study has shown that the incidence of retrobulbar hemorrhages was 0.4% with peribulbar blocks and 0.7% with retrobulbar blocks.
    2. The most significant complication from a retrobulbar hemorrhage is loss of vision secondary to a compressive optic neuropathy resulting from a compartment syndrome.
    3. There has been discussion about the discontinuation of antiplatelet and anticoagulation prior to retrobulbar anesthesia to prevent retrobulbar hemorrhages in regional blocks. However, there does not appear to be a significantly increased risk of sight-threatening complications with maintaining these medications.
    4. Patients with retrobulbar hemorrhages present with proptosis, chemosis, acute pain, and decreased vision.
    5. Signs upon examination include high intraocular pressure, conjunctival injection, limitation of extraocular movements, and resistance to retropulsion.
    6. Retrobulbar hemorrhage is an emergency, and treatment must be initiated immediately to prevent permanent vision loss. When retrobulbar hemorrhage is suspected, ophthalmology should be consulted immediately and treatment should not be delayed. The surgical treatment is divided into two steps: (1) a lateral canthotomy; and (2) a cantholysis. With the use of Westcott scissors and forceps (with heavy teeth), an incision is made across the full thickness of the lateral canthus. The inferior eyelid is then grasped at the lateral edge and pulled upward, while

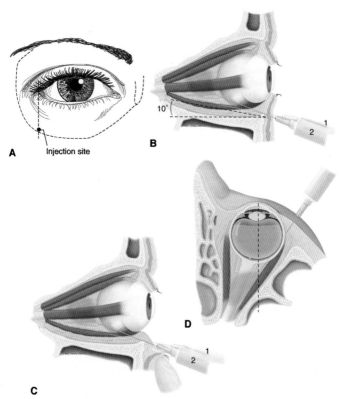

FIGURE 2.1 Retrobulbar block. A 1.25-inch, 25- or 27-gauge needle is inserted at the inferotemporal orbital rim at a point in line with the lateral limbus **(A)**. The needle is advanced tangential to the globe and parallel to the bony floor of the orbit, which inclines at an angle of 10 degrees from the transverse plane **(B1)**. Once the equator of the globe is passed, the needle is redirected upward and medially into the muscle cone **(B2)**. Either a transcutaneous **(B)** or transconjunctival **(C)** approach may be used. **D:** The midsagittal plane of the eye should not be crossed because the optic nerve lies on the nasal side of this plane. (Image Courtesy of American Academy of Ophthalmology.)

an incision is made medially toward the nose, until the canthal tendon is released, and the eyelid is free (Fig. 2.2).

b. Globe penetration and perforation
   1. Globe penetration and perforation can result in irreversible vision loss. The incidence of this result is approximately 0.2% following surgery.
   2. The most prominent risk factor for globe perforation following anesthetic infiltration is high myopia. Patients with posterior staphylomas are at increased risk of globe perforation because these patients have longer axial lengths, which increases their risk of perforation 30-fold.
   3. Other risk factors include enophthalmos, uncooperative patients, and prior scleral buckles.

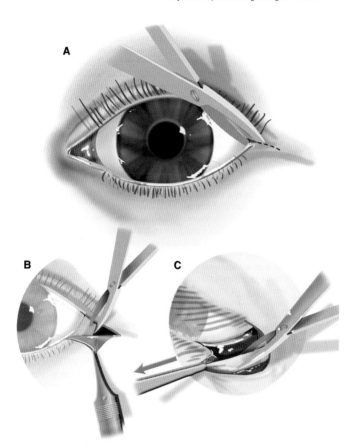

FIGURE 2.2 The figure demonstrates the surgical technique for a canthotomy **(A)** and cantholysis **(B** and **C)**. (From Ehlers JP, Shah CP, eds. *The Wills Eye Manual: Office and Emergency Room Diagnosis and Treatment of Eye Disease.* 5th ed. Philadelphia, PA: Lippincott Williams & Wilkins; 2008.)

4. Globe penetration and perforation present as severe eye pain and loss of vision. Upon examination, the intraocular pressure will be low and an entry and/or exit wound may be identified. However, many patients (up to 50%) may have no immediate symptoms. Ophthalmoscopy or ultrasound should be performed to assess the damage. Visual prognosis following globe penetration is often poor and retinal detachments may occur in conjunction with penetration, necessitating retinal surgery.

5. Ocular explosion/rupture of the globe is a very rare complication, which occurs when anesthesia is injected into the eyeball. Visual prognosis is poor, and patients often have light perception vision or worse.

c. Optic neuropathy
1. Injury to the optic nerve is a rare complication following regional anesthesia.

2. A postanesthetic optic neuropathy is thought to occur from direct needlestick injury to the optic nerve, resulting in pressure necrosis from the anesthetic solution or local hemorrhage within the nerve itself.

3. Risk factors for optic nerve damage include patients with small orbits, using a long needle, and the patient looking up during the time of the block (it is suggested that patients look straight ahead during retrobulbar blocks).

d. Muscle damage

1. Damage to extraocular muscles from orbital blocks can result in misalignment of the eyes resulting in binocular diplopia, ptosis, and entropion and/or ectropion (inversion or eversion of the eyelid).

2. Mechanisms for extraocular muscle damage include needle trauma to the extraocular muscle, ischemic pressure necrosis, and myotoxicity from the local anesthetic.

3. Transient double vision following peribulbar and retrobulbar blocks is relatively common and often resolves spontaneously. However, if diplopia or strabismus persists, then further evaluation is necessary. Often, in cases of permanent muscle damage, the inferior rectus is most susceptible.

4. Ptosis commonly follows ophthalmic surgery (whether performed with regional or general anesthesia) and, in 99% of cases, will resolve within 5 weeks. The mechanism of ptosis is likely levator dehiscence from the lid speculum or slight stretching during the surgical procedure.

e. Brainstem anesthesia

1. The sclera of the globe is contiguous with the optic nerve sheath surrounding the optic nerve. The optic nerve sheath is contiguous with the dura matter surrounding the CNS, thereby providing a continuous channel for local anesthetic to pass within the CNS if the integrity of the optic nerve sheath is disrupted.

2. Anesthetic spread within the CNS may occur if the needle punctures the optic nerve sheath when anesthetic is injected. A much less common mechanism is inadvertent injection within the orbital artery, and retrograde flow of anesthetic via the intracerebral arteries.

3. Symptoms often occur within the first 30 minutes following the injection. They can affect any part of the CNS, but most commonly result in decreased mental status, diplopia, amaurosis, focal neurologic signs, convulsions, and cardiopulmonary depression.

4. Treatment includes monitoring the patient and cardiopulmonary support as required. These patients should be monitored closely overnight to ensure CNS and cardiorespiratory stability.

Suggested Readings

American Academy of Ophthalmology. *Basic and Clinical Science Course, Fundamentals and Principles of Ophthalmology*. San Francisco, CA: AAO; 2009–2010.

American Academy of Ophthalmology. *Basic and Clinical Science Course, Lens and Cataracts*. San Francisco, CA: AAO; 2008–2009.

American Academy of Ophthalmology. *Basic and Clinical Science Course, Retina and Vitreous*. San Francisco, CA: AAO; 2008–2009.

Bryant JS, Busbee BG, Reichel E. Overview of ocular anesthesia: past and present. *Curr Opin Ophthalmol* 2011;22:180–184.

Ehlers JP, Shah CP, eds. *The Wills Eye Manual: Office and Emergency Room Diagnosis and Treatment of Eye Disease.* 5th ed. Philadelphia, PA: Lippincott Williams & Wilkins; 2008.

Eke T, Thompson JR. The national survey of local anesthesia for ocular surgery. II. Safety profiles of local anesthesia techniques. *Eye* 1999;13:196–204.

Kumar CM. Orbital regional anesthesia: complications and their prevention. *Indian J Ophthalmol* 2006;54:77–84.

Lip GYH, Durrani OM, Roldan V, et al. Peri-operative management of ophthalmic patients taking antithrombotic therapy. *Int J Clin Pract* 2011;65(3):361–371.

Schaller B. Trigeminocardiac reflex. A clinical phenomenon or a new physiological entity? *J Neurol* 2004;251(6):658–665.

3

Postoperative Care of the Thoracic Surgery Patient

Uma M. Sachdeva and
Christopher R. Morse

I. GENERAL CONSIDERATIONS

Patients who undergo thoracic surgery require close monitoring during the perioperative period and frequently spend the first postoperative night in the postanesthesia care unit (PACU) or surgical intensive care unit (SICU). Close attention must be paid to their respiratory, cardiac, fluid, and electrolyte status, because they are at risk for respiratory decompensation and cardiac arrhythmias that can result in significant morbidity and mortality if not recognized and treated early. In most institutions, patients who typically go to the SICU directly from the operating room for postoperative recovery include those who have undergone tracheal resection and reconstruction, esophagectomy, pulmonary decortication, or pneumonectomy. Most patients undergoing subtotal lung resection, including wedge resection, segmentectomy, or lobectomy, usually recover overnight in the PACU, which provides an increased level of care, and then transfer to the surgical floor on the first postoperative day. As such, these patients will be the focus of the remainder of this chapter.

II. PREOPERATIVE TESTING

Many patients undergoing pulmonary resection have multiple underlying comorbidities that increase their risk for complicated postoperative recovery, including chronic obstructive pulmonary disease (COPD), smoking, coronary artery disease, diabetes mellitus, and advanced age. Prior to surgery, it is essential that these patients undergo complete cardiac and pulmonary evaluation in order to develop appropriate anesthetic, operative, and recovery plans that are designed to minimize individual morbidity and mortality. Preoperative workup usually includes EKG, as well as echocardiogram and cardiac stress testing if there is history of coronary artery disease, heart failure, or other cardiac symptoms. Pulmonary function tests (PFTs) are routinely performed to predict postoperative residual respiratory capacity and dictate goals for recovery. PFTs are particularly important in patients undergoing pulmonary resection and contribute to determining the surgical approach. Often, routine PFTs are supplemented with ventilation/perfusion scanning and exercise testing in particularly marginal patients

Some data support that smoking cessation is best achieved 4 to 6 weeks prior to surgery in order to avoid a paradoxical increase in tracheobronchial secretions, which is thought to be caused by the regeneration of cilia that aid with mucous clearance. However, more recent studies have not found an optimal time frame for preoperative smoking cessation, but rather confirm that active smokers have a higher risk of pulmonary morbidity and mortality than those patients who had quit smoking preoperatively. It is therefore generally recommended that all patients attempt to quit smoking preoperatively, regardless of the time to surgery.

III. ANALGESIA

Adequate analgesia is critical to the postoperative recovery of lung function because inadequate pain control promotes atelectasis, mucous plugging, and inability to clear secretions, resulting in the development of life-threatening pneumonia. Most patients undergoing thoracotomy will have an epidural catheter placed preoperatively and receive a combination of local anesthetic and narcotic analgesia (most commonly 0.1% bupivacaine with 20 μg/mL hydromorphone or 2 μg/mL fentanyl) administered through both a continuous rate and a patient-controlled demand dose. In addition to improved pain control, thoracic epidural analgesia has been shown to improve clinical outcomes by reducing pulmonary morbidity, including atelectasis, hypoxia, and pneumonia, as well as reduce the rate of reintubation and the duration of mechanical ventilation if needed.

Although epidural analgesia is generally very well tolerated, the more common adverse reactions include pruritus, urinary retention, nausea, emesis, sedation, respiratory depression, and hypotension. High thoracic epidurals generally should not cause lower extremity weakness. If a patient does experience lower extremity weakness or tingling, the epidural infusion should be temporarily discontinued and leg strength assessed every 30 minutes. If the weakness does not improve, the anesthesia team must be immediately contacted due to concern for possible development of epidural hematoma or abscess. Pruritus will often improve with administration of antihistamines, but if persistent, can be treated by switching to an alternate opioid medication, administering the opioid agonist–antagonist nalbuphine hydrochloride, or removing the opioid entirely from the epidural infusion. Hypotension and sedation usually improve with decreasing the rate of epidural infusion, although it is not uncommon for patients to require low-dose vasopressor agents, usually phenylephrine, during the first 12 to 24 hours postoperatively. Urinary retention is prevented by placement of a urinary drainage catheter intraoperatively, which remains in place until the epidural catheter is removed. Epidural catheters are usually kept in place until removal of all thoracostomy tubes, or up to 5 days postoperatively.

Alternatives to epidural analgesia include paravertebral or intercostal nerve blocks or systemic opioid administration via patient-controlled administration (PCA) pumps. Patients who have undergone video-assisted thoracoscopic surgery (VATS) as opposed to open thoracotomy most commonly receive postoperative analgesia through PCA pump rather than epidural catheter. Nonsteroidal anti-inflammatory drugs such as ketorolac can also be given as an adjunct to opioids at doses of 15 to 30 mg every 6 hours if there is no concern for bleeding or renal insufficiency. Early and effective pain control is critical to improve pulmonary mechanics, minimize atelectasis, and allow for early patient mobilization, all of which have been shown to decrease morbidity, mortality, and length of hospital stay following pulmonary resection.

IV. PULMONARY TOILET AND EARLY AMBULATION

Promoting lung reexpansion and improving respiratory mechanics are critical during the postoperative period to prevent respiratory failure and pneumonia. Incentive spirometry should be taught early and encouraged regularly to minimize atelectasis. Chest physiotherapy, encouraging cough and deep breathing, and vibrational therapy can also assist with early mobilization and clearance of secretions. Early ambulation should be encouraged, and all patients should be walking by the first postoperative day. If possible, patients should be mobilized from bed to chair the night of surgery. Consultation with physical therapy is often helpful to assist with early mobilization and to assess discharge needs. In patients at risk for bronchospasm, scheduled nebulizer treatments with saline or bronchodilators, such as albuterol and ipratropium, can help promote deep breathing and air exchange. If there is concern for airway edema, steroids or racemic epinephrine nebulizer treatments can also be administered. If there is continued difficulty mobilizing thick or copious secretions, nasotracheal suctioning can be performed at the bedside or in the recovery room by an experienced provider. Early evaluation by respiratory therapists can be very effective for secretion management. Chest x-ray should be performed immediately postoperatively in the PACU, as well as daily throughout the postoperative course, in order to monitor lung reexpansion and to evaluate for pneumothorax, effusion, mucous plugging, or the development of pulmonary edema or pneumonia. If there is concern for declining respiratory status or increased secretions, workup should include arterial blood gas, chest x-ray, nebulizer treatments, evaluation by the respiratory therapist, and an immediate call to the thoracic surgeon or surgery team. Bedside bronchoscopy is sometimes required to assist with pulmonary toilet and remove inspissated mucous from the central airways.

V. FLUID BALANCE

In general, most patients undergoing pulmonary resection are kept with an even to minimally positive fluid balance in order to minimize postoperative pulmonary edema. Maintenance fluids are administered at a rate of 1 to 2 cc/kg/hour, with goal total fluid balance of no more than 1.5 L positive (20 cc/kg/day) during the initial 24 hours postoperatively. Almost all patients have a urinary catheter placed intraoperatively, and urine output is monitored closely within the first 24 hours postoperatively, with goal urine output roughly 0.5 cc/kg/hour. If urine output is adequate and there is no epidural in place, the urinary catheter is usually removed on the morning of the first postoperative day.

If hypotension is present, the patient should be assessed immediately for possible hemorrhage. Evaluation of the volume and character of the chest tube output, chest x-ray, and urine output is critical to determining whether a patient might be bleeding postoperatively. Output of over 200 cc of bloody fluid from the chest tubes for two consecutive hours often warrants return to the operating room for reexploration. If bleeding is suspected, complete blood count and coagulation studies (partial thromboplastin time, prothrombin time/international normalized ratio) should be followed, and blood products given as needed. If bleeding does not appear to be the cause of hypotension, and hypovolemia is still suspected, gentle fluid resuscitation may be undertaken. Fluid boluses should be low volume to prevent subsequent fluid overload and postoperative pulmonary edema, usually given as 250 cc boluses of normal saline or 5% albumin. If hypovolemia is not suspected to be the primary cause of hypotension, and the blood pressure does not improve with gentle fluid boluses and reduction of the epidural infusion rate (if present), patients may require temporary blood pressure support with vasopressors such as phenylephrine to ensure adequate tissue perfusion. In general, use of low-dose phenylephrine is preferred over excessive fluid administration in patients with postoperative low vascular tone. Maintaining an even to only slightly positive fluid balance minimizes postoperative lung injury, acute respiratory distress syndrome (ARDS), and pulmonary edema, as well as the development of postoperative atrial fibrillation (AF). On the night of surgery, oral intake is usually limited to clear liquids only, either as sips or ad lib. If the respiratory status is stable, diet advancement to a regular diet occurs on the first postoperative day, and intravenous fluids are discontinued as soon as oral intake is sufficient.

VI. CHEST TUBES

All patients undergoing pulmonary resection have at least one thoracostomy tube placed in the operating room prior to surgical closure of the chest.

The purpose of this drainage tube is to evacuate both air and residual fluid from the pleural space and to facilitate reexpansion of the remaining lung parenchyma. Chest tubes are placed to suction (usually –20 cm water) at the conclusion of the surgical procedure, and then transitioned to water seal when there is no longer evacuation of air from the pleural space. This may occur on the same postoperative day for smaller partial pulmonary resections, such as small wedge resections, where there is low concern for leak from the staple line. Alternatively, chest tubes may be placed to water seal on the first postoperative day following larger resections, such as larger wedge resections, segmentectomies, or lobectomies. Most chest tubes are removed on the first or second postoperative day if there is no residual air leak from the tubes when on water seal, output remains low, and the chest x-ray remains stable. Air leaks, if small, usually close spontaneously with time. If patients have a persistent or large air leak that does not resolve after several days with the thoracostomy tube to suction, further medical or surgical intervention may be required, such as chemical pleurodesis. Chest drains also serve to evacuate residual fluid or blood from the pleural space, and are important to monitor for postoperative hemorrhage during the initial postoperative period.

VII. DEEP VENOUS THROMBOSIS PROPHYLAXIS

All patients without a history of coagulopathy should receive prophylaxis for deep venous thrombosis (DVT) during the postoperative period. Prophylaxis is given subcutaneously with 5,000 units of unfractionated heparin twice daily if there is no concern for postoperative bleeding. This is continued throughout the hospital stay. Early ambulation is encouraged both to promote respiratory mechanics and to prevent development of DVT. If heparin is not tolerated or is contraindicated, an alternate anticoagulant can be given for prophylaxis, in addition to placement of compression stockings and pneumatic boots. DVT prophylaxis is particularly important in this patient population, because the development of pulmonary embolus that may accompany DVT can be serious and potentially life threatening in the setting of already-impaired respiratory capacity.

VIII. RESPIRATORY COMPLICATIONS

Respiratory failure is the most common complication following thoracic surgery and can be the result of airway edema, atelectasis, or inability to clear secretions. Adequate pain control and pulmonary toilet should be aggressively pursued to improve respiratory mechanics. If copious or thick secretions are unable to be cleared by these means or with nasotracheal suctioning, bedside bronchoscopy can be performed in the awake patient using topical analgesia (2% or 4% lidocaine via an atomizer or a nebulizer). If the patient is in distress, intubation may be necessary to maintain airway patency. Most patients undergoing larger pulmonary resections will have an arterial line placed preoperatively, and respiratory status can be closely monitored using arterial blood gas measurements if needed. As mentioned previously, if bronchospasm is suspected, albuterol and ipratropium nebulizer treatments should be administered. Racemic epinephrine or steroids can also be administered to decrease upper airway edema.

Pulmonary edema most commonly occurs with postoperative fluid shifts that occur 24 to 48 hours after surgery. Pulmonary edema can be diagnosed at any time by clinical exam and chest x-ray, and should be treated with diuresis as needed. As previously discussed, close attention to fluid balance within the first 24 hours after surgery is essential to minimize the likelihood of developing severe pulmonary edema that would result in significant respiratory compromise during the remainder of the hospital course. When pulmonary edema occurs postpneumonectomy, it is a critical and potentially life-threatening condition that must be treated aggressively within an ICU setting.

Rarely, patients can develop ARDS or acute lung injury following thoracic procedures. These conditions should also be treated in the ICU rather than the PACU or floor setting, because these patients need aggressive monitoring of their respiratory status and supportive measures that may include noninvasive ventilation or endotracheal intubation. The mortality associated with ARDS is 50% to 64% despite aggressive supportive measures, so if this condition is suspected, the airway should be secured and the patient transferred to the ICU immediately.

IX. CARDIAC COMPLICATIONS

Patients who undergo lung resection are at increased risk for postoperative cardiac events, most commonly arrhythmias, but also myocardial ischemia and infarction.

A. *AF* occurs following thoracic surgery at an incidence of 10% to 20% for lobectomy and up to 40% following pneumonectomy (Amar, 1998). Prolonged length of surgery, intrapericardial approach, bleeding, older age, and preexisting cardiovascular disease all increase the risk for postoperative AF. Prophylactic oral β-blockade can be given both pre- and postoperatively to decrease the incidence of postoperative AF, and has been shown in studies to decrease the rate of development of AF from 40% to 6.7%. Postoperative AF in a stable patient is usually treated with oral or IV rate-controlling agents, most commonly a selective β_1-receptor blocker, such as metoprolol. Calcium channel blockers such as diltiazem can also be used, and are first-line agents in patients with moderate to severe COPD or active bronchospasm. Digoxin can be used in combination with a β_1-blocker or calcium channel blocker if needed. Most patients will convert from AF back to sinus rhythm within 48 hours; however, a cardiologist should be consulted for refractory or persistent AF. If persistent, patients may be discharged home on a rate-controlling agent, with or without therapeutic anticoagulation. If patients become hemodynamically unstable with new-onset AF, they should undergo immediate electrical cardioversion and evaluation by a cardiologist. Electrical cardioversion can also be considered in patients with symptomatic AF within the first 24 hours of onset of tachyarrhythmia. Although amiodarone is an effective agent for management of postoperative AF, it is used only rarely in thoracic surgery patients given the higher incidence of ARDS, as well as the potential for worsening underlying pulmonary disease and development of pulmonary fibrosis with long-term use. Effort should be made to ensure that serum electrolytes, specifically magnesium and potassium, are also checked frequently and repleted as needed to a serum magnesium level of 2.0 mg/dL and a serum potassium level of 4.0 mEq/L.

B. *Myocardial ischemia* following thoracic surgery occurs at a rate of approximately 4%, with infarction incidence roughly 1.2%. Risk factors include a history of unstable angina, severe heart failure or valvular disease, or significant arrhythmias. If patients have these risk factors, they should undergo preoperative stress testing followed by angiography. Thoracic procedures are classified as high-risk procedures by the American College of Cardiology and the American Heart Association; therefore, it is extremely important to evaluate patients' cardiac status prior to surgery to minimize the chance of postoperative myocardial infarction. If a patient develops postoperative myocardial ischemia or infarction, these conditions must be recognized and treated immediately as per standard protocols.

C. *Cardiac tamponade* is a rare complication that may occur after open lobectomy because of unrecognized injury during operative retraction or dissection. More commonly, however, tamponade may occur following median sternotomy, such as undertaken for resection of a mediastinal mass. Suspicion should be raised in patients who develop hypotension following sternotomy or mediastinal dissection, or in postlobectomy patients who become hypotensive after administration of venodilating agents. Symptoms include low cardiac output, hypotension, elevated central venous pressure, and distant heart sounds. If there is suspicion for tamponade, patients should undergo emergent echocardiogram to evaluate for the presence of hemopericardium and to assess cardiac function. They should also undergo emergent chest x-ray, which may show cardiomegaly, or may identify an alternate source of bleeding, such as hemothorax. Treatment is emergent pericardiocentesis or placement of a pericardial drainage catheter, followed by surgical exploration to identify and repair the inciting injury.

D. *Cardiac herniation* is an extremely rare complication where the heart herniates through a surgically created defect in the pericardial sac. This complication has been reported following intrapericardial pneumonectomy or intrapericardial lobectomy. Symptoms include hypotension, jugular venous distention, ventricular fibrillation, or cardiovascular collapse, and suspicion should be raised in patients with sudden onset of superior vena cava syndrome and right-sided heart sounds. Treatment is either surgical closure or surgical enlargement of the pericardial defect to prevent recurrent herniation.

X. **BLEEDING**

Postoperative hemorrhage may be small and self-limited or may be larger and necessitate immediate return to the operating room for surgical exploration. VATS procedures have been reported to be associated with a slightly higher rate of postoperative hemorrhage (less than 2%) as compared with open thoracotomies (0.1% to 3%). This may be because of limitations in exposure provided by the minimally invasive technique (Iyer and Yadav, 2013; Peterffy and Henze, 1983; Sirbu et al., 1999; Krasna, Deshmukh, and McLaughlin, 1996; Yim and Liu, 1996). Nevertheless, this difference appears to be mitigated by the experience of the surgeon. Postoperative hemorrhage is assessed by closely monitoring the output of the chest tubes within the first several hours in the PACU. Drainage of more than 200 cc/hour for more than two consecutive hours or sudden drainage of a large volume of bloody output (more than 500 cc) is concerning for excessive hemorrhage that might necessitate surgical exploration. If bleeding is suspected, coagulation studies should be sent and any coagulopathy corrected with administration of fresh frozen plasma, coagulation factors, or blood products as needed. If bleeding persists after correction of coagulopathy, the patient should return to the operating room immediately for surgical exploration.

XI. **SUMMARY**

Overall, most patients who present to the PACU for recovery following thoracic procedures do quite well, and are able to transfer to the surgical floor on the first postoperative day. However, close attention must be paid to their fluid balance, respiratory status, pain control, and chest tube output during the first 24 hours after surgery. These patients are at higher risk for postoperative respiratory failure and cardiac events, so they must be monitored closely, with low threshold for transfer to the ICU if there is evidence of respiratory compromise, ARDS, or myocardial ischemia. Postoperative hemorrhage may necessitate return to the operating room for reexploration. Inability to clear tracheobronchial secretions may necessitate nasotracheal suctioning or bedside bronchoscopy. Most importantly, close communication between the PACU and surgical teams is essential during the early recovery period to address potential complications immediately and to develop effective treatment strategies that minimize in-hospital morbidity and mortality. Once patients have transferred to the surgical floor, recovery goals include chest physiotherapy, early ambulation, and treatment of AF and pulmonary edema if present. Patients are discharged home once all chest tubes are removed, pain is well controlled on an oral medication regimen, and cardiopulmonary status is stable.

Suggested Readings

Amar D. Cardiac arrhythmias. *Chest surgery clinics of North America*. 1998; 8(3): 479–93, vii.

Fleisher LA, Fleischmann KE, Auerbach AD, et al. 2014 ACC/AHA guideline on perioperative cardiovascular evaluation and management of patients undergoing noncardiac surgery: executive summary: a report of the American College of Cardiology/American Heart Association Task Force on practice guidelines. Developed in collaboration with the American College of Surgeons, American Society of Anesthesiologists, American Society of Echocardiography, American Society of Nuclear Cardiology, Heart Rhythm Society, Society for Cardiovascular Angiography and Interventions, Society of Cardiovascular Anesthesiologists, and Society of Vascular Medicine Endorsed by the Society of Hospital Medicine. *J Nucl Cardiol* 2015;22(1):162–215.

Frendl G, Sodickson AC, Chung MK, et al. 2014 AATS guidelines for the prevention and management of perioperative atrial fibrillation and flutter for thoracic surgical procedures. *J Thorac Cardiovasc Surg* 2014;148(3):e153–e193.

Iyer A, Yadav, S. In: Firstenberg M ed. *Principles and Practice of Cardiothoracic Surgery*. InTech; 2013:57–84.

Krasna MJ, Deshmukh S, and McLaughlin JS. Complications of thoracoscopy. *The Annals of thoracic surgery*. 1996;61(4):1066–9.

Kutlu CA, Williams EA, Evans TW, et al. Acute lung injury and acute respiratory distress syndrome after pulmonary resection. *Ann Thorac Surg* 2000;69(2):376–380.

Manion SC, Brennan TJ. Thoracic epidural analgesia and acute pain management. *Anesthesiology* 2011;115(1):181–188.

Peterffy A, and Henze A. Haemorrhagic complications during pulmonary resection. A retrospective review of 1428 resections with 113 haemorrhagic episodes. *Scandinavian journal of thoracic and cardiovascular surgery*. 1983;17(3):283–7.

Sirbu, H, Busch T, Aleksic I, Lotfi S, Ruschewski W, and Dalichau H. Chest re-exploration for complications after lung surgery. *The Thoracic and cardiovascular surgeon*. 1999;47(2):73–6.

von Knorring J, Lepantalo M, Lindgren L, et al. Cardiac arrhythmias and myocardial ischemia after thoracotomy for lung cancer. *Ann Thorac Surg* 1992;53(4):642–647.

Yim AP, and Liu HP. Complications and failures of video-assisted thoracic surgery: experience from two centers in Asia. *The Annals of thoracic surgery*. 1996;61(2): 538–41.

4

Vascular Patient

Elizabeth Turner

I. INTRODUCTION

A. Demographics of Vascular Patients

Every individual undergoes varying degrees of atherosclerotic changes to their arterial walls as they age. Whereas some individuals will never require vascular intervention, there are those with both unmodifiable risk factors (genetic predisposition) and modifiable risk factors (smoking) that will have progressive vascular disease requiring operative intervention.

B. Consideration of Patient Risk Factors

Risk factors for peripheral artery disease include, but are not limited to, increasing age, male sex, smoking, hypertension, hypercholesterolemia, diabetes, obesity, homocysteinemia, and a family history of vascular disease. Smoking and diabetes are the most influential risk factors in determining the severity of peripheral arterial disease.

C. Disposition from the Operating Room

Vascular surgery can range in complexity from day surgical procedures, such as a diagnostic angiogram, to more invasive peripheral artery revascularization and carotid endarterectomies, to the most complex open thoracoabdominal aneurysm repair, which can require a lengthy intensive care unit (ICU) stay. The majority of these patients have labile blood pressures, secondary to poorly controlled hypertension preoperatively, and may require close hemodynamic monitoring in the postoperative period. Depending on the resources available, these patients can be monitored in the PACU, in a step-down unit, or in the ICU.

II. MANAGEMENT OF COMMON POSTOPERATIVE PROBLEMS

A. Hemorrhage

1. Workup

Tachycardia, hypotension, and low urine output in the postoperative setting are the classic signs of hypovolemia, which could be secondary to under-resuscitation in the operating room and/or postsurgical hemorrhage. If bleeding is suspected as the cause of hypovolemia, a complete blood count should be drawn and the hemoglobin trend should be assessed. It is important to note that an initial hemoglobin drop may not be detected in a patient with acute blood loss anemia until there is sufficient time for appropriate hemodilution to occur.

2. Etiology

Postoperative hemorrhage is one of the most common complications in patients undergoing many vascular procedures secondary to the placing of stents within blood vessels, suturing blood vessels to graft and suturing blood vessels to each other.

3. Management

If the patient is unstable, has high sanguineous drain output, and is clearly bleeding at a high rate, the patient should be taken back to the operating room for direct control of the bleeding. Conversely, if the patient has a slow downward trend of hemoglobin over several days and is hemodynamically stable, further investigation can be performed to determine the source of bleeding.

A CT angiogram can be performed that can help determine the source and should help distinguish between a small amount of bleeding, which can be treated with normalization of the patient's coagulation factor levels, and a larger amount of bleeding from an anastomosis, which may require surgical intervention. In addition, bleeding that occurs during any abdominal or extremity surgery, such as from subcutaneous tissues or omental blood vessels, can also occur with vascular surgery.

B. Pain
1. Workup
The postoperative patient who is in pain may present with tachycardia and have difficulty explaining the location and characteristics of their pain.

2. Etiology
Although vascular operations can range from the very simple to the very complex, the underlying goal of all vascular operations is to restore perfusion to the extremities and the viscera. One of the most common sources of pain specific to vascular surgery is the pain that comes with reperfusion to previously ischemic tissue. This pain can be extremely difficult to control because reperfusion often leads to cramping, burning, and swelling of the extremity.

In addition, patients can also suffer from pain that is common to most surgical procedures, namely from the incision and stretching of the tissues.

3. Management
Patients who have thoracic, abdominal, or thoracoabdominal incisions will likely benefit from having an epidural placed preoperatively. Occasionally, however, epidurals placed preoperatively may not provide sufficient analgesia and the patient may have continued pain. Pain control by means of epidural should be assessed at the bedside, and it should be determined whether the patient has sensation in the targeted area. A test bolus of 3 to 5 cc of 2% lidocaine with epinephrine can be administered through the thoracic epidural to determine if it is functioning. In the case of a nonfunctioning epidural, the anesthesia team should be consulted to either replace the epidural or to recommend other forms of pain control, such as a patient-controlled analgesia (PCA).

A PCA allows the patient to administer pain medication in previously determined doses on demand at the push of the button. If the patient is not alert enough to use a PCA, the other option is to have the patient's nurse administer intravenous pain medications on demand at scheduled intervals.

C. Rhabdomyolysis
1. Workup
Rhabdomyolysis can occur in any patient who has had reperfusion to an ischemic extremity. The possibility of rhabdomyolysis should be considered early in the PACU, and preventative steps taken immediately to limit damage to the kidneys. The vascular patient with rhabdomyolysis will have had some degree of ischemia to their extremity and will present with pain in the affected extremity, **myoglobinuria** (seen as dark red–tinged urine), and a high **creatine kinase**.

Patients with rhabdomyolysis should have their creatine kinase trended. The creatine kinase can range from as low as 1,000 international units (IU)/L when the patient initially exhibits signs of rhabdomyolysis to as high as 100,000 IU/L. In addition to rising levels of creatine kinase in the serum, there will also be rising levels of myoglobin in the urine. The urine may appear pink tinged and a urine dipstick will be positive for blood, but will be negative for red blood cells.

In addition to an elevated creatinine kinase and urine myoglobin, the serum potassium level will also start to rise because of its release from dying muscle cells. The potassium level should be monitored as it may rise to toxic levels and, in the context of declining renal function, the patient may require dialysis to control the serum potassium level to avoid the development of cardiac dysrhythmias.

2. **Etiology**

Rhabdomyolysis is a frequent concern in vascular surgery. It results when the muscles do not receive blood flow and then the muscle cells die and release creatine kinase, myoglobin, and a variety of muscle cell enzymes and electrolytes. Any patient who has had ischemia to their extremities, such as ischemia that results from an embolus that blocks blood flow to the extremity, is at risk for rhabdomyolysis.

3. **Management**

The management of rhabdomyolysis has been the source of controversy in recent years. Initially, it was proposed that urinary alkalization improved outcomes because it prevented the formation of precipitates that occur in acidic urine, as it inhibited the reduction–oxidation pathway of myoglobin, and it prevented metmyoglobin-induced vasoconstriction that can occur in acidic environments. However, several recent meta-analyses have demonstrated that there is no significant difference between the outcomes of urine alkalization versus intravenous fluid hydration alone.

It has been firmly established that patients who are at risk for acute kidney injury secondary to rhabdomyolysis should undergo aggressive intravenous fluid hydration. The goal for urine output should be 3 cc/kg/hour. However, the benefit of diuretics in addition to intravenous fluid hydration in the treatment of rhabdomyolysis has been controversial. Several studies have failed to demonstrate a benefit between the use of diuretics and the use of intravenous hydration alone. The benefit of diuretics is thought to arise from increasing urinary flow, but this should be pursued only after it has been confirmed that the patient has been adequately resuscitated with intravenous fluids.

Recent interest has focused on the benefit of continuous renal replacement therapy (CRRT) for rhabdomyolysis. Although the Cochrane Database of Systematic Reviews found insufficient evidence that CRRT is effective at removing myoglobin, several other studies with insufficient power have found improved outcomes following the initiation of CRRT. It has also been suggested that myoglobin has a higher percentage removal with CRRT than with hemodialysis because of the size of the protein.

D. **Compartment Syndrome**

1. **Workup**

The upper and lower extremities are the most common sites of compartment syndrome in the vascular patient. Compartment syndrome most commonly occurs following trauma injury or reperfusion of a previously ischemic extremity. The names and numbers of compartments for the arms and legs are identified in Table 4.1.

The anterior compartment of the lower extremity exhibits signs of compartment syndrome earlier than other compartments. **Early** signs of compartment syndrome include pain out of proportion to

	Compartments of the Upper and Lower Extremities		
Forearm	**Arm**	**Lower Leg**	**Thigh**
Dorsal	Anterior	Anterior	Anterior
Lateral	Posterior	Lateral	Posterior
Deep Volar		Posterior Superficial	Medial
Superficial Volar		Posterior Deep	

expected findings and pain with passive movement. Later signs include a tense compartment to palpation, paresthesias, and persistent deep pain. **Late** signs include paralysis, diminished sensation, and lack of palpable pulses.

When compartment syndrome is suspected, compartment pressures should be measured. There are various methods and tools available that can be used to measure compartment pressures, such as the commonly used handheld manometer by Stryker. In the absence of an available handheld manometer, a pressure can be transduced by inserting an 18-gauge angiocath into the compartment, removing the inner needle, and connecting it to an arterial pressure monitor.

Normal compartment pressures are less than 8 mm Hg. Blood flow becomes impaired when the pressure within the compartment is within 30 mm Hg of the mean arterial pressure (MAP). Ischemia can occur when the pressure in the compartment becomes greater than the diastolic pressure of the patient.

2. **Etiology**

The most common theory of the etiology of compartment syndrome is hypoxia at the cellular level, which occurs when blood flow is impaired and the tissues in the compartment cannot be perfused. Venous outflow is also impaired and this results in edema and swelling of the tissues.

3. **Management**

When there is suspicion of developing compartment syndrome, the extremity should be examined frequently. The extremity should neither be elevated nor placed in a dependent position. When there is high suspicion for compartment syndrome, or when compartment syndrome is confirmed with measurement of compartment pressures, the patient should be taken to the operating room for fasciotomies to decompress all involved compartments.

E. **Hemoglobinuria**

1. **Workup**

Severe hemoglobinuria can occur following the use of the AngioJet device for thrombectomy. Following the use of the AngioJet, patients should be monitored for the development of hemoglobinuria, which has the appearance of deep red urine.

2. **Etiology**

Hemoglobin deposits in the kidney in a similar fashion to myoglobin, and can cause acute kidney injury in a similar fashion. Hemoglobin is released from hemolyzed red blood cells following AngioJet thrombectomy, whereas myoglobin is released from muscle cells following trauma or ischemia of the muscle. Heme deposition can injure the kidney through tubular obstruction, direct cell injury, and vasoconstriction.

3. **Management**

Like rhabdomyolysis, hemoglobinuria secondary to hemolysis is treated with aggressive intravenous resuscitation (see section on rhabdomyolysis for discussion of treatment). The goal urine output is 3 cc/kg/hour.

F. **Graft Thrombosis**

1. **Workup**

Patients who have undergone lower extremity bypass with either saphenous vein or prosthetic graft should be monitored in the initial postoperative phase for thrombosis. Patient should have their pulses palpated, their signals verified with Doppler, or their pulse volume recordings (PVRs) checked at regular intervals.

Changes in pulse, signal, or PVR exam should lead to evaluation of the graft for patency using further imaging. Grafts may be evaluated with ultrasound or, depending on the patient's renal function, a CT angiogram with run-off to the lower extremity.

2. **Etiology**

Graft patency in the initial postoperative period can be compromised by multiple factors. When a prosthetic graft is used, graft failure can occur as a result of anastomotic stenosis or positioning of the graft. When a saphenous vein graft is used, graft failure can occur because of positioning of the vein, anastomotic stricture, focal vein stenosis, valvulotome injury, retained valve leaflet, or intimal flap.

3. **Management**

When graft thrombosis is suspected, the patient should be taken back to the operating room for revision of the graft. Meta-analyses by the Cochrane Database of Systematic Reviews have shown that patients with saphenous vein grafts taking a vitamin K antagonist have improved patency over patients taking aspirin or aspirin and dipyridamole. Furthermore, there has not been a significant difference with regard to thrombosis in patients taking low-molecular-weight heparin (LMWH) and those taking unfractionated heparin. One trial showed improved patency in those individuals taking LMWH compared to those taking aspirin and dipyridamole.

Depending on the technical difficulty of the operation and the calibers of the vessels that were used in the anastomoses, the surgeon will weigh the risks and benefits of placing the patient on antithrombotic agents postoperatively to improve patency at the time of the operation.

III. **PITFALLS OF COMMON OPERATIONS**

A. **Angiogram**

The most common complication of an angiogram is bleeding from the sheath site. In cases where the sheath was placed in the femoral artery, this bleeding can manifest as a retroperitoneal bleed or a groin hematoma. Patients with retroperitoneal bleeding frequently complain of back or flank pain. If one suspects retroperitoneal bleeding, a CT angiogram of the torso with run-off to the extremities can assist in determining the source and location of the bleed.

In cases where the sheath was placed in the brachial artery, this bleeding can result in a brachial sheath hematoma. The medial brachial fascial compartment is a fibrous sheath that contains the brachial artery along with the radial and musculocutaneous nerves. If the patient exhibits swelling in the arm or has motor or sensory deficits, this is suggestive of the development of a brachial sheath hematoma. Development of a brachial sheath hematoma requires urgent return to the operating room for decompression, evacuation, and control of the bleeding. Compression of the microneural blood supply to the nerves requires pressures less than 30 mm Hg, and nerve injury can result long before the patient has a loss of radial or ulnar pulses.

B. Endovascular Aneurysm Repair

Endovascular aneurysm repair (EVAR) is used to describe the placement of a stent graft in the abdominal aorta, whereas thoracic endovascular aneurysm repair (TEVAR) is used to describe the placement of a stent graft in the thoracic aorta (see next section for TEVAR discussion). Access site hematomas can occur in either of these cases (see previous section for discussion). Other possible complications from placement of an endograft are intestinal ischemia, renal ischemia, pelvic ischemia, and lower extremity ischemia.

The colon tends to be the organ that is most frequently affected by ischemia after placement of an endograft likely secondary to the coverage of the inferior mesenteric artery. These patients may present with abdominal pain and bright red blood per rectum. A flexible sigmoidoscopy should be performed if colonic ischemia is suspected.

Renal ischemia can result from renal artery thrombosis, embolism, dissection, or encroachment of the graft into the orifice of the artery. Patients who have a rising serum creatinine and decreased urine output should be examined and the etiology investigated. Because patients who have undergone EVAR have also had a contrast load, it may be difficult to distinguish renal artery compromise from contrast-induced nephropathy. A renal artery ultrasound can be performed to evaluate flow in the renal artery. Contrast-induced nephropathy is a diagnosis of exclusion, and neither urinalysis nor fractional excretion of sodium is useful in identifying contrast-induced nephropathy as the source of acute kidney injury.

Extremity ischemia most often occurs as a result of endograft limb occlusion and requires a return to the operating room for repeat angiogram with thrombectomy or thrombolysis. In the case of failure of endovascular repair, the patient may require open femoro-femoral bypass. Other possible causes for extremity ischemia following EVAR are embolization and femoral artery injury or narrowing during femoral access. If the femoral artery has been narrowed or injured, this will require groin exploration with possible femoral endarterectomy and patch angioplasty.

Pelvic ischemia can result from coverage of the internal iliac artery orifice during placement of the stent graft. Erectile dysfunction and buttock claudication are the most common symptoms that occur after coverage or coil embolization of the internal iliac vessels.

C. Thoracic EVAR

The most severe complication of placement of a thoracic endograft is spinal ischemia. Whereas spinal ischemia following placement of an abdominal aortic endograft has rarely been reported, the incidence of spinal ischemia following placement of a thoracic endograft has been reported in as high as 12% of cases. The source of spinal cord ischemia is thought to be occlusion of the great radicular artery of Adamkiewicz by thoracic endograft. This artery originates from a left intercostal artery between T9 and T12 in 75% of individuals (Fig. 4.1). The remaining 25% of individuals have an artery that originates from the right side of the aorta.

Anterior spinal cord syndrome typically presents with bilateral lower extremity paralysis and urinary and fecal incontinence. Prophylactic spinal drains have commonly been used to control the spinal cord perfusion pressure (SCPP). It has been thought that increasing the patient's MAP and decreasing the patient's cerebral spinal fluid (CSF)

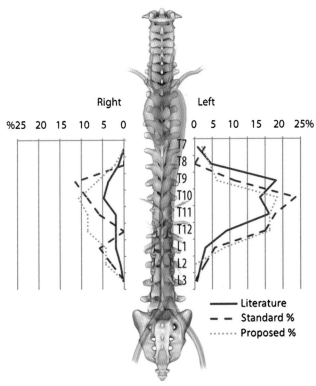

FIGURE 4.1 Percentage of Adamkiewicz artery (AKA) origin level in relation to the intercostal artery, its location, and method used. Note the higher left T9–T12 prevalence.

pressure through controlled drainage of their CSF (goal CSF pressure <mm Hg, 10 to 20 cc/hour CSF drainage, MAP 90 to 100 mm Hg) with a lumbar drain will improve SCPP (SCPP = MAP – CSF pressure). A recent systematic review has shown that pooled rates of spinal cord ischemia are similar between place groups that placed a prophylactic spinal drain and those that did not (3.2% vs. 3.5%, respectively).

D. Lower Extremity Bypass

Patients who have undergone lower extremity bypass grafts should be monitored closely for graft, which include frequent PVRs, continuous wave Doppler, and monitoring of the patient's pulse on physical exam.

PVRs are conducted by connecting blood pressure cuffs to a plethysmograph at four different levels of the leg. As seen in Fig. 4.2, PVRs are suggestive of occlusive disease if the upstroke is decreased and there is loss of the dicrotic notch.

Continuous wave Doppler can be used at the bedside to assess for changes in the blood flow to the distal extremities through the graft itself and is characterized as monophasic, biphasic, or triphasic. Triphasic signals are rare in patients with peripheral vascular disease. The character of the Doppler sound wave should be assessed for change following an operation. It is important to note

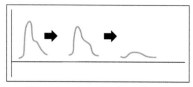

Normal → moderate → severe
obstruction to arterial inflow

FIGURE 4.2 Pulse volume recordings (PVRs) are used to detect occlusion of arteries. A PVR waveform is composed of a systolic upstroke followed by a downstroke with a dicrotic notch. Loss of the dicrotic notch occurs in moderate disease. In severe disease, the waveform is flattened. (Image Courtesy of the Division of Vascular Surgery at OHSU.)

the patient's blood pressure at the time of the exam, as variables in their hemodynamics will result in changes in the character of the continuous wave Doppler.

E. **Carotid Endarterectomy**

The most common postoperative complication in the patient who has undergone carotid endarterectomy is hemodynamic lability secondary to altered baroreceptor function.

A rare, but devastating complication of carotid endarterectomy is cerebral hyperperfusion syndrome. It occurs in only 1% to 3% of patients, but can result in irreversible deficits secondary to cerebral hemorrhage and edema. The earliest sign of hyperperfusion syndrome is severe unilateral headache on the same side as the carotid endarterectomy.

This syndrome ensues as a result of the cerebral compensation that occurs prior to the performance of the carotid endarterectomy. The normally smaller caliber cerebral vessels have dilated in order to compensate for the stenosed carotid artery, and after the stenosis is repaired with resultant increase in blood flow, these dilated small vessels are incapable of adequate vasoconstriction. In order to minimize the risk of hyperperfusion syndrome, rigid blood pressure control should be obtained by using vasoactive medications to maintain systolic blood pressure between 120 and 140 mm Hg.

F. **Hemodialysis Access**

The most common postoperative issues following placement of an arteriovenous fistula or graft are thrombosis and steal syndrome. The patient should be monitored in the PACU and the fistula or graft assessed for the presence of a thrill. Disappearance of a previously present thrill or lack of signal on continuous wave Doppler should raise suspicion for thrombosis of the graft or fistula and the patient will need to return to the operating room for revision.

Steal syndrome occurs when the patient has poor upper extremity perfusion preoperatively and the diversion of blood flow through the new graft or fistula results in hand ischemia. The symptoms of steal syndrome are hand pain, paresthesias, and coolness to the touch. It has been shown in several studies that the risk of steal syndrome is greater with proximal fistulas (e.g., brachiocephalic) than with distal fistulas (e.g., radiocephalic). Steal syndrome may be present in the PACU or, in the case of a fistula, it may develop over several weeks as the fistula matures. When steal syndrome is diagnosed in the PACU, the patient should be immediately taken back to the operating room for revision or ligation of the fistula.

IV. CLINICAL OUTCOMES OF VASCULAR OPERATIONS

The morbidity and mortality of most vascular procedures vary depending on the complexity and length of the operation in conjunction with the patient's underlying comorbidities. These patients should always be closely monitored for signs of cardiac and cerebral ischemia.

Suggested Readings

Brown C, Rhee P, Chan L, et al. Preventing renal failure in patients with rhabdomyolysis: do bicarbonate and mannitol make a difference? *J Trauma* 2004;56:1191–1196.

Brunicardi FC, ed. *Schwartz's Principles of Surgery*. 9th ed. New York, NY: McGraw Hill; 2010.

Geraghty AJ, Welch K. Antithrombotic agents for preventing thrombosis after infrainguinal bypass surgery. *Cochrane Database Syst Rev* 2011;(6):CD000536.

Greenberg RK, Lu Q, Roselli EE, et al. Contemporary analysis of descending thoracic and thoracoabdominal aneurysm repair; a comparison of endovascular and open techniques. *Circulation* 2008;118(8):808–817.

Hirsch AT, Haskal ZJ, Hertzer NR, et al. ACC/AHA 2005 Practice Guidelines for the management of patients with peripheral arterial disease (lower extremity, renal, mesenteric, and abdominal aortic): a collaborative report from the American Association for Vascular Surgery/Society for Vascular Surgery, Society for Cardiovascular Angiography and Interventions, Society for Vascular Medicine and Biology, Society of Interventional Radiology, and the ACC/AHA Task Force on Practice Guidelines (Writing Committee to Develop Guidelines for the Management of Patients With Peripheral Arterial Disease): endorsed by the American Association of Cardiovascular and Pulmonary Rehabilitation; National Heart, Lung, and Blood Institute; Society for Vascular Nursing; TransAtlantic Inter-Society Consensus; and Vascular Disease Foundation. *Circulation* 2006;113:e463–e654.

Kirkiziar O, Kendir M, Karaali Z, et al. Acute renal failure in a patient with severe hemolysis. *Int Urol Nephrol* 2007;39(2):651–654.

Melissano G, Bertoglio L, Civelli V, et al. Demonstration of the Adamkiewicz artery by multidetector computed tomography angiography analysed with the open-source software OsiriX. *Eur J Vasc Endovasc Surg* 2009;37(4):395–400.

Rayt HS, Bown MJ, Lambert KV, et al. Buttock claudication and erectile dysfunction after internal iliac artery embolization in patients prior to endovascular aortic aneurysm repair. *Cardiovasc Intervent Radiol* 2008;31(4):728–734.

Safi HJ, Winnerkvist A, Miller CC 3rd, et al. Effect of extended cross-clamp time during thoracoabdominal aortic aneurysm repair. *Ann Thorac Surg* 1998;66:1204–1209.

Setacci F, Sirignano P, De Donato G, et al. Endovascular thoracic aortic repair and risk of spinal cord ischemia: the role of previous or concomitant treatment for aortic aneurysm. *J Cardiovasc Surg* 2010;51(2):169–176.

Tiwari A, Haq AI, Myint F, et al. Acute compartment syndromes. *Br J Surg* 2002;89: 397–412.

Wong CS, Healy D, Canning C, et al. A systematic review of spinal cord injury and cerebrospinal fluid drainage after thoracic aortic endografting. *J Vasc Surg* 2012;56(5):1438–1447.

Zeng X, Zhang L, Wu T, et al. Continuous renal replacement therapy (CRRT) for rhabdomyolysis. *Cochrane Database Syst Rev* 2014;(6):CD008566.

Recovery of Patients Undergoing Radiologic Procedures with Anesthetic Management

John J. A. Marota

I. GENERAL CONSIDERATIONS

All radiologic procedures can be stratified as either diagnostic or interventional. The majority of these procedures are either **noninvasive** or **minimally invasive** and do not require patient management by a trained anesthesiologist. As such, the overwhelming majority of procedures in radiology are either performed without sedation or aided by conscious sedation provided by a trained nurse under the supervision of a qualified, nonanesthesiologist physician. These patients do not require recovery in a postanesthesia care unit (PACU).

Patients undergoing radiologic procedure may require management by an anesthesiologist for several reasons. These include the following:

A. **Airway management** is considered complex, i.e., maintaining a patent airway and mask ventilation is anticipated to be beyond the scope of practice of a nurse trained in conscious sedation.

B. Significant comorbidities (ASA physical status class III or IV) requiring management by a physician, i.e., cardiomyopathy, congestive heart failure, significant valvular heart disease, ongoing or potential cardiac ischemia, acute cerebral ischemia or elevated intracranial pressure (ICP), significant chronic obstructive lung disease, ongoing sepsis, multiorgan system failure, etc.

C. The patient cannot tolerate the position necessary for the procedure: prone, supine, lateral.

D. Pain from the procedure cannot be effectively alleviated with interventionist-provided local anesthesia, i.e., heat ablation of tumor.

E. Duration of procedure.

F. Altered mental status or developmental delay and cognitive impairment that prevent the ability to follow simple commands and remain immobile.

G. Significant tolerance to narcotic analgesics.

H. Patients requiring active resuscitation for life-threatening pathology, i.e., massive gastrointestinal hemorrhage, hemoptysis, septic shock.

These patients may require care after the procedure to recover from anesthetic management. Depending upon acuity, comorbidity, pathology requiring intervention, and outcome from the intervention, these patients may require intensive care for recovery.

It is beyond the scope of this chapter to discuss management of individual comorbidities that require management by an anesthesiologist. Rather, this chapter will discuss the acute circumstances associated with commonly encountered radiologic procedures that require anesthetic management and the impact of the procedure on postprocedure patient management.

II. CONTRAST AGENTS

A. **Contrast Media.** Intravenous or intra-arterial contrast media are frequently administered during diagnostic and interventional radiologic procedures to enhance imaging. Contrast media may be either ionic or nonionic; complexed gadolinium may be administered for both MRI and x-ray–based imaging. Hypo- and iso-osmolar iodinated media are considered less nephrotoxic compared to that of hyperosmolar. Contrast material can produce diuresis, necessitating either need to void or bladder catheterization after administration.

B. **Acute Contrast Media Reactions.** Serious and/or fatal reactions are infrequent, but remain unpredictable. These are not dose related and do not require repeat exposure. Although not IgE mediated, they are considered anaphylactoid because of anaphylactic features. Symptoms can develop within 5 to 30 minutes of exposure, but can occur several hours after administration; these reactions can occur in the PACU after completion of the procedure. Nonimmediate adverse reactions are defined as occurring greater than 1 hour after administration, but most occur within 6 to 12 hours and frequency varies from 0.5% to 23%.

1. Risk factors include history of previous adverse reaction, asthma, hay fever allergy requiring medical therapy, and concurrent use of β-blockers or interleukin-2.

2. Reaction presents as generalized skin reactions, and may progress to airway obstruction, angioedema, or cardiovascular collapse.

3. Treatment of acute reactions is supportive. Generalized anaphylactoid reactions should be treated with immediate administration of corticosteroids, H_1 and H_2 blockers. Oxygen, epinephrine, β_2-agonists may be necessary for more severe reactions. Intubation may be necessary to treat bronchospasm, laryngeal edema, or upper airway edema. Circulatory support includes IV fluids and vasopressors as necessary.

4. All interventionists do not support routine prophylaxis of all patients. Strategies commonly include prednisone 50 mg PO given 13, 7, and 1 hour prior to imaging, with 50 mg diphenhydramine 1 hour prior to contrast administration. Hydrocortisone 200 mg IV may be substituted for oral prednisone in patients who cannot take oral medications. Alternatively, methylprednisolone 32 mg is given orally 12 and 2 hours prior to contrast administration with or without antihistamine. For emergency procedures, treatment with 50 mg of diphenhydramine IV and 200 mg of hydrocortisone IV or 40 mg of methylprednisolone every 4 hours until the procedure is completed has been used successfully. Patients with methylprednisolone, aspirin, or NSAID allergies, especially if they have a coexisting diagnosis of asthma, should be pretreated with 7.5 mg of dexamethasone or 6 mg of betamethasone every 4 hours until the study has been completed. Prophylaxis is not 100% effective in preventing reaction with exposure.

III. **DIAGNOSTIC IMAGING PROCEDURES**
A. **CT, MRI, PET, PET/CT, ultrasound, and echocardiogram** all require some level of cooperation and varying degrees of immobility for a variable duration of time to acquire adequate diagnostic images. Anesthetic management may be necessary to provide both immobility and hemodynamic/respiratory support during the procedure. The majority of patients that require anesthetic management:

1. Altered mental status and/or inadequate intellectual capacity to remain immobile and follow simple commands.

2. Suffer from overwhelming anxiety associated with imaging conditions (claustrophobia).

3. Cannot tolerate positioning because of pain.

4. Possess significant comorbidity that interferes with adequate positioning to conduct the study, i.e., congestive heart failure or pulmonary hypertension significant enough to prevent assuming recumbent position.

Anesthetic management varies from mild sedation to full general anesthesia with instrumentation of the airway and mechanical ventilation depending upon the circumstances. Because there is minimal stimulation associated with imaging, only a light general anesthetic is required, sufficient to provide adequate conditions to obtain quality images. Recovery is usually rapid and requires only supportive care of comorbidities before discharge from the PACU.

Postimaging care for patients undergoing **PET** and **PET/CT** has a special concern because body fluid, mostly urine, may contain a **significant amount of radioactivity** as the PET isotope–labeled contrast is cleared from the body. Appropriate disposal and handling is required to ensure the safety of health care workers and other patients. Because disposal and caution over contact and exposure differ with isotope and contrast, it is recommended to contact the PET facility directly for instructions.

B. **Angiography** is generally a painless but invasive diagnostic procedure performed to visualize either the arterial or venous systems. Angiography can be performed to interrogate any vascular system, but is most commonly used to investigate the cerebral, abdominal, and peripheral vasculature and circulation. The process requires accessing the vascular system (arterial or venous) by placement of a cannula or sheath; this is performed most commonly under local anesthesia. Catheters are inserted through the vascular access and maneuvered into position for injection of contrast material. Once access is obtained, the process is painless, with patients doing well with only minimal sensation. The usual discomfort is frequently related to injection of contrast and may vary from minimal to painful depending upon location and quantity of injection.

1. Only children or uncooperative adults will require general anesthesia for angiography, although general anesthesia may be required for cases of potentially long duration.

2. Adult patients requiring general anesthesia for intracranial angiography may have depressed mental status because of elevated ICP, encephalopathy, recent stroke, or intracerebral hemorrhage. Spinal angiography may require several hours so that each vessel supplying the spinal cord can be identified and imaged.

3. At completion of the procedure, the vascular access may be removed. The site of penetration in the accessed arterial wall is closed by means of either a **"closure device"** that repairs the vessel wall or simple direct pressure on the area until bleeding stops. In either case, the accessed limb must remain straight and immobile for a period of time up to 6 hours to prevent hematoma formation at the site of vessel penetration. **Hematoma** formation with significant blood loss is an infrequent but potential complication. Hematoma formation requires immediate recognition and direct pressure at the access site. Occasionally, reversal of anticoagulation may be necessary and, more rarely, surgical exploration to repair the vessel. Hematoma formation is less likely after removal of venous cannula because of the lower venous pressure; time for immobilization is less.

IV. **INTERVENTIONAL PROCEDURES**

A. **Endovascular embolization** is performed for a wide variety of different pathologies of the arterial and venous systems of both the systemic and pulmonary vasculatures. Embolization is the intraluminal deposition of material (coils, balloons, particles, and solid or gel material) in order to obstruct blood flow in a vessel.

1. **Cerebral circulation:** to treat ruptured and unruptured cerebral aneurysms, interrupt blood supply to intracranial and extracranial arteriovenous (AV) fistulas and malformations, and interrupt blood supply of vascular tumors before surgery.

2. **Extracranial circulation:** to terminate the blood supply to vessels in the nose or pharynx producing epistaxis.

3. **Abdominal and pelvic circulation:** to identify and interrupt blood supply of both arterial and venous vessels producing active bleeding in organs within the abdomen and pelvis. These may include the gastrointestinal tract, liver, kidney, urogenital system, portal system, and gastric and esophageal varices. Uterine myoma may also be treated with embolization.

4. **Peripheral circulation:** to identify and interrupt blood supply to peripheral arterial and venous malformations and vascular tumors before surgical resection.

B. **Embolization,** as with angiography, requires obtaining access to the vascular tree, most commonly via the femoral artery. Similar to angiography, the **anesthetic goal** is to provide a still field during advancement of an intravascular catheter and deployment of the occlusive material. These procedures are relatively painless, with little stimulation from the procedure. The right internal jugular vein may be used for access to the portal system if a transjugular intrahepatic portosystemic shunt (TIPSS) is in place or is to be created (see below). Alternatively, the portal venous system may be accessed by direct percutaneous puncture.

V. PACU CONCERNS

A. **Hematoma** formation at the site of access or uncontrolled bleeding from the puncture site.

B. Hypertonic contrast agents may produce **diuresis;** bladder catheterization and fluid replacement may be necessary.

C. **Hypertension** should be avoided, particularly when the arterial system has been accessed, because it may increase the risk of hemorrhage at the site of access or the treated pathology. β-Blockers, calcium channel blockers, hydralazine, nitroglycerin, and sodium nitroprusside may be necessary to treat hypertension.

D. **Systemic anticoagulation** (heparin or argatroban) may be necessary during procedures to prevent thrombus formation on the catheter. Coil embolization of cerebral aneurysm may require anticoagulation to minimize propagation of thrombus from the embolization coils. Anticoagulation is monitored by activated clotting time, prothrombin time (PT) or activated partial thromboplastin time (APTT). Platelet inhibitors such as eptifibatide (Integrilin) may be administered by bolus and/or continuous infusion to minimize platelet aggregation. For some procedures, patients may receive aspirin and/or clopidogrel before or during the procedure. Reversal of anticoagulation may be necessary at the end of the procedure in order to prevent hematoma formation for removal of the vascular sheath. When patients are to remain anticoagulated, the vascular access sheath is usually left in place. When the vascular access sheath remains in the femoral artery, flexion at the hip is restricted, thus preventing the patient from being able to sit upright. This can present as a problem in patients with severe lung disease. Reverse Trendelenburg position may be helpful to aid in spontaneous ventilation. Alternatively, postprocedure mechanical ventilation may be necessary in severe cases until the sheath is removed and mobility at the hip is possible to prevent respiratory compromise or failure.

E. **Procedures and Potential Intra- and Postprocedure Complications**

1. **Intracranial procedures**

   a. **Rupture of an inadequately obliterated cerebral aneurysm, AV fistula, or malformation; dissection or rupture of a blood vessel; inadvertent occlusion of a blood vessel:** If intracranial hemorrhage is suspected, immediate placement of a ventriculostomy drain may be necessary to drain cerebrospinal fluid (CSF) and reduce ICP. Significant intracranial hemorrhage presents as sudden-onset headache and altered mental status, often associated with hypertension. ICP elevation may require emergent intubation to control the airway and initiation of hyperventilation. In addition, diuresis or pharmacologic maneuvers (propofol infusion) may be necessary to reduce ICP. Immediate CT scan may be necessary to determine the extent of hemorrhage, and emergency surgery may be required to remove the hematoma in order to decompress the brain.

   b. **Acute stroke from obstruction of a cerebral vessel:** This may be either thrombotic or embolic and related to the site of the procedure. Presentation is altered mental status and development of a focal deficit on neurologic exam. Effective treatment requires prompt diagnosis and potential return to the embolization suite for angiography and thrombolytic therapy. Deployment of an intravascular stent may be necessary after recannulization of the vessel to maintain vessel patency. Anticoagulation may be maintained in the postprocedure period.

2. **Embolization for control of epistaxis and extracranial vascular lesions** presents potential problems of postprocedure hemorrhage, hemodynamic instability, and large amounts of blood in the airway and stomach with risk of aspiration. Typed and cross-matched blood should be available to treat blood loss anemia. The nose and nasal pharynx may be packed to prevent further bleeding even after completion of the embolization. The branches of the external carotid artery are more commonly the bleeding source; nonetheless, traversing the carotid artery carries the potential for stroke or carotid artery dissection and rupture. Hematoma formation and sudden neurologic deterioration are signs of potential catastrophe.

3. **Embolization for gastrointestinal bleeding:** Arterial embolization is used to treat acute nonvariceal gastrointestinal hemorrhages of the upper or lower GI tract not accessible to endoscopic approach. Similarly, bleeding from gastric and esophageal varices is common with portal hypertension from cirrhosis and may require venous embolization or portal decompression with a TIPPS procedure (see below). Although this procedure can be performed under sedation, typically general anesthesia is required in cases of massive blood transfusion, obtundation, or risk of aspiration in patients with depressed mental status. Care should be taken concerning extubation because of aspiration risk with potentially large amounts of blood in the stomach. Hemodynamic resuscitation may require volume replacement with blood products to correct anemia and disorders of coagulation; vasopressors may be necessary to maintain perfusion pressure. Octreotide infusion is often administered to promote vasoconstriction of varices. Massive transfusion requires close attention to pH, calcium replacement, electrolytes, and maintaining body temperature; alterations may persist in the postprocedure period. Embolization

may not completely stop the hemorrhage; in such cases, resuscitation may continue in the postprocedure period.

4. **Embolization of pulmonary and bronchial vasculature**

    a. **Bronchial artery embolization** is an effective treatment for massive hemoptysis arising within cavitary pulmonary lesions (tuberculosis, abscess), bronchiectasis, and primary and metastatic pulmonary tumors. The angiographic approach is via the femoral artery; bronchial arteries arise from the thoracic aorta. Although these procedures may be performed with sedation, cases of ongoing or massive hemoptysis typically require general anesthesia and endotracheal intubation for airway control and pulmonary toilet. Lung isolation with a double-lumen tube or bronchial blocker may be necessary to maintain ventilation of the normal lung. Bronchoscopic examination of the airway may be necessary to confirm patency and suction under direct visualization to remove blood, thrombus, and embolic material before extubation. Patients may develop progressive decline in blood oxygen saturation in the postprocedure period because of a number of reasons including ongoing hemorrhage, retained thrombus or embolic material in the airway, and reaction to massive transfusion.

    b. **Pulmonary artery embolization** may be necessary in the event of hemoptysis from pulmonary artery rupture. The approach is from the internal jugular vein similar to placement of a pulmonary artery catheter. Concerns for recovery are similar to those for bronchial artery embolization. In addition, there may be significant loss of perfused lung from embolization that can contribute to postprocedure hypoxemia.

VI. **SPECIFIC NEURORADIOLOGIC PROCEDURES**

    A. **Trigeminal Neuralgia.** Percutaneous neurolysis of trigeminal ganglion and/or terminal nerves is effective therapy for management of this disorder of chronic pain. Frequently, patients may have multiple sclerosis as comorbidity. Although brief periods of general anesthesia (methohexital 0.5 to 1.0 mg/kg IV or propofol 1 to 2 mg/kg IV) are necessary for the actual ablation because of pain, ongoing neurologic examination and pain evaluation during positioning of the electrode require an awake and fully cooperative patient. Hypertension is common during lesion formation, and invasive blood pressure monitoring may be necessary in some patients. Postoperative concerns include hematoma formation at the tract of approach (infratemporal fossa) and lesion site (foramen ovale). Patients may also require pain medication depending upon the success of the procedure.

    B. **Lumbar puncture** is a procedure rarely requiring the need for anesthetic management. General anesthesia is necessary only in cases of uncooperative patients (dementia and/or delirium, encephalitis), profound anxiety, or pain with positioning that precludes a successful procedure. As with diagnostic imaging, postprocedure recovery concerns are related to the altered mental status of the patient population. Care should be taken with the decision to extubate, because these patients may have depressed gag reflexes or baseline obtundation because of depressed mental status. These patients are at risk for aspiration in the postprocedure period.

    C. **Balloon test occlusion** of the carotid artery is performed to determine whether permanent obstruction of the vessel will produce neurologic deficit. After angiography to interrogate the vascular supply, temporary obstruction of blood flow is performed by an endovascular approach with inflation of an intra-arterial balloon in the supplying vessel. If no deficit is elicited on neurologic examination, hypotension is induced and maintained for 20 to 30 minutes to further elicit signs of ischemia. Although sedation is appropriate during initial angiography and placement of the balloon, **a completely awake, nonsedated patient is necessary for neurologic testing during occlusion**; short-acting agents are preferred. **Hypotension is achieved with rapidly reversible agents** (nitroprusside or nitroglycerine). Consequently, these patients usually do not require recovery from anesthesia, and postprocedure concerns are similar to angiography. In some cases, a PET radioactive ligand is given during the period of interrupted blood flow because a PET scan is obtained immediately after the procedure. Accordingly, the patient's urine may be radioactive. Care should be taken in handling body fluids. Contacting Nuclear Medicine for details on disposal of body fluids is advisable.

D. **Vertebroplasty, kyphoplasty, and sacroplasty** are performed to treat painful vertebral body fractures that occur most commonly as a result of osteoporosis. Bone cement is injected under pressure via a trocar placed percutaneously in the fracture site within the vertebral body of the spine. Patients with multiple myeloma or metastatic cancers that are destructive to bone also undergo this procedure. Either monitored anesthesia care (MAC) or general anesthesia is appropriate, but sedation is often adequate. Patients remain supine for several hours afterward to permit the cement to harden completely. There is usually little discomfort after the procedure. Postprocedure complications may include desaturation from pulmonary embolism of bone cement injected under pressure into the bone and decreased respiratory function because of prone and then the supine position. Supplemental oxygen may be necessary. Kyphoplasty is similar to vertebroplasty except that a balloon is inflated within the vertebral body with the intention to expand the compression fracture and improve or restore normal anatomical alignment.

E. **Thrombolysis of acute stroke** is an emergency procedure performed to restore blood supply to cerebral vessels occluded by thrombus in patients with symptoms of acute ischemic stroke. Currently, IV thrombolytic therapy with tissue plasminogen activator is recommended in patients for up to 6 hours after onset of symptoms; endovascular mechanical disruption or retrieval of thrombus is recommended in patients for up to 8 hours after onset of symptoms. Angioplasty of atherosclerotic plaque and/or deployment of an intravascular stent may be necessary after recannulization of the vessel to maintain vessel patency. Anticoagulation and antiplatelet therapy may need to be maintained in the postprocedure period. Recannulization of the occluded vessels may not be complete and residual cerebral ischemia may persist at the end of the procedure. Although recent, retrospective studies suggest that patients undergoing general anesthesia for thrombolysis and mechanical clot disruption may have a higher rate of mortality after acute ischemic strokes, these studies do not effectively account for severity of stroke and postprocedural care.

1. Currently, sedation with MAC is preferred for angiography and therapeutic interventions. However, if the patient cannot remain immobile because of agitation, has a depressed level of consciousness, cannot protect and maintain the airway, has respiratory compromise, or cannot tolerate lying flat, general anesthesia with endotracheal intubation is required. Extubation at completion of

the procedure is preferable but is dependent upon the patient meeting extubation criteria.

2. There is concern that reperfusion in the setting of anticoagulation after prolonged ischemia may predispose to hemorrhage in the site of infarction after the procedure. Hemorrhage in a region of brain undergoing postischemic liquefaction necrosis is more likely to occur days later and is not an immediate postprocedure concern. Nonetheless, control of arterial blood pressure is a major goal of postprocedure therapy.

3. Damage to the carotid or vertebral arteries or the more distal cerebral vasculature by vessel dissection or rupture may occur during the procedure; vessel reocclusion may occur as well. Sudden change in mental status or onset of neurologic deficit should be investigated immediately with either CT or MRI diagnostic imaging.

F. **Cerebral vasospasm** is a common and potentially devastating late complication of subarachnoid hemorrhage. Patients may require angiography and local **intra-arterial infusion** of vasodilating drugs (**papaverine, verapamil, nicardipine, or milrinone**) or even angioplasty to increase the diameter of segments of cerebral blood vessels that are critically constricted. Medical management includes **hypervolemia, hemodilution, and hypertension** to increase blood flow through stenotic segments of feeding vessels; patients are often on large doses of vasopressors (phenylephrine, norepinephrine, or vasopressin) to achieve the elevated BP goal. ICP may be elevated from brain edema secondary to initial injury or evolving ischemic strokes. These patients are often critically ill and require intensive care management before and after the procedure.

1. **ICP monitoring** may be necessary to guide therapy because of intracranial hypertension, a common problem due to brain edema. Intraventricular catheter is preferable because it permits drainage of CSF to treat increased ICP; "Camino" bolt is adequate for monitoring, but CSF cannot be withdrawn.

2. Management goals are to optimize cerebral perfusion by **maintaining systemic hypertension and intracranial normotension,** maintain a hyperdynamic cardiovascular state, and provide a rapidly reversible general anesthetic so that neurologic examination can be performed after intervention to assess for ongoing ischemia. Patients may require postprocedure mechanical ventilation for control of ICP. Paralysis and mechanical ventilation may be necessary to control partial pressure of carbon dioxide. Propofol infusion may be necessary to keep the patient sedated to control the agitation and the ICP.

3. Because hyperglycemia may worsen consequences of cerebral ischemia, patients may be receiving an insulin infusion in conjunction with 5% dextrose in normal saline to maintain tight control of glucose.

4. Patients are often febrile, and normothermia can be maintained with surface cooling; hyperthermia may worsen consequences of cerebral ischemia.

VII. **SPECIFIC INTRA-ABDOMINAL PROCEDURES**

A. **Transjugular intrahepatic portosystemic shunt** decompresses the portal system in patients with decompensated portal hypertension. It is a less invasive technique that has replaced open portocaval and splenorenal shunts.

1. Patients may have advanced liver disease and severely compromised liver function including **hepatorenal** and **hepatopulmonary syndrome** and massive recurrent **ascites.** Often these patients present urgently

or emergently for actively bleeding esophageal varices. Oliguria from hepatorenal syndrome is common; some patients may have baseline hypoxemia from reduced lung volumes because of massive ascites and hepatopulmonary syndrome. Liver failure patients are frequently in a hyperdynamic state with low systemic vascular resistance because of AV fistulas in the liver and lung. Pre- and postprocedural hypoxemia may be multifactorial from $\dot{V}/\dot{Q}$ mismatch or hepatopulmonary syndrome with associated intrapulmonary vascular dilations. Patients with actively bleeding varices may be treated with continuous infusion of octreotide to reduce mesenteric blood flow. Hepatic encephalopathy can manifest as confusion and decreased mental status.

2. The procedure involves **cannulation of the right internal jugular**, after which a trocar is directed into a hepatic vein and passed through liver parenchyma to enter a portal vein to create a connection for egress of portal blood into systemic circulation; the conduit is dilated and patency is maintained with a stent.

3. Sedation under MAC with standard monitors may be sufficient in some patients, but general anesthesia is common because of the procedure length, discomfort, and comorbidities that preclude supine positioning. Significant hepatic encephalopathy will prevent cooperation necessary for MAC. Frequently, **paracentesis** to drain ascites improves conditions for the procedure by minimizing liver mobility. Rapid decompression of the portal system can produce hypotension during and after paracentesis. This is treated with volume replacement; **salt-poor albumin** may be necessary for volume replacement to maintain colloid oncotic pressure.

4. Postprocedure concerns relate to comorbidities of liver failure. **Hematoma** formation may occur at the jugular puncture site from elevated central venous pressure and impaired hemostasis. A compressive hematoma in the neck may compromise the airway. **Hypoxemia** may occur from reaccumulation of ascites; active bleeding in the abdomen and hepatic hematoma formation are rare. Patients with bleeding or ascites should be considered to have a full stomach even after the procedure and should receive a rapid-sequence induction, if urgent or emergent airway management in the postprocedure period is necessary. **Hepatic encephalopathy** can slow down recovery. Because portal blood now bypasses the liver and returns into the systemic circulation, patients may experience a significant increase in encephalopathy symptoms after a TIPSS procedure. These may necessitate reversal of the TIPSS.

B. **Balloon-occluded rotrograde transvenous obliteration (BRTO)** is a method to treat gastric varices in patients that are not candidates for TIPSS procedure. Balloon-occluded **sclerotherapy of gastric varices** is achieved through either a transjugular or transfemoral venous approach, using 3% sodium tetradecyl sulfate as the sclerosing agent. Although it is an effective treatment for gastric varices, BRTO can increase the risk of esophageal varices and ascites. This procedure can be performed under MAC or general anesthesia. The sclerosing material remains in place within the venous varices after the procedure, and the occlusive balloon is not removed or deflated for 24 hours. The concern in the postprocedure period is that sudden release of the sclerosing material into the systemic circulation may produce acute lung injury. Otherwise, concerns are similar as for TIPSS.

C. **Organ Biopsy**. Biopsy of specific organs, kidney, liver, pancreas, or adrenal, may be nonfocal or focal when a specifically identifiable lesion is targeted. In either case, a biopsy needle is directed percutaneously into the organ. Immediate postprocedure concerns are hemorrhage, which manifests as hypotension and tachycardia, and organ dysfunction, such as obstruction hydronephrosis from clot accumulation in the ureter or hematuria. In addition, the tract of the biopsy needle may produce complications including pneumothorax or hemothorax when the chest is violated during liver biopsy. These present as respiratory compromise. Bleeding from violation of great vessels is rare when biopsy is performed under imaging.

D. **Tumor Ablation**. Primary tumors of the liver, pancreas, kidney, and adrenal or metastatic lesions to these organs are all amenable to ablation. The process involves placement of an ablation probe in the lesion under imaging guidance. Tissue ablations are accomplished as **thermal ablation** by heating with radiofrequency or microwave, freezing with **cryoablation**, or cellular disruption by **percutaneous electroporation**. The probes are withdrawn after tumor destruction. Postprocedure concerns are related to patient comorbidity, particularly those associated with the specific tumor.

1. Postablation pain is common and related to the site of ablation; thermal ablation of the liver capsule or involvement of the diaphragm in liver dome lesions can be particularly painful.

2. Cryoablations are more commonly performed for painful lesions and usually lead to a significant reduction in pain after emergence from anesthesia. In the recovery period, lesions may still be frozen and the body surface over the lesion will be cold to touch.

3. Percutaneous electroporation requires profound muscle paralysis to prevent severe contractions during treatment. Postprocedure weakness may delay extubation, and recurarization is a potential concern when deep muscle relaxation is reversed with neostigmine.

4. After tumor ablation, some patients may develop a **postablation syndrome** characterized by fever, mild leukocytosis, and malaise related to necrosis of the tumor mass. This develops within 24 hours after ablation.

E. **Chemoembolization**. Site-specific, intra-arterial instillation of chemotherapeutic agents can be performed to treat some primary malignancies or metastatic disease with high-dose, highly toxic chemotherapy. This therapy targets the neoplasm, but spares systemic spread of the material. An angiogram is performed first to determine the arterial supply to the tumor and then chemotherapy is delivered via an intra-arterial catheter selectively to the perfusion territory involving the tumor. This procedure is performed more commonly for malignancy of the liver. Postprocedure pain may occur in the treated organ and may persist after infusion of chemotherapy; patient-controlled analgesia may be necessary to control discomfort.

F. **Percutaneous nephrostomy tube (PCN)** placement is performed for symptomatic hydronephrosis to create a pathway for urine flow. It involves placement of a flexible plastic catheter in the renal pelvis under fluoroscopic guidance. The catheter is placed through the renal parenchyma. This procedure is performed as an alternative to cystoscopy and ureteral stenting. Obstruction of urine flow from the calyxes into the bladder can be caused by a number of pathologies. Urgency of the procedure is determined by the degree of hydronephrosis, progression of renal impairment, and infection. Patients may be septic from systemic bacteremia from the infection. The procedure is performed with the patient either prone or lateral decubitus. The procedure can be performed under general anesthesia or sedation.

1. Postprocedure concerns relate to baseline comorbidities, underlying pathology, and degree of renal impairment. Patients may be fluid overloaded or hypovolemic at the time of presentation. Careful fluid resuscitation is required.

2. Bleeding may occur from penetration of the renal cortex with the catheter and trocar at the time of placement; occasionally, several passes with the needle through the renal parenchyma may be necessary before cannulation of the renal calyx. Anticoagulation status may be a factor in hemorrhage. Bleeding may not appear as hematuria, but is confined to a perinephric hematoma. Gross hematuria, tachycardia, hypotension, and a reduced hemoglobin occurring in the postprocedure period warrant investigation. Bedside ultrasound imaging can detect a hematoma.

3. In patients with a urinary tract infection and pyuria, placement of a PCN may precipitate significant **bacteremia** that may lead to septic shock. **Tachycardia with fever, rigors, or shaking chills** after placement of a PCN in the setting of pyuria and an elevated white cell count most likely represent systemic bacteremia caused by the procedure and should be treated with appropriate antibiotics and symptomatically; acetaminophen or ibuprofen is effective for fever, and small doses of meperidine to treat shaking chills. Some patients progress to **septic shock** with **hypotension** and **hemodynamic collapse**. It is not possible to predict which patients will progress to sepsis and which will recover from the bacteremia.

G. **Percutaneous biliary system drainage, stenting, and dilation** are performed in patients with obstruction within the intrahepatic biliary ducts, common bile duct, cystic duct, or ampulla of Vater that impede the flow of bile from the liver into the duodenum. A large number of pathologies can cause these obstructions; most common are stones, neoplasm, and postsurgical stricture. A percutaneous approach is performed when an endoscopic approach has failed or is not feasible. Similar in technique to percutaneous nephrostomy, a needle is introduced through liver parenchyma into a duct under image guidance. Frequently, the duct system is highlighted with contrast to establish the level of obstruction. The approach is through an **intercostal space** and does violate the lower thoracic cavity. A flexible tube is left in place attached to a bag to collect drainage. The procedure can be performed under local anesthesia and mild sedation or may require general anesthesia. Ducts narrowed by scarring, by neoplasm, or congenitally may be amenable to dilation similar to angioplasty. Although briefly stimulating, this can be extraordinarily painful and may require general anesthesia. Usually, a series of dilations are scheduled at weekly or biweekly intervals until the stenotic area improves.

1. Postprocedure concerns are related to patient comorbidity and underlying pathology that may have caused the obstruction. Frequently, patients are **jaundiced** and have an **elevated liver enzymes**. Liver function may be impaired; patients may have a coagulopathy and some element of **hepatic encephalopathy**. Patients with gastric outlet obstruction from neoplasms are considered a full stomach and at risk for aspiration.

2. Because the approach requires passing a needle through the liver, **hemorrhage** and **hepatic hematoma** formation can occur. **Hemothorax** is also possible because the tract traverses the chest. Bleeding may be occult, and a large volume may accumulate in the chest or abdomen before it presents as acute hypovolemia with tachycardia and hypotension, or respiratory difficulty and hypoxemia. Ultrasound evaluation at the bedside can detect hematoma.

3. **Pneumothorax** is also a potential postprocedure concern because the percutaneous puncture site is in the chest, and the tract violates the costal margins of the pleura.

4. Patients can present for biliary drainage with cholangitis complicating obstruction. Injection of contrast to highlight the duct system may precipitate systemic bacteremia, leading to profound sepsis. There may be sudden onset of fever, tachycardia, shaking chills, and rigors. Some patients may progress to hypotension and hemodynamic collapse with profound systemic sepsis. Immediate systemic appropriate antibiotic therapy and supportive therapy to treat symptoms and hypotension may be required.

5. **Intercostal nerve block** is an effective treatment for pain at the percutaneous puncture site. Blockade over two to five segments may be necessary to relieve pain.

6. **Balloon dilation** of a stricture and placement of a stent within the biliary duct system is a painful procedure that may require general anesthesia. Discomfort is short-lived and only occurs during the dilation process. Overtreatment with narcotics during the procedure may result in postprocedure obtundation and delayed recovery.

H. **Drainage of intra-abdominal, intrathoracic, or deep tissue abscess** is often performed under image guidance either by ultrasound or by CT. The procedure involves entering the abscess cavity with a needle and aspirating material for Gram stain and culture. A catheter is left in position to drain the cavity. Antibiotic therapy is initiated to treat the infection. Drainage can be accomplished under local anesthesia, with or without sedation depending upon the patient. General anesthesia may be necessary for painful lesions or because of ongoing sepsis or other comorbidities. Postprocedure concerns are similar to drainage of biliary or urinary systems in the setting of infection. A low index for suspicion must be kept for development of severe sepsis with hypotension and hemodynamic collapse recovery from the procedure. Patients already presenting with sepsis may suffer an acute exacerbation of symptoms because of bacteremia produced by the drainage process.

I. **Suprapubic urine drainage tubes** are placed in the bladder to drain urine when there is an obstruction to the urethra or there is incontinence that requires an indwelling Foley catheter. Placement of a urinary drainage catheter from a suprapubic approach is a short procedure that required filling of the bladder with fluid, usually saline, and then making a stab wound with ultrasound guidance to place the catheter. The procedure can be accomplished with or without sedation and use of local anesthetic to minimize discomfort. In patients with spinal cord injury above the lumbar region, distention of the bladder may precipitate severe **hypertension** from **autonomic dysreflexia**. This may require treatment with antihypertensives and may occur in the postprocedure period. Postprocedure concerns include bleeding and dislodgement of the catheter.

J. **Percutaneous insertion of gastrostomy and jejunostomy tube** rarely requires general anesthesia. Comorbid conditions may require aggressive medical management during procedures, necessitating the presence of an anesthesiologist to manage sedation or general anesthesia. Procedures are performed under fluoroscopy or CT guidance.

1. Patients with dysphagia or an inability to swallow often require gastrostomy and/or jejunostomy tube placement for nutritional support. This patient population often presents with depressed mental status, such as coma, marginal interaction, or dementia, as well as **head and neck cancers** or **amyotrophic lateral sclerosis** (ALS). Patients

with gastric outlet obstruction from abdominal malignancy may require a jejunostomy tube for nutritional support and a gastrostomy tube as a vent for stomach contents; such patients must be treated with full stomach precautions.

2. Comorbidities associated with tobacco and alcohol use include chronic obstructive pulmonary disease (COPD), coronary artery disease, hypertension, hepatic dysfunction, and alcohol withdrawal, which are common in oropharyngeal cancer patients and may complicate the postprocedure recovery. In particular, maintaining a supine position for the duration of the procedure may precipitate loss of lung volumes because of airway collapse and pooling of airway secretions. Persistent hypoxemia unresponsive to supplemental oxygen may require upright position, chest physiotherapy, and even tracheal suctioning in the postprocedure period.

3. Airway management is particularly important in this patient population because head and neck tumors, prior surgeries, and radiation may make mask ventilation and intubation potentially difficult. ALS is a degenerative neurologic disease with progressive profound muscle weakness that can affect respiratory function and swallowing. These patients often require constant positive airway pressure (CPAP) or bilevel positive airway pressure (BiPAP) for respiratory support and may require support postprocedure. Muscle relaxants are contraindicated in ALS because of uncertain duration of effect. Succinylcholine is contraindicated because of potential lethal hyperkalemia.

VIII. **SPECIFIC VASCULAR RADIOLOGIC PROCEDURES**

A. **Venogram and AV fistulogram** are performed to interrogate AV fistulas created for long-term hemodialysis. Occasionally, these otherwise high-flow fistulas develop stenosis or thrombus formation, which significantly diminishes flow. Angiography determines patency and location of stenosis, and provides a qualitative assessment of flow. After vascular access is attained, contrast is injected and vascular anatomy is visualized fluoroscopically.

1. These patients have renal failure and may have an interruption in their dialysis schedule because of the malfunctioning access. The major postprocedure concern is need for **dialysis** to correct electrolyte abnormalities. Careful attention is required for potassium level. If dialysis is not possible, treatment with insulin, dextrose, and calcium may be necessary.

2. Many of these patients are diabetic, and close attention to blood glucose is recommended.

3. Interrogation of the fistula is not a painful procedure and is amenable to sedation and infiltration of local anesthetic at the puncture site. Occasionally, general anesthesia is necessary for uncooperative patients.

4. **Angioplasty and stent placement** may be necessary in some cases to dilate a stricture and reestablish flow. When the stricture is in the upper extremity vasculature, this is tolerated well. Occasionally, dilation of a stricture within the chest is extremely stimulating and produces significant pain. General anesthesia may be necessary to control the discomfort.

5. Angioplasty may **dislodge thrombus** that has formed on the walls of the fistula, a common cause of fistula failure. After deflation of the angioplasty balloon, thrombus may migrate and form a **pulmonary embolism**. **Oxygen desaturation** may occur requiring supplemental oxygen. Oxygen requirements may persist in the postprocedure period.

B. **Vascular access** often requires image guidance for placement and to establish correct location, patency, and adequacy of flow. This procedure is performed in the vascular radiology suite, under ultrasound guidance, fluoroscopy, or both. There is usually minimal discomfort with access placement, and the procedure can be accomplished with infiltration of local anesthetic and little or no sedation. General anesthesia is required for uncooperative patients or those with significant comorbidity.

1. **Hemodialysis catheter** may be **tunneled** beneath the skin for a short distance beyond the entry site before accessing the vein or enter the vein directly, **nontunneled**. Most commonly, the internal or a branch of the external jugular is accessed. The goal is a large enough vessel to provide good flow and minimize thrombus formation around the end because of stasis. Alternatively, a femoral vein or subclavian vein may be used if the jugular vein is thrombosed or not available.

2. Venous access either by **infusion port or PIC line placement** is also a low-discomfort procedure accomplished quickly under ultrasound guidance to identify an adequate vein to access. Placement of an infusion port requires creating a pocket in the subcutaneous space for the device. Placement is typically in the upper chest.

3. Postprocedure concerns relate to comorbidity that requires establishment of long-term access. Hematoma formation at the site is a concern, particularly in the setting of anticoagulation or in patients with a coagulopathy from renal or liver failure.

IX. **SPECIFIC THORACIC PROCEDURES**

A. **Percutaneous lung biopsy** under CT guidance is a relatively painless procedure amenable to procedural sedation with MAC; blockade of the intercostal nerves at the site of entry and one or two segments above and below may provide good anesthesia for the procedure. The pleura is richly innervated, and penetration with a needle may be painful. Patients may be positioned prone or supine and must remain immobile, preferably with shallow regular respirations during needle placement and biopsy because the target lesions are small and subject to excursion with respiration. On removal of the needle, the patient is repositioned immediately to lie on the puncture site in order to minimize the incidence of pneumothorax.

1. The major postprocedure concern is respiratory compromise from development of a **pneumothorax, tension pneumothorax, hemothorax,** or ongoing **hemorrhage** from the biopsy site into the airways to produce hemoptysis; any of these may be present at the time of removal of the needle or develop and progress in the postprocedure period. Prone positioning and requirement to remain motionless after the procedure for a minimum of 2 hours may further compromise respiratory function and produce atelectasis. Coughing and clearing of the airway is discouraged because of concern for development of pneumothorax. After 2 hours, radiograph of the chest is obtained to detect pneumothorax, bleeding, or airway consolidation.

2. **Oxygen desaturation** is a common problem from a wide variety of potential causes. Several factors can contribute to progressive oxygen desaturation including baseline COPD and tumor burden. Oxygen desaturation may worsen with progression of atelectasis; supplemental oxygen may be necessary.

3. A **chest tube** may be necessary in cases of pneumothorax and hemothorax to maintain or improve respiratory function.

4. Emergency airway management with intubation and positive pressure ventilation may be necessary for pulmonary toilet, to treat hemoptysis, or to recruit lost lung volume. Patients with severely compromised gas exchange may require postprocedure mechanical ventilation to maintain oxygenation after biopsy when positioned prone and to prevent coughing.

5. Placement of a double-lumen endotracheal tube or a bronchial blocker may be necessary for significant **hemoptysis**; emergency surgery may be necessary to treat hemorrhage.

B. **Percutaneous radiofrequency ablation of lung tumors** is similar to the biopsy, but a larger puncture device is used to insert a probe for ablation into the tumor; the actual ablation may be painful. Several ablations may be necessary for one tumor with repositioning of the probe.

1. As with biopsy, at conclusion of the procedure, the probe is removed and the wound immediately covered to prevent a sucking chest wound and pneumothorax. This necessitates turning the patient prone or supine, depending upon the insertion site, immediately after removal of the electrode. **Pneumothorax and tension pneumothorax** are a valid concern even after the completion of all procedures involving penetration through the chest wall. All patients receive a chest x-ray after recovery to identify significant pneumothorax.

2. Hemoptysis is also a concern with vascular lesions adjacent to large airways. Placement of a double-lumen endotracheal tube or bronchial blocker to preserve ventilation may be necessary in the event of active bleeding.

X. **SPECIFIC MUSCULOSKELETAL INTERVENTIONAL PROCEDURES**

A. **Biopsy** of a lesion within bone or muscle under image guidance is similar in practice to organ biopsy within the abdomen, the major difference being the drilling process that occurs through the bone to reach the target lesion. The procedural concerns are similar, which are specifically pain management and issues related to positioning. The anesthetic management can either be sedation or a general anesthetic, depending upon the individual circumstances of the patient. Typically, the most sensitive portion of the bone is the periosteum. Injection of local anesthetic directly on the periosteal layer is effective at providing analgesia for the procedure itself as well as in the postprocedure period. Postprocedural concerns are pain at the site of biopsy and potential for bleeding and hematoma formation.

B. **Ablation of bony tumors** with either radiofrequency lesioning or cryolesioning (freezing the tissue) carries the same concerns as ablation of soft tissues (see above). Anesthetic management is necessary because of painfulness of the lesion, difficult positioning, and duration of the procedure. The indication for ablation of metastatic lesions to bone is often unremitting bone pain. These patients may be on large dose of narcotics at home and may have developed tolerance to opioid medications. Postprocedure pain is not uncommon, but pain associated with the target lesion may be significantly reduced after treatment and may improve with time.

C. **Aspiration of a joint or soft-tissue abscess** is performed when a **septic process** is suspected. This may be painful and require some degree of anesthetic management. **Overwhelming sepsis** is uncommon from these procedures. A drain may be left in place to facilitate treatment of the infection. Postprocedure concern is development of **bacteremia and sepsis**, potentially progression to shock. This is treated symptomatically and with antibiotics.

D. Instillation of bone cement is used to treat lytic lesions of bone from neoplasms. Painful osteolytic destruction of the vertebral body or other weight-bearing bones by metastases from cancers, multiple myeloma, and lymphomas is a source of pain and disability. Cement injection allows fast consolidation, resulting in effective pain relief. Complications due to cementoplasty are mainly due to cement leakage. Cortical destruction, extension in the paraosseous soft tissues, and highly vascularized tumors are likely to increase the rate of complications. Venous intravasation of cement can cause filling of the epidural or paravertebral veins, resulting in epidural cement leakage or pulmonary embolism.

XI. ANESTHESIA FOR PROTON BEAM THERAPY AND RADIATION THERAPY

A. **Proton beam radiation therapy** is used to treat AV malformations, pituitary tumors, retinoblastomas, and an expanding number of other tumors. Irradiation is painless, but planning sessions and creation of molds may take many hours, whereas each individual therapy session is much shorter. During irradiation, the target area must remain in a fixed position using a stereotactic frame locked to a positioning device.

1. **In adults**, placement of small pins or screws in the skull can be performed under local anesthesia with 2% lidocaine with epinephrine. If "ear bars" are used, a satisfactory ear block can be performed by subcutaneous injection of 3 mL of 2% lidocaine with epinephrine in the outer ear canal. Sedation is usually not recommended because patient cooperation is required.

2. **For children**, a general anesthetic is usually administered in order to ensure immobility. The procedure commonly is performed daily for about 4 weeks. Typically, an implanted Broviac or Hickman catheter is placed and a propofol induction and maintenance infusion is used to provide immobility. Spontaneous ventilation is permitted whenever possible. Radiation is provided with the patient's head positioned in a custom-made plaster mold formed to maintain the head in the correct position for treatment and maintain a patent airway; laryngeal mask airway (LMA) is considered if a natural airway cannot be maintained.

B. **Radiation Therapy.** Children or noncooperative adults with developmental delay or cognitive impairment receiving radiation therapy often require general anesthesia.

1. Typical treatment course is 3 or 4 times a week for 4 weeks. It is desirable to choose an anesthetic that allows rapid recovery with minimal risk of nausea and vomiting.

2. The first radiation procedure may be time-consuming (one to several hours) because measurements must be performed and molds made of the patient. Subsequent treatments are typically less than 30 minutes.

3. Many patients have indwelling venous access for chemotherapy. An IV induction and maintenance with propofol infusion is a suitable technique. Intramuscular injection of a combination of midazolam, glycopyrrolate, and ketamine may be useful in children with difficult venous access.

C. Posttherapy and recovery concerns are similar to any other anesthetic. Radiation changes to the skin and significant tissue edema may occur at the therapy site; this can compromise swallowing function if the pharynx is irradiated. With progression of therapy for head and neck cancers, trismus may result with shortening of the temporalis muscle. This compromises the ability to instrument the airway. Mucositis can occur in the pharynx, which can necessitate placement of a gastrostomy tube to maintain nutritional support. Pain at the site of therapy may lead to prolonged opioid use and development of tolerance. Use of a fentanyl patch with oral therapy for breakthrough pain is common.

Suggested Readings

Fusco MR, Ogilvy CS. Surgical and endovascular management of cerebral aneurysms. *Int Anesthesiol Clin* 2015;53(1):146–165.

Gómez E, Ariza A, Blanca-López N, et al. Nonimmediate hypersensitivity reactions to iodinated contrast media. *Curr Opin Allergy Clin Immunol* 2013;13(4):345–353.

Guercio JR, Nimjee SM, James ML, et al. Anesthesia for interventional neuroradiology. *Int Anesthesiol Clin* 2015;53(1):87–106.

Hsu L, Li H, Pucheril D, et al. Use of percutaneous nephrostomy and ureteral stenting in management of ureteral obstruction. *World J Nephrol* 2016;5(2):172–181.

Janne d'Othée B, Walker TG, Marota JJ, et al. Splenic venous congestion after balloon-occluded retrograde transvenous obliteration of gastric varices. *Cardiovasc Intervent Radiol* 2012;35(2):434–438.

Kidwell CS, Jahan R. Endovascular treatment of acute ischemic stroke. *Neurol Clin* 2015;33(2):401–420.

Landrigan-Ossar M. Common procedures and strategies for anaesthesia in interventional radiology. *Curr Opin Anaesthesiol* 2015;28(4):458–463.

Papanagiotou P, White CJ. Endovascular reperfusion strategies for acute stroke. *JACC Cardiovasc Interv* 2016;9(4):307–317.

Schmidt U, Bittner E, Pivi S, et al. Hemodynamic management and outcome of patients treated for cerebral vasospasm with intraarterial nicardipine and/or milrinone. *Anesth Analg* 2010;110(3):895–902.

6

Postoperative Care of the Orthopedic Patient

Benjamin Hollingsworth
and Joseph Schwab

INTRODUCTION

The postoperative management of patients who have undergone orthopedic surgery is unique from most other surgical patients owing to the relatively higher risk of venous thromboembolism (VTE) as well as issues related to mobilization and weight bearing. Bone healing and bone quality are also important considerations in the postoperative setting, particularly after fracture treatment or bone instrumentation. There are several other important complications that occur more commonly in orthopedic patients such as fat embolism and compartment syndrome. The purpose of this chapter is to highlight issues that are more commonly encountered in patients who have undergone an orthopedic procedure.

VENOUS THROMBOEMBOLISM

VTE is a major cause of morbidity and mortality after orthopedic surgery. Many patients who have an orthopedic operation, such as total hip arthroplasty, are of an advanced age and are relatively immobile after surgery, which are known risk factors for VTE. Pelvic and lower extremity fractures are risk factors even in the absence of an operation. Other mitigating factors pertaining to VTE include prior VTE, stroke, myocardial infarction, obesity, congestive heart failure, and hypercoagulable states.

FACTORS CONTRIBUTING TO VTE RISK AFTER ORTHOPEDIC SURGERY

1. Stasis—increased cell to vessel wall contact time prevents mixing of natural anticoagulants and increased stasis.
2. Coagulation—many orthopedic procedures lead to the release of tissue debris and fats into the bloodstream, which serve as antigens that promote clotting.
3. Damage to vessel walls—during physical manipulation of tissues, the damage to intracellular bridges releases substances that promote clotting.

Most deep venous thromboses (DVTs) form in the thigh and calf. Interestingly, less than one-third of patients present with the classic signs of pain, edema, and foot pain. Clinical signs such as calf tenderness are neither sensitive nor specific enough to be used to diagnose DVT. Venous duplex ultrasonography studies are recommended to diagnose DVT. Contrast-enhanced imaging modalities are the most sensitive diagnostic tool, particularly when one is concerned about a proximal DVT. The American Academy of Orthopedic Surgery strongly recommends against routine screening for DVT using duplex ultrasonography and instead recommends using these studies only when there is a high index of suspicion for the presence of a DVT.

DVTs can cause pain and swelling and, in extreme cases, compartment syndrome. However, the most feared complication is that of a pulmonary embolism (PE), which can be fatal.

Early mobilization exercises and mechanical compression devices should begin as soon as possible after total hip and knee replacement. The use of chemical prophylaxis to prevent DVT is controversial in that there is not one preferred pharmacologic agent currently available. Each agent carries its own set of independent risk factors, with postoperative bleeding as one of the most feared risks. There is the known link between postoperative hematoma and subsequent infection. Furthermore, although many pharmacologic agents have been shown to prevent DVT and PE, it is very difficult to show that chemical prophylaxis prevents fatal PE owing to the extreme rarity (0.01%) of the event. Closer examination of available data demonstrates that mechanical compression devices with or without aspirin are noninferior to other forms of chemical anticoagulation after hip and knee replacement. For this reason, pharmacologic agents and/or mechanical compressive devices after total hip and knee replacement are recommended. Mechanical compression should be used alone when patients are at an increased risk for postoperative hemorrhage. In some cases, a filter device may be placed in a large vessel to prevent migration of clots; however, their efficacy is disputed.

VTE prophylaxis in other areas of orthopedics follows similar logic, and the balance between the risks and benefits of chemical anticoagulation must be determined. That is, a patient who has multiple bony fractures after a motor vehicle accident would be at increased risk for VTE; however, if that patient has a cerebral bleed at the same time, then the risks of causing worsening bleeding would have to be closely considered and may outweigh the benefits of using chemical anticoagulation for VTE prophylaxis.

COMPARTMENT SYNDROME

Compartment syndrome occurs when the pressure within a fascial compartment is greater than the perfusion pressure of the compartment, leading to tissue damage. Compartment syndrome is usually associated with bony fractures; however, it can occur in the absence of fracture. In the postoperative setting, one might discover compartment syndrome after a long tourniquet time, poor patient positioning, or if an infusion is mistakenly infiltrated into an extremity. Recognizing compartment syndrome early facilitates prevention of permanent muscle damage. The signs of compartment syndrome include the "six Ps":

1. Pain
2. Pallor
3. Pulselessness
4. Paresthesia
5. Paralysis
6. Poikilothermia

These may be difficult to ascertain, especially when one may not be anticipating the onset of compartment syndrome. Two major risk factors for failure to diagnose compartment syndrome are an obtunded patient and the use of regional anesthesia.

When compartment syndrome is suspected, compartment pressures should be obtained to help provide objective data, which will influence the surgeon's decision on whether or not to open the fascial compartments. The compartment pressure should be at least 30 mm Hg below the diastolic blood pressure. If the difference in pressures is less than 30 mm Hg, then operative release of the compartment should be considered.

FAT EMBOLI

Fat emboli occur in most patients with long bone fractures. Studies have demonstrated that 54% to 96% of trauma patients at autopsy who have suffered long bone fractures will have associated fat emboli. However, the triad of skin, brain, and lung dysfunction, also known as the fat emboli syndrome, only occurs in 1% to 30% of trauma patients. Risk factors for fat embolism include young age and multiple, closed fractures. From a surgical procedure standpoint, reaming of the intramedullary canal in order to place an intramedullary nail or long-stemmed arthroplasty prosthesis is a known risk factor. Typical signs and symptoms may include respiratory and cerebral dysfunction along with a petechial rash. The treatment of fat emboli syndrome is mostly supportive therapy to maintain adequate blood pressure. Corticosteroids are controversial in this setting.

PAIN MANAGEMENT

Appropriate management of postoperative pain can lead to earlier mobilization, a shorter length of stay, reduced costs, and improved patient perceptions. The pain management plan should not be a standard protocol but rather adjusted to meet the needs of the individual patient. The specific pain medication regimen should be created based on the patient's preoperative level of pain mediation usage; age; medical, physiologic, and psychological status; as well as the operative procedure.

The goal should be to adequately manage pain with the minimal dosing possible. Often this is best performed with multimodal agents and preemptive action. If a pain service/team is available, they may be useful for formulating an effective plan, particularly in complicated patients.

Orthopedic surgery patients may receive a peripheral nerve block or catheter, which delivers local anesthetic to anesthetize the nerve supply. Parenteral opioids may be the most efficient means of immediate postoperative pain management. Morphine, hydromorphone, and fentanyl are among the most common narcotics used for pain relief. These medications may be ordered in a patient-controlled pump fashion. Eventual transition to oral pain medications should be made, usually by postoperative day 2. Common agents here may include oxycodone, hydromorphone, controlled-release and/or immediate-release morphine, and methadone in chronic pain cases. Tylenol should be administered where it is not contraindicated. Typically nonsteroidal anti-inflammatory drugs (NSAIDs) are avoided in the postoperative orthopedic patient with fractures or bone revisions, as these medications are thought to interfere with new bone growth, which will impair healing.

FLUID MANAGEMENT

Intraoperative intravascular volume optimization has been shown to improve outcomes and shorten hospital length of stay. Early mobilization is crucial and depends on hemodynamic stability in the postoperative period. In many instances, the postoperative orthopedic patient is perceived as frail and of high cardiac risk given their age and comorbidities and thus is under-resuscitated in the perioperative period because of fear of creating a state of heart failure owing to fluid overload and left ventricular failure. Under-resuscitation may result in hypotension and hypoperfusion of organ systems.

DRAIN MANAGEMENT

Surgical wound drains are used in orthopedics to decrease tissue edema, lessen hematoma and seroma formation, and aid in reduction of infection. The use of wound drainage is somewhat controversial. Some believe the drain itself may provide a portal for bacteria into a wound. Studies have shown that blood transfusions occur at higher rates in patients with surgical drains. Timing of removal is also an important factor to consider as it has been shown that bacterial contamination found on a drain tip increases after 24 hours. The use of closed suction drains in elective surgery may not be recommended; however, in the open, contaminated, and/or infected wounds, there may be some utility for wound drainage.

MOBILIZATION

Improvement in surgical techniques, implants, and protocols in the current practice of orthopedic surgery has accelerated rehabilitation. Implementation of multimodal pain management, early multidisciplinary involvement, surgical methods, and fluid management has shortened the time to mobilization of the postoperative patient. Many patients experience postoperative nausea (up to 10%). This can be a hurdle to ambulation and patient satisfaction. Minimizing blood loss and preventing anemia may contribute to increased readiness from a hemodynamic standpoint to ambulate and perform rehabilitation. Pain must be controlled early; control of pain leads to improved willingness to participate and ability to endure physical therapy treatments. This early and aggressive therapy after surgery is essential for accelerating to a rehabilitation center. Attempts to minimize restrictions on patient weight-bearing and mobility should be made to facilitate early mobilization. Shortening of the postoperative stay is a combined effort addressing such matters as patient expectations, postoperative nausea and anemia, poor pain management, urinary retention, and difficulty mobilizing.

BONE HEALING

Healing of a fracture is a physiologic process where the bone heals to transfer force loads. Secondary bone healing advances through five stages:

1. Hematoma formation
2. Inflammation
3. Formation of the callus
4. Transition to the hard callus
5. Reformation of bone

   In contrast, primary healing occurs when there is rigid fixation. Cutting cones, also known as tunneling osteoclasts, followed by osteoblasts, extend across the fracture to form new bone. These are distinct intracellular processes, and many factors can disrupt this progression of bone healing.
Each patient's inherent comorbidities can play a deleterious role in bone healing. Fracture callus in the setting of diabetes mellitus can be up to 30% weaker than normal. Anemia reduces levels of oxygen and iron that are dependent for healthy callus and bone formation. Nutrition should be optimized with vitamin and mineral supplementation. Peripheral vascular disease reduces blood flow and oxygen to the tissues. Hypothyroidism inhibits the endochondral ossification and impairs the repair of fracture because of thyroxine deficiency.

   NSAIDs have been shown to interfere with prostaglandin function and blood flow across the fracture site itself. Corticosteroids used for greater than 7 consecutive days have been shown to cause osteoporosis, and their inherent anti-inflammatory activity results in inhibition of IGF-1 and TGF-β.

   Antibiotics such as ciprofloxacin and rifampicin have been associated with the risk of fracture nonunion.

SPINAL SURGERY

Dural tears can occur both during elective spinal surgery and during surgical intervention following a trauma. Treatment may include primary repair, closed subarachnoid drainage, laser tissue welding, muscle fat or fascia grafts, blood patch, fibrin adhesive, or cyanoacrylate. Traditional symptoms of a dural tear include headache after surgery, photophobia, nausea and vomiting, or wound drainage. Gel foam installation and bed rest are options for management.

Perioperative vision loss is a rare but devastating complication that can occur after spine surgery. The main causes of visual loss are retinal vascular occlusion and ischemic optic neuropathy. Risk factors may include: obesity, male sex, Wilson frame use in the OR, long anesthetic duration, and large volume blood loss. Unfortunately, postoperative vision loss is usually not reversible.

CONCLUSIONS

Postoperative care of the orthopedic patient is similar to that of the general surgery patient with a few caveats. Close attention should be paid to the neurovascular exam of the affected extremities. Typically, early mobilization not only demonstrates a benefit in the patient's overall recovery time, it also is associated with a decrease in postoperative complications. The patient should be closely monitored for signs and symptoms of postoperative hemorrhage. Postoperative pain must be maintained at acceptable levels, which will vary with regard to the procedure itself as well as the patient's level of pain tolerance. Any concerns should be relayed to the orthopedic service promptly for evaluation.

Suggested Readings

Bulger EM, Smith DG, Maier RV, et al. Fat embolism syndrome: 10 years review. *Arch Surg* 1997;132:435–439.

Cain J, Dryer R, Barton B. Evaluation of dural tear closure techniques. Suture methods, fibrin adhesive sealant, and cyanoacrylate polymer. *Spine* 1988;13:720–725.

Christian CA. General principles of fracture treatment. In: Canale S, ed. *Campbell's Operative Orthopedics*. St Louis, MO: Mosby; 1998:1993–2041.

Georgopolous D, Bouros D. Fat embolism syndrome: clinical examination is still the preferable diagnostic method. *Chest* 2003;123:982–983.

Haggis P, Yates P, Blakeway C, et al. Compartment syndrome following total knee arthroplasty: a report of seven cases. *J Bone Joint Surg Br* 2006;88(3):331–334.

Kelly DJ, Ahmad M, Brull SJ. Preemptive analgesia I: physiological pathways and pharmacological modalities. *Can J Anaesth* 2001;48:1000–1010.

Lombardi AV, Berend KR, Adams JB. A rapid recovery program: early home and pain free. *Orthopedics* 2010;33:656.

Mancuso CA, Salvati EA, Johanson NA, et al. Patients' expectations and satisfaction with total hip arthroplasty. *J Arthroplast* 1997;12:387–396.

Mckibbin B. The biology of fracture healing in long bones. *J Bone Joint Surg Br* 1978;60:150–162.

Mithofer K, Lhowe D, Vrahas M, et al. Clinical spectrum of acute compartment syndrome of the thigh and its relation to associated injuries. *Clin Orthop Relat Res* 2004;425:223–229.

Ong CK, Lirk P, Seymour RA, et al. The efficacy of preemptive analgesia for acute postoperative pain management: a meta-analysis. *Anesth Analg* 2005;100:757–773.

Shen Y, Drum M, Roth S. The prevalence of perioperative visual loss in the United States: a 10 year study from 1996 to 2005 of spinal, orthopedic, cardiac, and general surgery. *Anesth Analg* 2009;109:1534–1545.

Shoemaker WC, Appel PL, Kram HB, et al. Prospective trial of supranormal values of survivors as therapeutic goals in high risk surgical patients. *Chest* 1988;94:1176–1186.

Todd CJ, Freeman CJ, Camilleri-Ferante C, et al. Differences in mortality after fracture of hip: the East Anglian Audit. *BMJ* 1995;310:904–908.

Waugh TR, Stinchfield FE. Suction drainage of orthopedic wounds. *J Bone Joint Surg Am* 1961;43:939–946.

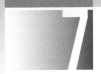

Postoperative Care of the Neurosurgical Patient

Joanne E. Baker and Ala Nozari

POSTOPERATIVE CARE OF THE NEUROSURGICAL PATIENT

A hospitalized patient can present following a number of neurosurgical procedures that can vary significantly depending on location and invasiveness of the surgery performed. For many of the neurosurgical patients, postoperative monitoring is expected to take place in the intensive care unit (ICU) to allow for more rapid recognition and treatment of complications that may arise quickly, and to act swiftly, in order to prevent permanent loss of function.

This chapter will give a broad overview of the postoperative care for the common neurosurgical procedures including: craniotomies, cerebral and spinal vascular repair (including coiling), spinal surgery (laminectomies, fusions, tumor removal), and minimally invasive procedures (biopsies, placement of deep brain stimulators). As the care of these patients is reviewed, it is important to focus on the similarities in the management of these patients, most notably, the importance of neurologic assessments and physiologic monitoring with the goal to optimize the perioperative cerebral perfusion and oxygenation.

THE IMMEDIATE POSTANESTHESIA CARE

Recovery from anesthesia is a stress period that is often characterized by a transient surge in sympathetic output. Emergence from general anesthesia and tracheal extubation induce a major sympathetic stimulation that is associated with an increased oxygen consumption, catecholamine secretion, tachycardia, and hypertension. Control of hypertension is of utmost importance for the neurosurgical patient, given the increased risk for intracranial bleeding in the setting of elevated blood pressure.

Neurologic assessment should be performed as soon as possible in the postoperative phase. As with any patient, if perfusion and ventilation are adequate and extubation criteria are met, then early extubation is optimal to decrease the discomfort and agitation caused by the endotracheal tube and to allow for more accurate neurologic exams to be performed. If patients are slow to wake, it may be difficult to distinguish if the cause is residual pharmacologic sedation or a neurologic event. Early assessment and identification of surgical complications is key to allow for intervention in order to prevent progressive injury and decrease the possibility of irreversible deficits. If a deficit is identified, then this may require emergent neuroimaging using computed tomography to assess for hemorrhagic complications or mass effect, or magnetic resonance imaging to assess the surgical resection, edema, or ischemic injury.

- Hypertension is caused by a variety of mechanisms including but not limited to pain, anxiety, delirium, hypothermia, hypercarbia, hypoxia, emergence excitement, and other triggers of catecholamine release. Treatment of the hypertension must be immediate and patient specific, and should target its often multifactorial etiology. A balanced approach to analgesics to reduce perioperative pain while avoiding excessive sedation, maintaining normothermia, and ensuring adequate oxygenation and ventilation is imperative and can help in the management of postoperative hypertension. Medical treatment of hypertension often includes intravenous administration of β-blocking agents (e.g., labetalol) or calcium channel blockers (e.g., nicardipine), both of which are readily found in the infusion formulation.

- As in any postsurgical patient, hypotension is also a common finding after neurosurgical procedures and may require optimization of the volume status or administration of vasopressors. Common causes include large perioperative blood loss and hypovolemia from other volume losses such as vomiting (seen often with brain tumors) and urinary losses associated with diabetes insipidus or cerebral salt wasting. If volume resuscitation is required, it is important to avoid hypotonic solutions (e.g., 0.45% saline), which could worsen the intracranial swelling and raise the intracranial pressure (ICP). Isotonic crystalloids (normal saline or lactated ringers) are typically used, but hypertonic saline and colloids are also sometimes used, with the aim to minimize the risk of worsening edema and intracranial hypertension.

- Similar to other postsurgical patients, tachycardia after neurosurgery can be a response to hypovolemia, pain, and withdrawal from medications (most notably benzodiazepines, nodal agents). It may be managed by treating the underlying cause or through pharmacologic rate control with β-blockers or calcium channel blockers. Given the prolonged time of immobility and inability to use deep venous thrombosis prophylaxis during the immediate postoperative period, it is important to consider pulmonary embolism as a potential etiology, particularly in patients with associated hypoxemia or chest pain. In the setting of an acute stress response, patients with underlying cardiac disease and electrolyte abnormalities (i.e., secondary to excessive diuresis or after brain relaxation therapy) are at higher risk for developing dysrhythmias and should be managed carefully through correction of the underlying conditions and administration of antiarrhythmic agents.

- Postoperative nausea and vomiting (PONV) is common, especially following infratentorial craniotomies and resection of acoustic neuromas. In the general population, the predictors of PONV include female gender, history of motion sickness or PONV, duration of surgery, use of postoperative opioids, and a nonsmoking status. In the case of neurosurgical procedures, this complication may be augmented by the stimulation of the chemoreceptor trigger zone, which is located in the infratentorial compartment. In addition to the usual antiemetic agents such as ondansetron, prochlorperazine, and low-dose haloperidol, prophylactic dexamethasone has been reported to reduce the incidence of PONV.

- Postoperative neurosurgical patients usually stay in the ICU for a few hours to a few days depending on the pathophysiology of their underlying disease, intervention performed, intraoperative or immediate postoperative events, their comorbid conditions, and the efficacy of their pharmacologic treatment. An accurate and comprehensive baseline medical and neurologic evaluation is important to minimizing the ICU time and improving patient outcome. An accurate and timely medication reconciliation and reintroduction of the patient's home regimen is also important to the postoperative hemodynamic management.

THE POSTCRANIOTOMY PATIENT

Craniotomies are performed for diagnosing, removing, or treating tumors; clipping or repairing an aneurysm; removing blood or clot; controlling hemorrhage; repair of vessels; drainage of brain abscess; relieving pressure in the skull; and biopsy, among others. Most complications requiring reoperation occur in the first 6 hours after a craniotomy. It is important to establish a baseline preoperative neurologic exam, and to outline any anticipated neurologic deficits associated with the surgery.

Decompressive craniectomy, a craniotomy aiming for the decompression of the supratentorial space without reinsertion of the bone flap, may be performed in patients with traumatic brain injury or ischemic hemispheric stroke at risk for refractory intracranial hypertension and herniation. These patients require intensive physiologic monitoring and ICP management in the ICU setting, with frequent neurologic checks and often multimodal neuromonitoring. In the setting of a cerebrovascular accident, systemic pressures, temperature, and the blood glucose need to be closely monitored and controlled to prevent progression of the injury (see management earlier in the chapter).

In addition to the aforementioned conditions, common postoperative complications specific to the neurosurgical patients undergoing intracranial procedures include cerebral edema, seizures, neurovascular injury, and postoperative hemorrhage. Other complications can be patient- and procedure specific, and related to the surgical resection of eloquent regions of the brain or associated with the underlying neurologic disease. Many tumor beds contain vessels that are susceptible to injury and may bleed easily after resection. Agitation and discomfort must be treated rapidly and appropriately, e.g., with titrated doses of a short-acting opioid such as fentanyl, to allow for decreased interference with neurologic monitoring. Postoperative delirium may present with hypoactive signs or agitation, and should be managed with measures aimed at treating the underlying conditions and, when appropriate, neuroleptic agents. Benzodiazepines are typically avoided in the postneurosurgical patient.

A feared complication of certain intracranial procedures is occlusion of the venous system, leading to cerebral edema and potential hemorrhage. Meningioma surgery located near venous sinuses is one example. Arterial infarcts can also occur after traumatic laceration or sacrifice of an artery for hemostasis, and the neurologic injury can evolve during the immediate postoperative period.

Postoperative hemorrhage can occur in the parenchymal, epidural, or subdural spaces. This can occur from reperfusion, debulking tumor, cerebrospinal fluid (CSF) drainage or hyperosmolar therapy that causes a shift of parenchyma, and coagulation abnormalities. Hematomas usually occur within the first 6 hours of surgery, especially following posterior fossa surgery or emergency craniotomy. These patients may rapidly deteriorate and often require emergency airway management and surgical intervention.

Pneumocephalus is an important postoperative complication that can occur after intracranial procedures. Pneumocephalus is usually benign but is a well-described cause of postoperative delirium, and is treated with high-flow oxygen for 24 to 48 hours. It is important to consider tension pneumocephalus in patients with neurologic deterioration after skull base fracture or transsphenoidal procedures that require positive pressure mask ventilation.

Seizures may be associated with many neurologic conditions and are seen after neurosurgical procedures, in particular in patients with traumatic brain injury (TBI) and subdural empyema, and after epilepsy surgery and glial resection near the motor cortex. Rapid control with antiepileptic drugs, benzodiazepines, and, when needed, adjunctive therapies and burst suppression may be needed to terminate the seizure and prevent permanent neurologic injury.

In the postoperative period, it is important to consider certain complications that are more likely to occur with specific pathophysiologic conditions or after particular neurosurgical procedures. For instance, following glioma removal, it is not unusual to see worsening cerebral edema. Following epilepsy surgery, hemiplegia can develop if the anterior choroidal artery is injured. Word-finding difficulties can develop with injury to the left temporal lobe. Diabetes insipidus, neuroendocrine disorders, CSF leaks, and hyponatremia can develop following pituitary and transsphenoidal surgery. Air embolism is more likely to occur after posterior fossa surgery.

Patients with a subarachnoid hemorrhage (SAH) remain at risk for cerebral vasospasm and delayed neurologic injury. Hemodynamic management after clipping of the aneurysm should focus on optimizing the cerebral perfusion, which frequently involves administration of fluids and vasopressors to increase the systemic pressures and improve the blood rheology. Treatment of vasospasm may also include calcium channel blockers such as nimodipine.

Patients with SAH may develop associated cardiovascular abnormalities such as Takotsubo cardiomyopathy, and their hemodynamic management may hence require invasive monitoring of the filling pressures, sometimes using a pulmonary artery catheter. Hydrocephalus can develop after SAH from obstruction of CSF flow, and may require the placement of an external ventricular drain. Seizures are a risk after rupture of cerebral aneurysms, and these patients are therefore placed on prophylactic antiseizure medications. Hyponatremia is not uncommon, and may be caused by cerebral salt wasting or syndrome of inappropriate antidiuretic hormone (SIADH). Starting a mineralocorticoid such as fludrocortisone can be helpful to reduce the renal loss of sodium.

Postoperative infection most commonly presents as meningitis, subdural empyema, or cerebral abscess. Meningitis is more common following posterior fossa surgery than other intracranial procedures because of the likelihood of CSF leakage. Subdural empyemas and abscesses are more likely to occur with infected bone flaps. These will require reoperation for evacuation of abscess and washout. Surgical site infections affect the subgaleal space, subdural space, cranial bone, or brain. Early and goal-directed antibiotic administration continues to be a mainstay of treatment for infective processes.

CSF leak can develop after a dural tear and is more likely to occur with surgery to the posterior fossa. Symptoms include a headache and change in mental status. After pituitary surgery, patients' CSF leaks may present with postnasal drip or runny nose. A CSF leak may require surgical intervention, but is commonly first managed conservatively or via placement of a lumbar drain.

POSTOPERATIVE CARE AFTER CAROTID SURGERY

Carotid artery disease can be symptomatic, usually notable for dizziness, light-headedness, syncope, and neurologic deficits; or it can be asymptomatic. The stenotic artery can be repaired either by endarterectomy (carotid endarterectomy [CEA]) or stenting. The benefits of stenting versus endarterectomy for treatment of carotid artery stenosis remain controversial, but the International Carotid Stenting Study (ICSS) as well as the Carotid Revascularization Endarterectomy Versus Stenting (CREST) trials showed that perioperative myocardial infarction is more prevalent after CEA, whereas the risk of perioperative stroke is greater with stenting. Stenting is therefore often considered for patients with severe cardiovascular comorbidities, in addition to those with contralateral carotid occlusion or restenosis after a prior CEA. Patients with contralateral laryngeal nerve palsy and previous radiation to the neck may also benefit from stenting. CEA is more effective than medical therapy alone in reducing the incidence of stroke in patients with symptomatic stenosis.

Postoperatively, patients that have undergone CEA or stenting are commonly monitored closely in the postanesthesia care unit or in an ICU for strict blood pressure control, monitoring of the neurologic exam, and evaluation of the surgical site for bleeding. In addition to stroke and other cardiovascular events, other postoperative complications after CEA include: cranial nerve injuries, wound hematoma, hyperperfusion syndrome, intracerebral hemorrhage, seizures, and recurrent stenosis.

Wound hematomas are relatively common. Small hematomas can be uncomfortable, but are usually not of clinical concern. Large hematomas can, on the other hand, rapidly evolve, causing compression or deviation of the airway, with risk for airway compromise and death. Airway compromise in the setting of a large hematoma is, therefore, an emergency, requiring immediate intubation of the trachea and decompression and drainage of the hematoma. An emergent surgical airway may be needed if orotracheal intubation cannot be accomplished.

Poorly controlled hypertension can increase the risk of bleeding and developing a hematoma, and the development of cerebral hyperperfusion syndrome (CHS). CHS is more common in patients with diminished cerebrovascular reserve and is typically characterized by ipsilateral headache, hypertension, seizures, and focal neurologic deficits. Preoperative risk factors include advanced age, hypertension, high-grade stenosis, poor collateral flow, and slow flow in the middle cerebral artery territory seen on angiography. Strict control of blood pressure in patients who are at risk for developing CHS can prevent or mitigate the symptoms and improve outcome. If not appropriately managed, CHS can result in severe cerebral edema, intracerebral hemorrhage or SAH, and death.

Hypotension can also occur after CEA, and these patients may require short-term vasopressor support, usually with phenylephrine infusion. If hypotension persists for longer than 24 hours, the patient should have a more extensive cardiovascular evaluation to rule out hypovolemia, myocardial ischemia, or dysfunction or causes of low vascular tone.

ENDOVASCULAR INTERVENTIONS

Interventional neuroradiology is a relatively new approach for the nonsurgical treatment of cerebral aneurysms, SAH, arteriovenous malformations, and stroke.

Many endovascular procedures are performed under general anesthesia, but some outcome data suggest that general anesthesia (likely due to hypotension during anesthesia) may be associated with worse outcomes in patients who require endovascular treatment for acute ischemic stroke.

For patients with cerebral aneurysms, endovascular interventions may be used for coiling or embolic obliteration of the aneurysm, depending on the size and location. Postprocedural care is commonly provided in the ICU, where in addition to close neurologic monitoring, the access site can be assessed for local bleeding, and perfusion checks of the lower extremity can be performed. The extremity corresponding to the access site should be inspected for distal pulses, change in color (pallor), and temperature.

Blood pressure control is also crucial to prevent rebleeding.

FUNCTIONAL NEUROSURGERY

Deep brain stimulation (DBS) is an increasingly common procedure for the treatment of advanced Parkinson's disease. Electrical stimulation of the internal segment of the globus pallidus and subthalamic nucleus or the pedunculopontine nucleus can mitigate symptoms without destroying tissue. Postoperative complications of DBS are infrequent, but there is a risk of intracerebral hemorrhage. Transient confusion, infection, seizures, and pulmonary embolism are also among the reported complications.

SEIZURE AND EPILEPSY SURGERY

Epilepsy surgery is performed for resection of epileptic focus or of lesions causing epilepsy. Epilepsy surgery is usually performed as an awake craniotomy. This enables communication with the patient in order to assess functioning during the cortical mapping for surgical precision. Postoperative care is similar to that of patients undergoing a craniotomy, with the added importance of monitoring for postoperative seizures.

CONCLUSION

Given the increasing complexity and diversity of the neurosurgical procedures, strict neurologic and hemodynamic monitoring is of utmost importance during the postoperative period to allow for early identification of complications and to minimize the risk for developing irreversible neurologic sequelae. Though many of the risks and complications are procedure specific, key focus points for any patient postneurosurgical for postoperative management also include airway control and adequate oxygenation, controlling seizures, temperature and blood glucose management, decreasing cerebral oxygen consumption, managing cerebral perfusion pressure and preventing cerebral edema, and minimizing risk for infection. Postoperative care of neurosurgical patients requires a thorough knowledge of the cerebral physiology and is essential for minimizing secondary or delayed neuronal damage, and optimizing functional neurologic recovery.

Suggested Readings

Bederson JB, Awad IA, Wiebers DO, et al. Recommendations for the management of patients with unruptured intracranial aneurysms: a statement for healthcare professionals from the Stroke Council of the American Heart Association. *Circulation* 2000;102:2300–2308.

Biller J, Feinberg WM, Castaldo JE, et al. Guidelines for carotid endarterectomy: a statement for healthcare professionals from a Special Writing Group of the Stroke Council, American Heart Association. *Circulation* 1998;97:501–509.

Bruder N, Stordeur JM, Ravussin P, et al. Metabolic and hemodynamic changes during recovery and tracheal extubation in neurosurgical patients: immediate versus delayed recovery. *Anesth Analg* 1999;89:674–678.

Chiang H-Y, Kamath AS, Pottinger JM, et al. Risk factors and outcomes associated with surgical site infections after craniotomy or craniectomy. *J Neurosurg* 2014;120: 509–521.

Dashti SR, Baharvahdat H, Spetzler RF, et al. Operative intracranial infection following craniotomy. *Neurosurg Focus* 2008;24(6):E10.

Zacko C, LeRoux P. Preoperative neurosurgical critical care. In: *2013 Neurocritical Care Society Practice Update.*

Postoperative Care of the Endocrine Surgery Patient

Yufei Chen and Roy Phitayakorn

Endocrine surgery is a subspecialty of general surgery that focuses predominantly on diseases of the thyroid, parathyroid, and adrenal glands. Understanding the pathophysiology of endocrine disease and its surgical management is important for providing optimal postoperative care.

I. THYROID AND PARATHYROID SURGERY

A. Thyroidectomy

1. The thyroid is a bilobed gland located in the anterior central neck, deep to the platysma, sternohyoid, and sternothyroid muscles. The two lobes are connected by a median isthmus that is usually anterior to the second to fourth tracheal rings. The primary functions of the thyroid are to produce thyroid hormone, an important metabolic hormone, and calcitonin, a regulatory hormone for calcium and phosphorus metabolism.

2. Indications for thyroid surgery include both benign (Graves' disease, multinodular goiter) and malignant (papillary thyroid cancer, follicular thyroid cancer, medullary thyroid cancer, anaplastic thyroid cancer, and metastatic cancers) disease.

3. There are two main types of thyroid surgery: a hemithyroidectomy and isthmusectomy, where a unilateral lobe and the isthmus are resected, and a near or total thyroidectomy, where almost the entire gland is removed.

4. Depending on the indication, the thyroid resection may also be accompanied by lymph node dissection. This is most commonly performed in the central neck (Level VI), but modified radical neck dissections in the lateral compartments (Levels II, III, and IV) are done for lymph nodes that are clinically or radiographically positive for metastatic cancer.

5. Nearly all thyroid surgery and lymph node dissections can be performed through a single transverse cervical incision, but a separate lateral incision may be necessary for very high (Level II) lateral neck dissections.

B. Parathyroidectomy

1. The parathyroid glands are small glands that are typically closely associated with the posterior aspect or surgical capsule of the thyroid gland. There are usually two parathyroid glands on each side of the thyroid gland (superior and inferior), although ectopic (unexpected anatomical location) or supernumerary (more than four) glands can occur in 6% to 16% and 2.5% to 13% of patients, respectively. The parathyroid glands secrete parathyroid hormone (PTH), which regulates serum levels of calcium through effects on the bone, kidney, and intestines.

2. Indications for parathyroid surgery are usually primary hyperparathyroidism (HPT; autonomous oversecretion of PTH) from a parathyroid

adenoma (80% to 85% of patients with primary HPT), parathyroid hyperplasia (10% to 15% of patients), or rarely parathyroid carcinoma (<1% of patients with primary HPT). Operations for secondary HPT (physiologic increase in PTH secretion secondary to hypocalcemia) typically due to renal failure occur much less frequently since the development of calcimimetic therapies that increase the sensitivity of calcium-sensing receptors of the parathyroid glands.

3. Approaches to parathyroid surgery include standard bilateral exploration where all four glands are visualized or minimally invasive single-gland exploration that requires positive preoperative localization.

4. Parathyroid surgery is performed through either a single central or lateral transverse cervical incision.

C. Standard Postoperative Care

1. Recovery after thyroid and parathyroid surgery is usually rapid, and patients are typically provided a regular soft diet by the morning after surgery. Patients typically complain of throat pain with swallowing, but incisional pain is usually minimal because of disruption of the small cervical sensory nerves around the incision, and nausea can be well controlled with the use of antiemetics. Patients are monitored carefully for signs of recurrent laryngeal nerve (RLN) damage, hematoma, and hypocalcemia. Select patients may be suitable for outpatient surgery where they follow clear postoperative care pathways and are discharged home after a short period of monitoring in the postanesthesia care unit (typically around 4 hours of monitoring).

2. Hypothyroidism is expected following total thyroidectomy and can also occur in 15% to 50% of patients after hemithyroidectomy. Patients are usually given thyroid hormone replacement with levothyroxine at a dose of 1.4 to 1.8 μg/kg/day, with a slightly higher dose used in men and in patients with known malignancy to suppress thyroid-stimulating hormone.

II. COMPLICATIONS FOLLOWING THYROID AND PARATHYROID SURGERY

A. RLN Injury

1. RLN is a branch of the vagus nerve that innervates all intrinsic muscles of the larynx, with the exception of the cricothyroid muscle. As the RLN comes off the vagus, the right RLN travels down and courses behind the right subclavian artery and the left RLN courses behind the aortic arch before ascending in bilateral tracheoesophageal grooves and entering the larynx just under the inferior constrictor muscles.

2. Injury to the RLN may occur following thyroid surgery and, to a lesser extent, parathyroid surgery. Rates vary in the literature depending on the definition but typically average around 1% in large series.

3. The mechanism of injury to the RLN can vary from a transient stretch injury to inadvertent or deliberate transection of the nerve. Risk factors for RLN injury include invasive malignancy, nonidentification of the RLN, anterior displacement, excessive manipulation or dissection around the nerve resulting in traction or ischemia, and a reoperative field.

4. **Signs and symptoms**

   a. Symptoms of unilateral RLN injury vary from being completely asymptomatic to dysphagia and voice compromise.

   b. The most common symptom of unilateral RLN injury is dysphonia, or hoarseness. Other symptoms of unilateral RLN injury include an increased risk of aspiration with thin liquids, dysphagia, and resulting dyspnea.

  c. Bilateral RLN injury is a surgical emergency because it has the greatest impact on respiration and can present with stridor or respiratory distress because both vocal cords may be nearly closed.

5. **Diagnosis**
  a. The gold standard for diagnosis of RLN injury is by fiberoptic laryngoscopy. Depending on practice patterns, this can be performed routinely or selectively following thyroid surgery.
  b. RLN injury results in the cord lying in the paramedian position (Fig. 8.1). The most common explanation is the Wagner and Grossman theory, which states that injury to the RLN will lead to overrepresentation of the innervated cricothyroid muscle, which acts to adduct the cord.
  c. The extent of vocal symptoms is usually related to the distance of the paralyzed cord from the midline.
  d. Other diagnostic tools such as laryngeal electromyography and video stroboscopy are typically utilized in the later outpatient setting.

6. **Management**
  a. Unilateral injury
    1. Early management of a patient with identified RLN injury should be to maintain aspiration precautions. Postural strategies such as chin tuck when drinking thin liquids can help reduce the risk of aspiration. Patients should also be instructed to use more force when speaking.
    2. Transient injury should resolve by 3 months postoperatively. If the patient's voice or ability to swallow liquids has not fully recovered by then, the injury may be permanent, which can have a significant impact on the patient's quality of life and ability to work. Therefore, patients with suspected permanent nerve injury should be referred to a laryngeal surgeon for laryngoscopy and likely vocal cord medialization (thyroplasty or vocal cord injection).
  b. Bilateral injury
    1. If the patient develops acute stridor and respiratory distress in the immediate postoperative period, bilateral RLN injury should be suspected and immediate fiberoptic laryngoscopy should be done to confirm the diagnosis.
    2. Emergent reintubation or a surgical airway (cricothyrotomy or preferably tracheostomy) may be required.

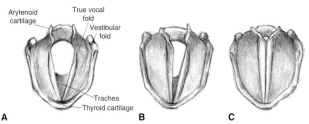

FIGURE 8.1 Vocal cord positions during normal respiration following recurrent laryngeal nerve injury. **A:** Normal position, **B:** Unilateral right RLN injury, and **C:** Bilateral RLN injury.

7. **Differentials**
   a. Alternative causes of postoperative hoarseness include superior laryngeal nerve injury, direct cricothyroid muscle injury, or intubation trauma leading to vocal fold injury or arytenoid dislocation.

B. **Hypoparathyroidism**
   1. Hypoparathyroidism is the most common complication following thyroid and parathyroid surgery. The definition of postoperative hypoparathyroidism varies in the literature, but usually always involves the identification of low serum calcium levels after surgery. It is the most common cause of prolonged hospitalization following neck surgery and is the leading cause of readmission.
   2. Hypoparathyroidism can be temporary or permanent, with the latter usually defined as no recovery of the parathyroid glands 6 months after surgery. Quoted rates of temporary hypoparathyroidism are 15% to 30%, with rates of permanent hypoparathyroidism being 1% to 2%.
   3. The mechanism of hypoparathyroidism is due to either direct or indirect injury to the parathyroid glands. This can be due to excessive manipulation, inadvertent removal, or devascularization of one or more glands. Strategies such as parathyroid reimplantation into the sternocleidomastoid muscle are utilized intraoperatively to help reduce the incidence of permanent hypoparathyroidism. Injury to the parathyroids leads to an inadequate release of PTH to maintain calcium homeostasis with resulting hypocalcemia and its subsequent clinical manifestations.
   4. Factors that increase the risk of postoperative hypoparathyroidism include more extensive surgery, central neck dissection (usually results in removal/ischemia of both inferior parathyroid glands), neck reoperation, and Graves' disease.
   5. Serum intact PTH levels may be drawn at the end of thyroid or parathyroid operations, with levels <15 pg/mL suggestive of increased risk of developing postoperative hypoparathyroidism.
   6. **Signs and symptoms**
      a. Acute hypocalcemia leads to neuromuscular irritability. The earliest symptoms of mild hypocalcemia include perioral or digital paresthesia and numbness as well as muscle cramping. It is important to differentiate digital paresthesia versus postanesthesia muscle cramping because of patient positioning or residual neuromuscular blockade. Unlike postanesthesia paresthesia, digital paresthesia secondary to hypocalcemia typically occurs in the fingers or toes *bilaterally*.
      b. Historical signs of hypocalcemia included Chvostek's sign (ipsilateral facial twitching elicited by tapping over the facial nerve, which is also present in up to 20% of normocalcemic individuals) and Trousseau's sign (carpal spasm elicited by inflating a blood pressure cuff around the arm above systolic pressure for 3 minutes). These signs are not reliable and should not be used for diagnosis.
      c. Late and more severe signs of acute hypocalcemia include tetany, altered mental status, bronchospasm, laryngospasm, and heart failure. The hallmark ECG change of hypocalcemia is prolongation of the QTc interval.
   7. **Diagnosis**
      a. Serum calcium, ionized calcium, and albumin levels should be drawn when there is suspicion for postoperative hypoparathyroidism, although this is often checked routinely in many institutions.

b. If ionized calcium levels are not available, serum calcium levels should be corrected for hypoalbuminemia (normal albumin 4 g/dL).
   1. Corrected Ca = Serum Ca + 0.8 × (Normal albumin − Patient albumin)
c. Note that serum PTH levels often take several days to be analyzed, so they are unlikely to be helpful for immediate diagnosis of hypoparathyroidism.
d. Many surgeons give routine postoperative calcium supplementation (1,250 mg calcium carbonate [500 mg elemental Ca] 2 to 4 times a day) to reduce the risk of developing hypocalcemia.
e. In patients that develop mild symptoms or who have mild hypocalcemia, extra oral doses of calcium carbonate can be given.
   1. Calcium carbonate benefits from an acidic environment for absorption and is best taken with meals. Calcium citrate should be considered in patients with altered gastric acid production (e.g., patients on proton pump inhibitor, previous gastric surgery).
f. Patients with more severe symptoms or severe hypocalcemia (serum <7.5 mg/dL or ionized calcium <0.8 mmol/L) may require IV calcium repletion.
   1. Unless the hypocalcemia is life-threatening, slow repletion of calcium is preferred and accomplished by adding 11 g of calcium gluconate (equivalent to 990 mg of elemental Ca) diluted in 1,000 mL of normal saline or 5% dextrose water and should be infused starting at 50 mL/hour. Concurrent oral calcium and vitamin D therapy should be initiated per surgeons' preferences and the calcium drip can be titrated according to new lab values.
   2. Calcium gluconate is preferred over calcium chloride as $CaCl_2$ carries a significant risk of tissue necrosis if extravasation occurs and should only be administered centrally.
   3. Calcitriol (0.25 μg BID or TID either orally or IV), an activated form of vitamin D, can also be given to patients with hypoparathyroidism to improve calcium absorption from the gut and calcium conservation in the kidney.
   4. Concurrent hypomagnesemia should also be corrected because low serum magnesium levels decrease PTH secretion and also induce PTH resistance.

C. Hematoma
1. Postoperative hematoma after thyroid and/or parathyroid surgery occurs in approximately 1% to 2% of cases. It most commonly occurs in the immediate postoperative period (within the first 3 to 6 hours), but can also be delayed (2 to 7 days postprocedure). It can be located either superficial or deep to the infrahyoid (strap) muscles or can be a combination of both.
2. Risk factors for postoperative hemorrhage include larger tumor size, substernal goiter, postoperative hypertension, lymph node dissection, Graves' disease, and a reoperative neck. The routine placement of drains has not been effective in reducing the incidence of postoperative hematoma.
3. **Signs and symptoms**
   a. Swelling and firmness over the neck are typically the first signs of postoperative hemorrhage. Superficial hematomas will often manifest with ecchymosis and oozing from the suture line or saturation of the dressing.
   b. Obstructive symptoms occur more commonly in deep hematomas and include dysphagia and stridor. Respiratory compromise

occurs secondary to venous congestion and laryngopharyngeal edema because of high neck compartment pressures secondary to the hematoma.

4. **Management**

   a. Small hematomas that do not progress or cause significant symptoms can often be managed expectantly. Ultrasound can be used to see if there is active flow into the hematoma. Regardless, the surgical team should be notified immediately.

   b. Airway compromise or expanding hematomas will require immediate evacuation and wound exploration. In the setting of imminent airway compromise, opening of the wound at the bedside and evacuation of the hematoma should be performed. Avoid laying the patient flat because this can worsen the patient's symptoms.

   c. When there is suspicion for a postoperative hematoma, an experienced practitioner should always be available to intubate the patient if required. These patients will often have significant vocal cord and laryngeal edema, so advanced airway techniques should be readily available, including video laryngoscope and fiberoptic tools.

   d. If there continues to be significant edema despite hematoma evacuation and endotracheal intubation cannot be performed, cricothyrotomy or tracheostomy through the prior cervical neck incision may be necessary.

D. **Thyrotoxic Storm**

1. A rare but potentially life-threatening complication of thyroid surgery seen in patients with Graves' disease or toxic thyroid nodules. The hyperthyroid state in combination with a precipitating event such as surgery can result in a sudden disassociation of thyroid hormone and lead to high circulating levels of free thyroid hormone.

2. The risk of developing thyrotoxic storm can be minimized through optimal preoperative management of the patient's antithyroid medications. Those who have persistent symptoms of thyrotoxicosis should be on β-blockade preoperatively and in the immediate postoperative period.

3. **Signs and symptoms**

   a. The features of thyrotoxic storm are those of a hypermetabolic state. Patients will develop fever, tachycardia, arrhythmias, and subsequent high-output cardiac failure. Neurologic symptoms include agitation, delirium, and even seizures and coma. Hepatic dysfunction and diarrhea associated with jaundice and abdominal pain can also develop.

4. **Management**

   a. Thyrotoxic storm is a clinical diagnosis, and identification or suspicion of this condition should prompt monitoring of the patient in an intensive care setting.

   b. Acetaminophen is given to address the patient's pyrexia, although care must be taken if the patient is known to have significant hepatic dysfunction.

   c. β-Blockade is initiated to reduce sympathetic stimulation. Most commonly, propranolol is utilized either IV (1 to 2 mg/minute) for hemodynamically unstable patients or orally (60 to 80 mg q4h). Propranolol has advantages over other types of β-blockers because it also decreases the peripheral conversion of levothyroxine (T_4) to the more metabolically active triiodothyronine (T_3).

   d. Steroids such as hydrocortisone (100 mg intravenous q8h) are given to prevent iodine uptake and the peripheral conversion of T_4 to T_3.

e. Antithyroid medications including methimazole (20 to 30 mg PO q6h) or propylthiouracil (200 to 400 mg PO q6h) have a later onset of action, but should be initiated early to prevent thyroid hormone synthesis, with the latter also inhibiting peripheral conversion.

f. Inorganic iodine with potassium iodide (SSKI) or Lugol's solution (5 drops q6h) can be used to block new thyroid hormone synthesis and release.

E. Infection

1. Surgical site infections are uncommonly seen after thyroid or parathyroid surgery given its clean nature and the high vascularity of the neck. Therefore, perioperative antibiotics are rarely used.

2. **Signs and symptoms**

   a. Typical features of a surgical site infection include fevers, redness, swelling, pain, and purulent drainage. It is important to note that skin flap devascularization/ischemia may be mistaken for erythema, especially in reoperative fields.

   b. Patients who develop a deep space infection may develop an acute inability to swallow with obstructive symptoms such as dysphagia, drooling, or stridor.

3. **Treatment**

   a. Superficial cellulitis should be treated with antibiotics typically targeting skin flora.

   b. Deep space infections are surgical emergencies and require urgent computed tomographic imaging to localize and drain. Drains are typically placed percutaneously and patients are treated with broad-spectrum intravenous antibiotics that are eventually tailored to culture results. If surgical drainage is necessary, a careful inspection of the aerodigestive tract should be done to rule out inadvertent esophageal or laryngeal injury as the source of infection.

F. Pneumothorax

1. Pneumothorax and pneumomediastinum are rare complications after thyroid and parathyroid surgery, but can occur in patients who also undergo an extensive neck dissection or those with large retrosternal goiters or ectopic parathyroid glands that require extensive dissection toward the mediastinum.

2. **Signs and symptoms**

   a. Most pneumothoraces are asymptomatic and have minimal clinical significance and as a result go largely undetected.

   b. A large pneumothorax can present with shortness of breath and decreased breath sounds. Patients who develop a tension pneumothorax can have tracheal deviation away from the affected side, distended neck veins, and hemodynamic collapse.

3. **Management**

   a. Patients should be placed on 100% oxygen to accelerate pleural air absorption.

   b. Small, asymptomatic pneumothoraces can be managed expectantly with serial chest radiographs to monitor for stability or resolution.

   c. Larger, symptomatic pneumothoraces can be treated with simple aspiration, although the majority, particularly those with tension physiology, will require tube thoracostomy placement connected to an underwater seal drainage system.

III. ADRENAL SURGERY

A. Adrenal Glands

1. The adrenal glands are paired endocrine organs located above the kidneys in the retroperitoneum. The gland consists of an outer cor-

tex and an inner medulla. The outer cortex has three distinct layers; the zona glomerulosa, zona fasciculata, and zona reticularis, which secrete mineralocorticoid, glucocorticoid, and sex hormones, respectively. The adrenal medulla contains chromaffin cells that secrete catecholamines including norepinephrine, epinephrine, and dopamine.

B. **Indications for Surgery**

1. Indications for adrenal surgery include both benign and malignant disease. Benign adrenal lesions include nonfunctional adrenal adenomas as well as hormonally active aldosteronomas (Conn's syndrome), cortisol-secreting adenomas (Cushing's syndrome), and pheochromocytomas (although 10% of these are also malignant).

2. Other malignant lesions include primary adrenocortical carcinoma and secondary metastases (most commonly from lung, breast, and gastrointestinal cancer).

3. Bilateral adrenalectomy is also considered for patients with refractory Cushing's disease despite transsphenoidal surgery, patients with ectopic adrenocorticotropic hormone (ACTH) production, and those with bilateral pheochromocytoma (often seen in patients with multiple endocrine neoplasia type 2 or Von Hippel–Lindau disease).

C. **Approaches to Surgery**

1. There are a variety of approaches to adrenal surgery depending on patient, tumor, and surgeon factors. The gold standard and traditional method is an open procedure, which can be performed via an anterior, posterior, or thoracoabdominal approach.

2. Minimally invasive techniques are now the most common management approach for adrenalectomy, given its benefits of rapid recovery and minimal postoperative pain. This can be performed laparoscopically or via retroperitoneoscopic method with or without the assistance of robotics.

3. Open techniques are still predominantly utilized for larger tumors (>7 cm) and adrenocortical carcinomas.

4. Cortical-sparing adrenalectomy has also been advocated by some surgeons as an approach for bilateral adrenal tumors in order to prevent the need for lifelong steroid replacement. The outcomes of this approach with regard to recurrence rates and long-term survival are as yet unclear.

IV. **COMPLICATIONS FOLLOWING ADRENAL SURGERY**

A. **Bleeding**

1. Postoperative hemorrhage can occur after any surgery and can be immediate or delayed. It is important to keep in mind the laterality of the adrenal resection and surgical approach in order to identify potential sources of bleeding. The adrenal glands have a rich blood supply that generally involves a plexus of arteries from branches of the inferior phrenic artery, renal artery, and aorta that drain through a single adrenal vein.

2. The right adrenal is closely associated with the inferior vena cava (IVC) and liver, with the right adrenal vein draining directly into the IVC. The left adrenal vein drains into the left renal vein and is closely associated with the spleen, stomach, and pancreas. Injuries to the liver and spleen from a right and left adrenalectomy, respectively, need to be considered as sources of postoperative hemorrhage.

3. **Signs and symptoms**

   a. Postoperative hypotension and tachycardia should raise concern for hemorrhage. Patient may complain of abdominal or back pain and on exam there may be significant ecchymosis (Grey Turner's sign is typically a late finding) or peritonitis.

4. **Diagnosis**
   a. The diagnosis of immediate postoperative hemorrhage is often one of clinical suspicion because hemoglobin levels and hematocrit may remain unchanged in acute hemorrhage.
   b. Serial hematocrits are useful in quantifying slower bleeding often seen from venous oozing or visceral injuries and provide a guide for transfusion requirements.
   c. If time permits, axial imaging with computed tomography and IV contrast can often help localize the source of the bleeding.

5. **Management**
   a. Immediate management should focus on ensuring there is adequate access with ideally two large-bore IV cannulas. Hemodynamically unstable patients should be transfused blood following the principles of permissive hypotension, and in the early postoperative period, return to the operating room for reexploration and surgical control of the bleeding should be considered.
   b. Delayed hemorrhage can often be managed by transfusion, correcting coagulopathy, and monitoring serial blood counts. Should there be continued bleeding despite these measures or if the patient becomes unstable, operative reexploration or endovascular approaches with coil embolization or covered stent placement have been described.

B. **Complications after Pheochromocytoma Resection**
   1. Functional pheochromocytomas secrete varying amounts of catecholamines including epinephrine, norepinephrine, and dopamine. These agents have profound sympathetic effects on the autonomic nervous system. The preoperative preparation of these patients with α- and β-blockade is necessary to prevent postoperative complications, but can also cause postoperative hemodynamic instability.
   2. Larger tumor size and higher preoperative urinary metanephrine and catecholamine levels have been correlated with an increased risk of postoperative complications.
   3. **Signs and symptoms**
      a. Hemodynamic instability can result from the higher levels of circulating catecholamines and prolonged effects of preoperative α-blockade. This can range from prolonged hypotension to uncontrolled hypertension as well as cardiac arrhythmias.
      b. Postoperative hypoglycemia can manifest as decreased alertness, seizures, or even coma in the early postoperative period. The mechanism is related to rebound hyperinsulinism after loss of the catecholamine inhibitory effect on β_2 receptors located on pancreatic islet cells and glycogen store depletion.
   4. **Management**
      a. All postoperative patients should be kept on cardiac monitoring, and most patients will have an arterial line in the perioperative period for close hemodynamic monitoring. Patients with pheochromocytoma may be intravascularly volume depleted because of venous dilation, so hypotension should be treated with a combination of volume resuscitation and vasopressor agents such as phenylephrine. Hypertension should be managed with short-acting vasodilators including nitroprusside or β-blockers such as esmolol.
      b. Blood sugar should be monitored regularly during the first 24 hours postoperatively, particularly the first 4 to 6 hours. Any patient with a depressed mental status following pheochromocytoma resection should have their glucose checked. Treatment

of hypoglycemia is typically with intravenous dextrose-containing solutions, and some patients may require admission to the ICU for a prolonged dextrose infusion.

C. Complications after Aldosteronoma Resection

1. Excessive mineralocorticoid secretion, principally aldosterone, is the primary feature of Conn's syndrome. This can be due to a solitary adenoma or bilateral adrenal hyperplasia, although the latter is mainly treated medically with mineralocorticoid receptor antagonists such as spironolactone. Aldosterone is a major regulator of extracellular fluid volume and acts on the distal tubules of the kidneys to reabsorb Na^+ and excrete K^+ and H^+.

2. Patients with Conn's syndrome will often present with hypertension secondary to an expanded extracellular fluid volume and are treated preoperatively with spironolactone or eplerenone, and hypokalemia is treated with potassium supplementation.

3. Postoperatively, a transient hypoaldosteronism can develop and as a result patients should not be administered potassium-containing fluids.

4. **Signs and symptoms**
   a. Hypoaldosteronism can result in a rapid loss of Na^+ and subsequent hypotension from loss of intravascular volume.
   b. Patients should be monitored for the development of hyperkalemia, which can present with nonspecific symptoms of malaise and muscle weakness. These patients are also at risk for developing cardiac arrhythmias and sudden cardiac death. ECG changes in hyperkalemia include peaked T-waves and widening of the QRS complex.

5. **Management**
   a. Most antihypertensives and potassium supplements should be discontinued after surgery. Serum electrolytes should be monitored routinely for the development of hyperkalemia.
   b. Patients who do develop severe hypoaldosteronism may require a short course of mineralocorticoid replacement such as fludrocortisone (0.1 mg/day).
   c. Treatment of hyperkalemia depends on its severity. Mild hyperkalemia without ECG changes can be treated with cation exchange resins such as polystyrene sulfonate (Resonium or Kayexalate). More severe hyperkalemia and those with ECG changes will require urgent treatment with IV calcium gluconate for myocardial stabilization, transcellular shifting of potassium with IV insulin, dextrose, and/or albuterol, and occasionally removal of excess potassium with dialysis.

D. Complications after Cortisol-Producing Adenoma Resection

1. Cushing's syndrome describes the clinical picture of prolonged exposure to excessive cortisol. This can be exogenous or endogenous from excessive ACTH stimulation of the adrenals or primary secretion from the adrenal glands. The latter is typically from a functional adrenal adenoma or more rarely from bilateral macronodular adrenal hyperplasia. Certain adrenocortical carcinomas can also produce excess cortisol.

2. Although any unilateral adrenal resection for any etiology can eventually lead to adrenal insufficiency, patients who had a functional cortisol-secreting tumor are at much higher risk because the contralateral gland is often chronically suppressed.

3. Patients with Cushing's syndrome are also at increased risk of developing venous thromboembolic complications for unclear reasons.

4. **Signs and symptoms**
   a. Symptoms of adrenal insufficiency include abdominal pain, nausea, vomiting, refractory hypotension, and hypoglycemia.
   b. These features often overlap with many other common postoperative complications, and a high degree of clinical suspicion is needed. A short ACTH stimulation test can be performed to confirm the diagnosis, but critically ill patients should be treated empirically.
   c. Signs of potential venous thromboembolic complications include calf pain and swelling, shortness of breath, pleuritic chest pain, and hypoxia.
5. **Management**
   a. All patients undergoing adrenal resection for Cushing's syndrome should receive stress dose steroids perioperatively. A typical regimen is 50 to 100 mg of hydrocortisone IV q8h, which is weaned to maintenance over the next few postoperative days. Once the patient can adequately take oral medications, this is converted to PO hydrocortisone or prednisone.
   b. Supplemental steroid therapy is given until the hypothalamic–pituitary–adrenal axis recovers (can take up to 6 to 12 months and is usually coordinated by the endocrinologist using an ACTH stimulation test).
   c. Basal physiologic steroid requirements are approximately 5 to 10 mg of prednisone or 10 to 20 mg of hydrocortisone daily, with increased doses needed in times of physiologic stress.
   d. Prevention of venous thromboembolic complications utilizes perioperative low-molecular-weight heparin and early mobilization. Patients who do develop a deep vein thrombosis or a pulmonary embolus should be systemically anticoagulated once safe from a surgical perspective.

Suggested Readings

Domi R, Sula H, Kaci M. Anesthetic considerations on adrenal gland surgery. *J Clin Med Res* 2015;7(1):1–7.

Phitayakorn R, McHenry CR. Perioperative considerations in patients with adrenal tumors. *J Surg Oncol* 2012;106(5):604–610.

Randolph GW. *Surgery of the Thyroid and Parathyroid Glands.* 2nd ed. Philadelphia, PA: Saunders; 2012.

Roh JL, Park CI. Routine oral calcium and vitamin D supplements for prevention of hypocalcemia after total thyroidectomy. *Am J Surg* 2006;192(5):675–678.

Rosato L, Avenia N, Bernante P, et al. Complications of thyroid surgery: analysis of a multicentric study on 14,934 patients operated on in Italy over 5 years. *World J Surg* 2004;28(3):271–276.

Terris DJ, Snyder S, Carneiro-Pla D, et al. American Thyroid Association statement on outpatient thyroidectomy. *Thyroid* 2013;23(10):1193–1202.

9 Gastrointestinal, Abdominal, and Anorectal Patient

Elizabeth Turner

I. INTRODUCTION

A. Demographics of Gastrointestinal, Abdominal, and Anorectal Patients

There are a wide variety of operative procedures for treating gastrointestinal (GI), abdominal, and anorectal diseases. The circumstances of the operation can range from the emergent exploratory laparotomy for bowel obstruction to electively scheduled laparoscopic sigmoid colectomy for diverticulitis. The rate of complications can vary from 2% to 90% depending on the baseline health of the patient and on whether the surgery is elective or emergent. The surgical procedure may be more complex, such as a laparoscopic total proctocolectomy for ulcerative colitis, or less complex, such as a day surgery for hemorrhoidectomy. The patient can be young or elderly, and their baseline health can vary greatly.

B. Consideration of Patient Risk Factors

Patients undergoing emergent operations are not medically optimized and are at increased risk of perioperative complications. Patients undergoing an emergent operation for bowel obstruction, for example, tend to be dehydrated and require increased resuscitation.

The nutritional status of patients undergoing GI, abdominal, and anorectal surgery can also vary widely. Patients with poor preoperative nutritional status are at greater risk for anastomotic leak. Baseline nutritional status can be determined by looking at both longer term indicators of nutritional status, such as albumin (half-life 20 days), and shorter term indicators of nutritional status, such as pre-albumin (half-life 2 to 3 days).

Patients with cardiac risk factors undergoing elective GI, abdominal, and anorectal surgery should be medically optimized according to the American College of Cardiology/American Heart Association (ACC/AHA) Guidelines on Perioperative Cardiovascular Evaluation and Management of Patients Undergoing Noncardiac Surgery. β-Blockers should be continued in patients receiving β-blockers prior to surgery, or should be started in patients with intermediate- and high-risk factors according to the ACC/AHA guidelines, if they are not already taking them preoperatively. Patients undergoing emergent GI, abdominal, and anorectal operations are at increased perioperative cardiovascular risk.

There are multiple risk score calculators that can help determine the risk of postoperative pulmonary complications for patients undergoing GI, abdominal, and anorectal surgery. Patients at higher risk of pulmonary complications include, but are not limited to, those with chronic obstructive pulmonary disease (COPD), asthma, smokers, obstructive sleep apnea (OSA), obesity, heart failure, pulmonary hypertension, poor general baseline health, and the elderly.

C. Disposition from the Operating Room

Following surgery, patients undergoing GI, abdominal, and anorectal procedures are commonly admitted to the postanesthesia care unit

(PACU). Patients undergoing more minor procedures such as hemorrhoidectomy, sphincterotomy, pilonidal cyst excision, or perirectal abscess drainage are generally discharged home from the PACU following a short period of observation. It is important to ensure that these patients are discharged with adequate pain medication because these procedures can be very painful.

Patients with multiple comorbidities who undergo emergent surgery often need the increased level of care provided by the intensive care unit (ICU). These unstable patients will proceed directly from the operating room to the ICU, and will not go to the recovery room postoperatively.

II. MANAGEMENT OF COMMON POSTOPERATIVE PROBLEMS

A. Hemorrhage

1. Workup

Postoperative bleeding after GI, abdominal, and anorectal surgery may present either *early* in the PACU or *later* on the floor. There are multiple possible etiologies for bleeding in the GI, abdominal, and anorectal patient. These include, but are not limited to, anastomotic bleeding, large vessel injury, splenic laceration, and presacral bleeding.

The signs of postoperative bleeding include tachycardia, hypotension, and low urine output. If there is concern for bleeding, an abdominal exam should be performed, vital signs and urine output should be assessed, and a complete blood count should be obtained.

Hypovolemia causing hypotension and tachycardia may result from underresuscitation, but this is a diagnosis of exclusion, and bleeding should be excluded. The amount of resuscitation the patient received in the operating room should be assessed, in order to determine whether it was appropriate for the duration of the patient's operation, recorded estimated blood loss, and predicted insensible losses.

A patient who has had a large amount of bleeding in a short period of time may have a "stable" hemoglobin because the hemoglobin has not had time to equilibrate.

2. Management

Once it has been confirmed that there is bleeding, the source of the bleeding needs to be identified. Knowledge of intraoperative events can help to determine the source of the bleeding. For example, mobilization of the splenic flexure during an extended left colectomy or low anterior resection (LAR) would make splenic laceration more likely. Presacral bleeding that was temporized with sterile tacks intraoperatively would make a recurrence of this bleeding more likely.

Hemodynamically unstable patients with persistent transfusion requirements should return to the operating room for definitive management. Anastomotic bleeding may present as GI bleeding or intra-abdominal bleeding depending on the location of the bleeding relative to the GI lumen. If the bleeding is intraluminal, colonoscopy can be performed to control the bleeding.

If the patient remains hemodynamically stable, but there is evidence of ongoing bleeding, the source of bleeding can be further investigated with radiologic imaging. Endovascular angiography can serve as an effective alternative to surgical intervention for GI bleeding in some cases.

B. Pain

Pain is a common postoperative complication after GI, abdominal, and anorectal surgery.

The nature of the surgical procedure will determine the location and characteristics of the pain. Patients who undergo laparotomy primarily experience incisional pain, whereas patients who undergo laparoscopy commonly experience shoulder pain that is referred from irritation of the diaphragm. Perianal procedures can result in significant pain and discomfort. The most common reason a post-hemorrhoidectomy patient presents to the emergency room is insufficient pain control.

1. **Management**

Several meta-analyses have investigated the benefits of epidural anesthesia for pain control in both laparoscopic and open colorectal surgery. The results of these studies have been mixed. Some studies report improved outcomes with decreased lengths of stay and complications, whereas others have shown the exact opposite with increased lengths of stay and a higher incidence of urinary tract infections.

An alternative to epidural analgesia is patient-controlled analgesia (PCA). In addition, adjuncts such as intravenous (IV) acetaminophen and, when the risk of bleeding has decreased, IV nonsteroidal anti-inflammatory drugs (NSAIDs), can result in significant improvement in postoperative pain control. Patients who have a history of chronic pain may require substantially increased doses of medication to achieve adequate postoperative pain control. For these patients, consultation of the acute pain service may be beneficial.

C. **Enterotomy and Anastomotic Leak**

Anastomotic leak is most commonly a delayed postoperative complication, occurring most often during the second postoperative week or, in some cases, up to a month following surgery. Although anastomotic leak presents later in the postoperative course, this does not exclude enterotomy or primary failure of the staple/suture line, both of which can present much earlier. Hypotension, tachycardia, low urine output, and peritoneal signs are all suggestive of a possible enterotomy or anastomotic leak.

When a leak is suspected, it can be further investigated with imaging. Computed tomography with PO contrast is the most common choice; however, fluoroscopy with either PO or rectal contrast is also an option, depending on the location of the suspected leak (Fig. 9.1).

1. **Etiology**

Multiple patient factors increase the risk of anastomotic leak, including male sex, obesity, coronary artery disease, pulmonary disease, diabetes, anticoagulation, decreased preoperative albumin, complications during the surgery, and high ASA score. The etiology of the anastomotic leak can vary. No difference has been found between the rates of anastomotic leak in open versus laparoscopic operations.

Leaks that occur within the first 24 to 48 hours of an operation are because of failure of the suture line or staple line. Studies have shown that surgeons are unable to predict on the basis of the intraoperative course whether or not a patient will have an anastomotic leak. Multiple scoring systems have been developed in an attempt to predict the risk of anastomotic leak, most with limited validation. The strongest predictors for anastomotic leak are poor baseline nutrition and obesity.

2. **Management**

Treatment of an anastomotic leak or enterotomy depends on the timing of presentation and whether the leak is controlled or uncontrolled. Primary anastomotic failure or enterotomy is likely to be uncontrolled and will present in the first 24 to 48 hours after surgery. These patients should be taken back to the operating room for exploration and repair.

The anastomosis is weakest in the second postoperative week, and anastomotic leaks most commonly occur during this interval. Leaks occurring in this period may be controlled because the bowel

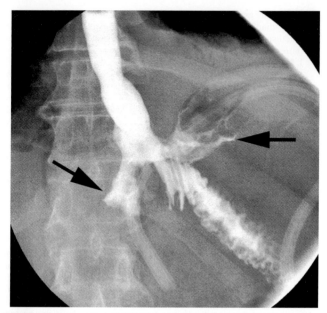

FIGURE 9.1 Anastomotic leak following bariatric surgery. Fluoroscopic spot image shows the leakage of contrast (*arrows*). (From Maheshwary RK, Hartman MS, Daffner RH. Gastrointestinal imaging. In: Daffner RH, Hartman MS, eds. *Clinical Radiology: The Essentials*. 4th ed. Philadelphia, PA: Wolters Kluwer Health; 2014:284.)

has had a chance to heal around the leak. If the leak is "controlled," that is, GI contents are not freely leaking into the abdominal cavity, but are localized to one area, interventional radiology (IR) drainage is an effective management strategy. The patient is made nil per os (NPO), and drain output can be monitored. Once the drainage stops, the drain can be removed.

If the leak is not contained and the patient is exhibiting signs of diffuse peritonitis, the patient should return to the operating room for exploration and revision of the anastomosis.

D. Wound Infection

1. Workup

The combination of an unclean environment, major surgery, and debilitated patients creates a situation that is associated with a very high incidence of wound infection. Patients with wound infections can present with a wide variety of symptoms, including fever, tachycardia, hypotension, and low urine output. Patients who begin to have fevers following a GI, abdominal, or anorectal operation should have their wound assessed for erythema, fluctuance, and drainage.

Wound infections may be superficial and involve only the skin and subcutaneous tissue, or they may be deep and involve the fascial and muscle layers or drain freely into the peritoneal cavity (Fig. 9.2).

The wounds of patients who have undergone GI, abdominal, and anorectal surgery range from clean contaminated to dirty. These wounds tend to be polymicrobial and may be difficult to treat.

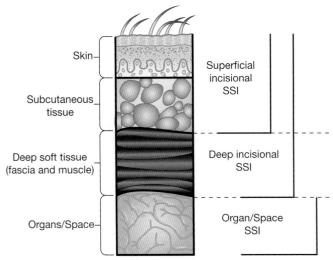

FIGURE 9.2 Definition of superficial, deep, and organ/space surgical site infections (SSIs). (Redrawn from Horan TC, Gaynes RP, Martone WJ, et al. CDC definitions of nosocomial surgical site infections, 1992: a modification of CDC definitions of surgical wound infections. *Infect Control Hosp Epidemiol* 1992;13(10):606–608.)

2. Management

Once a wound infection has been identified, the wound should be opened to allow for drainage. This may involve removing some or all of the staples or sutures holding the wound together. Once the wound has been opened, it may be packed with slightly moistened sterile gauze (known as "wet-to-dry") or, if the wound is very small, left to drain spontaneously.

The addition of systemic antibiotics is not necessary, but should be started if there are systemic signs of infection, including significant erythema, induration, fever, elevated white blood cell, and/or tachycardia. The choice of antibiotics will vary depending on the expected pattern of resistance in the area, but should include gram negative and anaerobic coverage in the case of wound infections following lower GI tract operations.

E. Ileus

1. Workup

Ileus occurs from hypomotility of the GI tract in the absence of mechanical bowel obstruction. Although ileus has numerous causes, the postoperative state is the most common setting for the development of ileus. Postoperative ileus can be divided into expected physiologic ileus and pathologic ileus. A physiologic ileus is broadly defined in the literature as 0 to 24 hours for the small intestine, 24 to 48 hours in the stomach, and 48 to 72 hours in the colon. In the absence of evidence of mechanical obstruction or intra-abdominal process responsible for the continued ileus, the ileus can be considered a prolonged physiologic ileus, which can last upward of 6 days.

Prolonged postoperative ileus can result from electrolyte derangements, such as hypokalemia, hypomagnesemia, and uremia. Pancreatitis and cholecystitis can also produce an ileus. Other pathologic

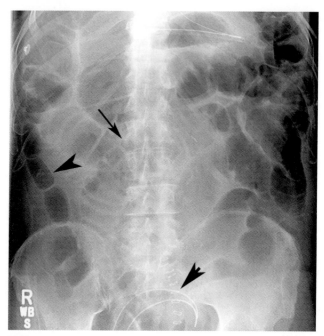

FIGURE 9.3 Plain supine abdominal radiograph of a patient with ileus. Air–fluid levels are present in the small intestine (*thin arrow*). Gas is seen in the colon (*thick arrowhead*). These findings are characteristic of, but not specific for, ileus. Surgical drains in the pelvis and skin staples (*short arrow*). (From Soybel DI, Santos AP. Ileus and bowel obstruction. In: Mulholland MW, Lillemoe KD, Doherty GM, et al, eds. *Greenfield's Surgery: Scientific Principles and Practice.* 6th ed. Philadelphia, PA: Wolters Kluwer; 2017:800.)

causes of ileus are intra-abdominal abscess, anastomotic leak, small bowel obstruction, and internal hernia. Certain risk factors such as a large tumor burden or peritoneal metastases make a mechanical bowel obstruction more likely.

The diagnosis of a prolonged benign physiologic ileus is one of exclusion, and patients should undergo evaluation after 3 to 5 days of no evidence of bowel function to rule out possible pathologic causes of the ileus. A plain abdominal radiograph is commonly obtained to look at the pattern of air–fluid levels, the degree of dilation of the small bowel, and whether or not there is evidence of air in the rectal vault (Fig. 9.3).

In the absence of concerning findings on abdominal radiograph, a CT abdomen/pelvis may be obtained to look for evidence of pathology such as fluid collections or anastomotic leak that may be the cause of the persistent ileus. Clinical exam and laboratory findings such as fever, tachycardia, hypotension, and leukocytosis may heighten the concern for anastomotic leak or abscess.

2. **Management**

In the absence of evidence of concerning clinical signs of perforation or intra-abdominal sepsis, a prolonged ileus can be managed conservatively. A nasogastric tube should be placed to low continuous wall suction for proximal decompression, and the patient should be made NPO and administered continuous IV fluids. Serial abdominal exams should be performed, and the vital signs and nasogastric tube output should be assessed regularly for signs of resolution.

Should the patient exhibit signs of peritonitis on abdominal exam or have worsening tachycardia and hypotension, this is evidence that the patient will require operative exploration.

F. High Ostomy Output

The colon is responsible for the reabsorption of water, and patients who have a diverting loop ileostomy, an endileostomy, or a proximal colostomy can have problems with dehydration, electrolyte abnormalities, and nutrition. On clinical exam, dehydration may manifest as dry mucous membranes, postural hypotension, tachycardia, and low urine output.

Following the creation of an ostomy, the patient's ostomy output should be monitored and his or her bowel regimen adjusted according to the ostomy output (see "Management" section below). Electrolytes should be monitored daily until the ostomy output has stabilized. The average ileostomy output is between 500 and 1,500 cc/day. Patients should be instructed to recognize the symptoms of dehydration and rehydrate accordingly. On average, patients with an ileostomy require increased fluid intake of 500 to 1,000 cc/day.

During the initial postoperative phase, the patient's ostomy output should be titrated to between 500 and 1,200 cc/day. This is accomplished by adding a combination of stool thickeners and antimotility agents to the patient's bowel regimen. Antimotility agents such as loperamide can be titrated to the patient's stool output from a dose of 1 mg to a dose of 16 mg daily divided into four daily doses. Tincture of opium may be given 0.3 to 1 cc up to 4 times daily. Diphenoxylate with atropine, a central nervous system depressant, may also be added to the regimen to slow bowel motility and should be given 30 minutes prior to meals. Psyllium wafers without the use of water intake can be used to add bulk to the patient's stool and slow down transit time.

In addition, those with a diverting loop ileostomy will also have issues with skin care around the ostomy site because a diverting loop ileostomy empties closer to the skin surface, and the GI contents will cause burns and erosions of the skin around the ostomy.

III. PITFALLS OF COMMON OPERATIONS

A. Colectomy

During a colectomy, care should be taken to avoid injuring adjacent structures. As the distal portion of the right colon or left colon is mobilized, the ureter should be identified. This may be difficult in cases where the colon is stuck to the pelvic side wall, such as with perforated colon cancer, diverticulitis, prior pelvic operations, or inflammatory bowel disease. The rates of ureteral injury have been reported in the literature to be as high as 10%.

Ureteral injuries not identified in the operating room may present early in the postoperative period, as in the case with transection, or late, up to more than a month later, as in the case with ureteral stricture. Patients with ureteral injuries may present with fever, flank pain, hematuria, abdominal distension, ileus, abdominal tenderness, or peritoneal signs.

Injury to the duodenum can also occur during mobilization of the proximal right colon, causing serious complications such as uncontrolled leak and proximal fistula. These duodenal injuries can result in uncontrolled leak and intra-abdominal sepsis and are associated with high morbidity.

B. Low Anterior Resection

Patients who have undergone a LAR with total mesorectal excision (TME) are at risk for a number of complications, including the following:

1. Urinary retention and voiding trials following catheter removal should be closely monitored.

2. Coloanal anastomoses are associated with increased risk of anastomotic leak (~15%) when compared with other intestinal anastomosis (~1.5%). Anastomotic leak may present as a contained leak or a free intraperitoneal leak. A contained leak with a small abscess less than 3 cm may be managed conservatively with IV hydration and antibiotics. In the case of abscesses greater than 3 cm, drainage is generally needed.

3. Patients may also present in a delayed manner with anastomotic stricture. Signs of stricture include abdominal distension, pain, and constipation. Patients with stricture should undergo colonoscopy for dilation and to assess for ischemia and evidence of malignant stricture. If dilations of the anastomosis are not effective, surgical revision of the anastomosis is often needed.

4. Creation of the colonic anastomosis during LAR requires mobilization of splenic flexure to allow the colon to reach the pelvic outlet. During this process, tearing of the splenic capsule can occur, resulting in bleeding. This bleeding is identified frequently during the operation and controlled at that time. However, postoperatively bleeding from the spleen should always be considered a potential source of hemorrhage in the patient after undergoing LAR.

C. Abdominoperineal Resection

Abdominoperineal resection (APR) involves removal of the anus, therectum, and part of the sigmoid colon along with creation of acolostomy. Of great concern for the postoperative patient who has undergone APR is the avoidance of a perineal wound infection.

Perineal wound infections without evidence of intraperitoneal abscesses can be managed conservatively with local wound control, debridement of nonviable tissue, packing or the use of a wound VAC (vacuum-assisted closure) device. Those with evidence of intraperitoneal abscesses greater than 3 cm should undergo placement of abdominal drains by IR.

Like the patient who undergoes an LAR, the patient who undergoes an APR is also at increased risk of urinary retention due to the degree of pelvic dissection.

D. Total Proctocolectomy with Ileal Pouch–Anal Anastomosis

Patients who undergo total proctocolectomyare at risk of high stool output and need titration of antimotility agents in a similar fashion to the patient with an ostomy (see "High Ostomy Output" section above).

An additional problem that frequently plagues patients with an ileal pouch is pouchitis. The incidence of pouchitis is thought to be as high as 60%. The cause of pouchitis is uncertain, but current hypotheses include the immune system's response to a change in the mucosal bacteria of the intestine. Patients with pouchitis will present with increased bowel frequency, urgency, tenesmus, abdominal pain, and cramps. Lower endoscopy often shows ulcerations, diffuse erythema, and exudates. The treatment of pouchitis includes 10 to 14 days of antibiotics such as ciprofloxacinand metronidazole.

E. Anorectal Procedures

One of the most common complaints of patients who have undergone an anorectal procedure is pain. After anorectal procedures, patients benefit from education about methods for maintaining an adequate bowel regimen to keep their stools soft and easy to pass. A variety of stool softeners and laxatives can be used to accomplish this. Oral narcotics should be used sparingly, and adjuncts should include use of acetaminophen or ibuprofen if not contraindicated.

Suggested Readings

Brunicardi FC, ed. *Schwartz's Principles of Surgery*. 8th ed. New York, NY: McGraw Hill; 2005.

Delacroix SE, Winters JC. Urinary tract injuries: recognition and management. *Clin Colon Rectal Surg* 2010;23:104–112.

Fleisher LA, Fleischmann KE, Auerbach AD, et al. 2014 ACC/AHA guideline on perioperative cardiovascular evaluation and management of patients undergoing noncardiac surgery: a report of the American College of Cardiology/American Heart Association Task Force on Practice Guidelines. *J Am Coll Cardiol* 2014;64:e77.

Frasson M, Flor-Lorente B, Rodriguez JL, et al. Risk factors for anastomotic leak after colon resection for cancer: Multivariate analysis and nomogram from a multicentric, prospective, national study with 3193 patients. *Ann Surg* 2015;262:321–330.

Halabi W, Jafari M, Nguyen V, et al. A nationwide analysis of the use and outcomes of epidural analgesia in open colorectal surgery. *J Gastrointest Surg* 2013;17:1130–1137.

Ju MH, Cohen ME, Bilimoria KY, et al. Effect of wound classification on risk adjustment in American College of Surgeons NSQIP. *J Am Coll Surg* 2014;219:371–381.

Liu H, Hu X, Duan X, et al. Thoracic epidural analgesia (TEA) versus patient controlled analgesia (PCA) in laparoscopic colectomy: a meta-analysis. *Hepatogastroenterology* 2014;133:1213–1219.

Mangram AJ, Horan TC, Pearson ML, et al. Guideline for prevention of surgical site infection, 1999. Hospital infection control practices advisory committee. *Infect Control Hosp Epidemiol* 1999;20:250–278.

Mirnezami A, Mirnezami R, Chandrakumaran K, et al. Increased local recurrence and reduced survival from colorectal cancer following anastomotic leak: systematic review and meta-analysis. *Ann Surg* 2011;253(5):890.

Tsujinaka A, Konishi F. Drain versus no drain after colorectal surgery. *Indian J Surg Oncol* 2011;1:3–8.

Management of the Genitourinary Surgical Patient

Rebecca I. Kalman, Elisabeth M. Baker, and Heather Renzi

Given the multitude of genitourinary procedures, this chapter focuses on those procedures with expected blood loss and anticipated inpatient stay. In this chapter, we review the prevalence and clinical significance of genitourinary malignancies in the U.S. population, discuss surgical management of nephrolithiasis and benign prostatic hypertrophy (BPH), and highlight preoperative considerations and postoperative risk reduction strategies for open surgical and minimally invasive urologic procedures.

PREVALENCE AND CLINICAL SIGNIFICANCE OF GENITOURINARY MALIGNANCIES

Renal cell carcinoma (RCC) is the seventh most common cancer in men and the ninth most common in women. RCC is approximately 50% more common in men than in women. Associated risk factors include tobacco use, obesity, hypertension, occupational exposures, polycystic kidney disease, chronic hepatitis C infection, long-term analgesic use, and genetics. RCCs are classified according to cell type and extent of metastasis, with clear cell tumors being more common and carrying a better prognosis than granular cell or spindle tumors. Clinical manifestations include hematuria, flank pain, and in the some cases, a palpable mass in the abdomen or flank. Treatment includes surgical removal (open radical nephrectomy vs. laparoscopy), radiofrequency ablation, and/or chemotherapy/radiation therapy.

Prostate cancer is the second most common malignancy among men. Prostate cancer occurs more often in African American men than in men of other races. Risk factors include genetics, first-degree relatives with prostate cancer, tobacco use, and high-fat diet. More than 95% of prostate neoplasms are adenocarcinomas, and clinical manifestations include bladder outlet obstruction (different from symptoms of BPH in that symptoms do not remit) and rectal obstruction. Bone pain is often associated with advanced disease. Treatment considerations include the stage of the cancer, life expectancy, general health of the individual, age, and anticipated effects of treatment. Surgical options include radical prostatectomy (with either a retropubic or perineal approach), transurethral resection of the prostate (TURP), cryosurgery, or laparoscopy (done manually or via robotic approach). Other options include chemotherapy, radiation therapy, hormone therapy, or no treatment.

Bladder cancer is the fourth most common malignancy among men and is 3 times more common in men than in women. Although bladder cancer is considered a disease of the elderly, the disease is more prevalent in Caucasians than in African Americans and Hispanics. Associated risk factors include tobacco use, pelvic irradiation, and exposure to cyclophosphamide, aromatic amines, diesel exhaust, and chemicals used in aluminum, rubber, or leather making industries. Although nonpapillary tumors tend to be less common, they are more invasive and carry worse prognoses when compared to papillary tumors. Although certain individuals may be asymptomatic, a common clinical manifestation includes painless hematuria. Treatment options include transurethral resection of the bladder tumor or laser treatment with neodymium:yttrium aluminum garnet for superficial tumors, intravesicular BCG or interferon for carcinoma in situ, or cystectomy for invasive bladder cancer and/or chemotherapy/radiation therapy.

NEPHROLITHIASIS

Across both genders, Caucasians have the highest prevalence of nephrolithiasis, with males 2 to 3 times more affected than females. Calcium-containing stones are the most common stone type and account for 70% to 90%, followed by uric acid, struvite, cystine, and xanthine stones. The larger the stone type, the more invasive the procedure. Percutaneous nephrolithotomy is often reserved for stones greater than 1.5 to 2.0 cm because shock wave lithotripsy and ureteroscopy may not be as effective for larger stones. Indications for immediate urologic evaluation and/or hospitalization include obstruction (especially in individuals with solitary kidney or transplanted kidney), urosepsis, intractable pain, and/or acute renal failure.

BENIGN PROSTATIC HYPERTROPHY

According to the *National Institute of Diabetes and Digestive and Kidney Diseases*, BPH affects about 50% of men between the ages of 51 and 60 and up to 90% of men older than 80. Clinical manifestations include increased hesitancy and straining, weak urine stream, dribbling, incomplete bladder emptying, increased urgency, dysuria, nocturia, and/or frequent urination. Treatment options for BPH include surveillance, medical therapy, minimally invasive therapies, or surgery. TURP is the most common procedure performed to treat BPH with significant lower urinary tract symptoms. Other transurethral procedures such as ablation, laster enucleaton, and photoseclective vaporization are also available. This chapter mainly focuses on postoperative management after TURP.

PREOPERATIVE CONSIDERATIONS

Patients presenting for urologic procedures are often elderly and have comorbid medical conditions including preexisting cardiopulmonary disease and renal impairment. This must be taken into account when evaluating and caring for this patient population.

Transurethral Resection of the Prostate

Individuals with cardiopulmonary disease carry greater perioperative risk. Large volumes of irrigation solution used during the procedure can be absorbed via prostatic venous sinuses. Thus, preoperative consideration should be made to individuals with poor cardiopulmonary function. Individuals with limited cardiac reserve may require invasive monitoring with arterial catheter placment, and in certain cirucmstances placment of central acess for monitoring and administration of vasoactive medications. A baseline hematocrit is helpful because blood loss is often obscured by increases in intravascular volume. Spinal anesthesia is ideal in patients undergoing TURP because it reduces the risk of pulmonary edema, decreases blood loss, and allows for detection of mental status changes associated with "TURP syndrome."

TURP and other percutaneous urologic procedure use large volumes of irrigation solution. Non-electrolye solutions of mannitol, sorbitol, or glycine aretypically used. Saline solutions are not compatible with electrosurgical devices. Use of sterile water is not feasibe as it is hypotonic and causes hemolysis and hyponatremia when absorbed.

Percutaneous Nephrolithotomy

Although percutaneous nephrolithotomy is often reserved for stones greater than 1.5 to 2.0 cm, other indications include removal of ureteral stones that cannot be treated by ureteroscopy, stone-encrusted stents, diverticular stones, and renal stones in individuals with ileal loops or other forms of genitourinary reconstruction. If the entire stone is unable to be fragmented with percutaneous nephrolithotomy and/or the stone burden is so large that it would require multiple procedures, conversion to an open surgical approach may be required. Contraindications for percutaneous nephrolithotomy include an inability for individuals to lie in a prone position, anticoagulation, existing urinary tract infection, or anatomic challenges (namely, the kidney cannot be accessed without going through other adjacent organs). Perioperative pain control with paravertebral block can be helpful for these procedures.

Laparoscopic Procedures

Of the common laparoscopic genitourinary procedures performed, this section focuses on laparoscopic nephrectomy and partial nephrectomy for RCC.

Relative indications (based on surgical experience) for laparoscopic radical nephrectomy include tumors <12 cm, tumors not extensively involving the hilum, and no tumor in main renal vein or inferior vena cava. Absolute indications for patients undergoing partial nephrectomy for RCC include individuals with a solitary kidney or bilateral tumors. Relative indications are individuals with hereditary RCC or the contralateral kidney is at risk for dysfunction because of stones, diabetes, hypertension, reflux, or renal artery stenosis. Elective indications are individuals with normal contralateral kidney function and whose tumor is less than 4 cm in size.

At the minimum, a baseline type and screen, complete blood count, and basic metabolic panel should be obtained preoperatively. For nephrectomies (whether laparoscopic or open surgical approach), preoperative consideration should be made in individuals with cardiopulmonary disease, diabetes, hypertension, and any degree of renal impairment. The hemodynamic changes that can occur with laparoscopy should be taken in to account. These include increased mean arterial pressure, increased systemic vascular resistance, decreased venous return, decreased functional residual capacity, and worsening $\dot{V}/\dot{Q}$ mismatch. Individuals with limited cardiac reserve may require more invasive monitoring with arterial catheter, central venous line, and in some cases, pulmonary artery catheter.

Open Surgical Procedures

Of the common open genitourinary procedures performed, this section focuses on radical cystectomies for bladder cancer, radical and partial nephrectomies for RCC, and open radical retropubic prostatectomy for prostate cancer.

At the minimum, a baseline type and screen, complete blood count, and basic metabolic panel should be obtained preoperatively. As always, patients underlying comorbidities must be assessed. Those wih poor cardiopulmonary function may benfit from more inasive monitoring. General anesthesia is the anesthetic of choice in this patient population.

In patients undergoing an open radical cystectomy or open radical retropubic prostatectomy, epidural anesthesia as an adjunct to general anesthesia may help to decrease postoperative pain. Transvers abdoinis plane, (TAP) blocks may be useful in certain patients for post operative pain relief. Multimodal recovery programs combining epidural analgesia, early mobilization, and oral nutrition help improve patient outcomes.

Robotic Surgical Procedures

This section focuses on robotic-assisted prostatectomy for prostate cancer. General anesthesia is the anesthetic of choice in this patient population, as with those individuals undergoing open radical retropubic prostatectomy. Preoperative consideration should be made in individuals with cardiopulmonary issues, in addition to those with a history of stroke or cerebral aneurysm or elevated intracranial pressure because the procedure requires prolonged Trendelenburg positioning. Unlike open radical retropubic prostatectomy in which exposure may prove difficult, robotic-assisted prostatectomy provides improved visualization, and reduced blood loss.

POSTOPERATIVE COMPLICATIONS

Transurethral Resection of the Prostate

TURP has distinct postoperative complications in that the procedure requires large volumes of nonelectrolyte irrigating fluid as part of the surgical resection. Because of this, in approximately 5% of cases, systemic absorption of the irrigation fluid can lead to TURP syndrome, causing cardiovascular, central nervous system, and metabolic changes. Early signs include lethargy, apprehension, restlessness, complaint of headache, bradycardia, hypotension, postoperative nausea, vomiting, and abdominal distention (because of absorption of the irrigating fluid through perforations in the prostatic capsule). Conversely, patients may develop hypertension and reflex tachycardia as a result of rapid volume expansion. Late signs include visual disturbances, focal or generalized seizures, and altered consciousness because of hyponatremia. To put it into perspective, systemic absorption of 1 L of irrigation within 1 hour corresponds to a decrease in the serum sodium concentration of 5 to 8 mmol/L. Severe TURP (as defined by a drop in serum sodium concentration to <120 mmol/L) may result in coma, permanent brain damage, respiratory arrest, brain stem herniation, or death. Moreover, irrigation solutions containing glycine may lead to absorption, and its metabolic product, ammonia, may cause hyperammonemia. Postoperative fluid balance must be monitored, and attention should be paid to the amount of irrigation used and the volume recovered. Treatment includes supportive care and (in severe cases) ventilatory management and intravenous anticonvulsants. Individuals with severe hyponatremia should be treated with 3% hypertonic saline. Diuretic therapy with lasix and mannitol may also be used. Special attention should be made to monitoring sodium plasma concentrations so as to avoid rapid overcorrection and/or central pontine myelinolysis.

Other immediate postoperative complications include hypothermia (which can be minimized with warm irrigating/intravenous solutions and warming blankets), bacteremia (minimized by appropriate antibiotic therapy), bleeding (which increases with the duration of surgery), and extravasation of fluids because of perforation (individuals with bladder perforation may develop peritoneal signs, and hiccups may be the result of diaphragmatic irritation). Visual impairments and transient blindness have been reported after TURPs when glycine was used, because glycine is also an inhibitory neurotransmitter in the retina, and therefore, large absorption leads to delayed transmission of impulses. Long-term complications associated with TURP include urinary incontinence, impotence, and retrograde ejaculation.

Peroneal nerve injury because of lithotomy positioning can occur, leading to foot drop.

Percutaneous Nephrolithotomy

Complications include inability to pass a rigid nephroscope into the kidney, bleeding, creation of an arteriovenous fistula or pseudoaneurysm, infection, impaired renal function, pneumothorax (air trapped in chest causing lung collapse), urinothorax (accumulation of urine in the pleural space), hydrothorax (accumulation of serous fluid in the pleural space), damage to adjacent organs, or retained stone fragments. Should surgical entry into the thorax result, chest tube placement may be necessary. Early complications include fever, hematuria, or drainage from the surgical incision site. In certain circumstances, individuals may require discharge with a nephrostomy tube. In addition, after the removal of renal stones one must always maintain a high clinical suspicion for spread of infection and development of sepsis, which may first present in the post operative care unit.

Laparoscopic Nephrectomy and Partial Nephrectomy

Compared to open nephrectomy, benfits of laparoscopic nephrectomy include decreased blood loss, decreased pain, shorter hospital stay, earlier return to activities, and a better cosmetic result. Following laparoscopic nephrectomy, the Foley catheter is often removed on postoperative day 1, early ambulation is encouraged, and diet is advanced more quickly. Patients are typically discharged home on postoperative day 1 or 2.

Although the indication for laparoscopic partial nephrectomy is the same as open, it is a less painful procedure with a faster recovery time. However, laparoscopic partial nephrectomies are more technically challenging and have more complications compared to open partial nephrectomies. Common postoperative complications associated with laparoscopic partial nephrectomies including hemorrhage and urine leak, in some circumstances, may require ureteral stent placement. Following laparoscopic partial nephrectomy, a Foley catheter is left in place and is typically removed on postoperative day 1 or 2. A Jackson–Pratt drain is left in situ, and any increased sanguineous drainage should prompt the provider to suspect hemorrhage. Similarly, any increased serous drainage should prompt the provider to suspect a urine leak (in which a ureteral stent may be needed). Therefore, the Jackson–Pratt drain should be removed only after the Foley catheter is removed. Early ambulation is encouraged, and diet is advanced from clears to regular postoperatively. Patients are typically discharged home on postoperative day 1 or 2.

Open Radical Nephrectomy

As with percutaneous nephrolithotomy, pneumothorax may occur secondary to surgical entry into the thorax, necessitating chest tube placement. Therefore, in the recovery room, a chest x-ray should be obtained. Early complications related to open radical nephrectomy include infection, bleeding, postoperative pneumonia, ileus, and pulmonary embolism/deep vein thrombosis. Late complications include development of an incisional hernia or permanent renal failure.

Radical Cystectomies

Aside from invasive carcinoma of the bladder, other indications for urinary diversion include pelvic malignancies (and secondary involvement of the bladder), intractable radiation cystitis, and end-stage interstitial cystitis. Options for treatment include urinary diversion with an ileal conduit, continent urinary diversion, or neobladder.

Early complications related to ileal conduit include ureterointestinal anastomotic disruption/obstruction, sepsis, wound infection/dehiscence, ileus, and conduit bleeding. Late complications include ureterointestinal anastomotic obstruction, parastomal hernia, stomal issues (including stenosis and retraction), pyelonephritis, higher risk of stone formation, urinary tract infections, metabolic acidosis, volvulus, conduit enteric fistula, loop stricture, and transitional cell carcinoma (TCC) recurrence in the upper tract.

Management of early or late ureterointestinal anastomotic leak requires radiographic evaluation and interventional radiology stenting, drain placement, or reoperation. Sepsis management includes early initiation of supportive care and early goal-directed therapy. Ileus often includes conservative management versus nasogastric tube placement and, in some cases, initiation of total parenteral nutrition. In certain circumstances, management of parastomal hernia and stomal issues necessitates stomal relocation. Stomal stenosis or stricture may lead to stomal ischemia, and signs of necrosis require urgent reexploration. Management of stones requires aggressive metabolic management and, in certain circumstances, laser lithotripsy versus extracorporeal shockwave lithotripsy. Under certain conditions, management of urinary tract infections includes empiric treatment while awaiting urine culture speciation. Ureterointestinal fistula requires interventional radiology for placement of catheter in loop versus stent placement. Strictures are often evaluated by intravenous pyelogram, CT scan, or loopogram, and treatment includes endoscopic balloon dilation versus open surgical repair. Upper tract TCC recurrence is monitored with cytology, loopograms, and CT/MRI scans, and gross hematuria should be evaluated with catheterized loop specimen for culture.

Complications associated with continent cutaneous diversion include metabolic (acidosis, malabsorption/steatorrhea, and vitamin B_{12} deficiency), incontinence, stomal stenosis, recurrent infection, difficulty with catheterization, and pouch stones. In certain circumstances, chronic metabolic acidosis is treated with sodium bicarbonate replacement tabs, malabsorption is treated with cholestyramine, and B_{12} deficiency is treated with injections. Incontinence or difficulty with catheterization sometimes requires open revision of catheterizable segment, and in cases of reservoir perforation, surgical repair is warranted and may require conversion to a conduit. Pouch stones are caused by metabolic abnormalities, chronic bacteriuria, and recurrent infections (e.g., from use of metal staples), and treatment includes percutaneous versus open removal.

Lastly, complications associated with orthotopic neobladder include poor emptying, ureteral stricture, fistula, incontinence, and infection. In these patients, incontinence is sometimes treated with an external clamp, bulking agents, and an artificial urinary sphincter.

Robotic Radical Prostatectomy

Potential risks associated with robotic radical prostatectomy include injury to surrounding organs, need to convert to an open surgical approach, rectal injury, incontinence, and erectile dysfunction. The usual postoperative course for males undergoing robotic radical prostatectomy is that they are discharged with a urinary catheter (which is typically removed 7 to 10 days postoperatively), and the recovery period is usually 4 to 6 weeks. The majority of patients are discharged on postoperative day 1 or 2. Although most patients experience some degree of incontinence following robotic prostatectomy, most patients quickly regain control by 3 to 6 months following surgery.

Suggested Readings

Aglio LS, Street JA, Allen PD. Anesthesia for urogenital surgery. In: Loughlin KR, ed. *Complications of Urologic Surgery and Practice: Diagnosis, Prevention, and Management*. 1st ed. Boca Raton, FL: CRC Press; 2007:35–47.

Campbell MF, Walsh PC, Retik AB, eds. *Campbell's Urology*. 8th ed. Philadelphia, PA: Saunders; 2002.

Hawary A, Mukhtar K, Sinclair A, et al. Transurethral resection of the prostate syndrome: almost gone but not forgotten. *J Endourol* 2009;23(12):2013–2020.

Liedberg F. Early complications and morbidity of radical cystectomy. *Eur Urol Suppl* 2010;9:25–30.

McCance KL, Huether SE, eds. *Pathophysiology: The Biologic Basis for Disease in Adults and Children.* 5th ed. St Louis, MO: Elsevier Mosby; 2006.

Mills RD, Studer UE. Metabolic consequences of continent urinary diversion. *J Urol* 1999;161:1057–1066.

Pasero C. Epidural analgesia for postoperative pain, part 2: multimodal recovery programs improve patient outcomes. *Am J Nurs* 2003;103(11):43–45.

Sabatine MS, ed. *Pocket Medicine.* 3rd ed. Philadelphia, PA: Lippincott Williams & Wilkins; 2008.

Salami SS, George AK, Rais-Bahrami S. Outcomes of minimally invasive urologic surgery in the elderly patient population. *Curr Transl Geriatr Exp Gerontol Rep* 2013;2:84–90.

Willis DL, Gonzalgo ML, Brotzman M, et al. Comparison of outcomes between pure laparoscopic vs robot-assisted laparoscopic radical prostatectomy: a study of comparative effectiveness based upon validated quality of life outcomes. *BJU Int* 2012;109:898–905.

11

Patient Care: Trauma Patient

Matthew Tichauer, Craig S. Jabaley, and D. Dante Yeh

I. In the United States, **trauma** is the leading cause of death for patients 1 to 44 years of age and the third overall leading cause of death for all age groups. It accounts for more deaths in individuals aged 1 to 34 than all other causes combined.

II. **Assessment** of the trauma patient must rapidly identify life-threatening injuries and initiate appropriate supportive therapies. Strict adherence to **Advanced Trauma Life Support** (ATLS) guidelines ensures efficient management of the trauma patient. The primary survey, resuscitation, secondary survey, definitive treatment or transfer of care, and tertiary survey are the principal steps of ATLS. Of note, assessment of the trauma patient is **dynamic**. Clinical deterioration should prompt a return to the primary survey.

A. The **primary survey** includes the evaluation of airway, breathing, circulation, disability, and exposure (**ABCDE**). Providers should be familiar with the Glasgow Coma Scale (GCS) and normal hemodynamic values as outlined in Tables 11.1 and 11.2, respectively. A detailed approach to the primary survey is reviewed in Table 11.3.

1. The Focused Assessment with Sonography for Trauma (**FAST**) exam or Extended-FAST (**eFAST**) has become an integral part of the primary survey. Serial FAST examinations following nonoperative management of trauma are commonplace. Indications for FAST examination in the postoperative setting include hemodynamic instability, changes in physical examination (e.g., increasing abdominal tenderness or distention, decreased breath sounds, chest pain, etc.), persistent anemia despite transfusions, and sudden-onset dyspnea.

B. Following appropriate interventions to address life-threatening injuries discovered during the primary survey, as well as managing hemodynamic instability, the **resuscitation phase** commences.

C. Following resuscitation, ATLS then calls for a **secondary survey**, which involves a thorough evaluation of the patient, including a history and comprehensive physical evaluation. Radiographic studies are often used as adjuncts to the secondary survey. Of note, the **secondary survey** may have been deferred or only completed partially if emergent operative intervention was required. Communication with the surgical team is important to ascertain the extent to which a secondary survey was completed to facilitate completion and timely acquisition of pending diagnostic studies.

D. The **tertiary survey** seeks to identify any **missed injuries** after initial resuscitation and operative intervention. A thorough review of the patient's history, medical record, diagnostic studies, and a repeat physical examination are all elements of the tertiary survey.

III. The **disposition** of trauma patients from the OR must account for the complex and resource-intense nature of their care.

A. Admission to the **postanesthesia care unit** (PACU) should be considered only for well-resuscitated patients with limited trauma burden who

TABLE 11.1	Glasgow Coma Scale					
	1	2	3	4	5	6
Eyes (open to)	None	Pain	Verbal command	Spontaneous		
Verbal	None/intubated	Incomprehensible sounds	Inappropriate/ incomprehensible words	Disoriented conversation	Oriented conversation	
Motor (response to painful stimuli)	None	Extensor posturing	Flexure posturing	Withdrawal	Localizes	Obeys verbal commands

TABLE 11.2   Normal Hemodynamic Values by Age Group

Age Group	Respiratory Rate	Heart Rate	Minimum Systolic Blood Pressure
Newborn	40–60	100–170	50
3 mo	30–50	100–170	50
6 mo	30–50	100–170	60
1 y	30–40	110–160	70–90
1–2 y	25–35	100–150	80–95
2–5 y	25–30	95–140	80–100
5–12 y	20–25	80–120	90–110
>12 y	15–20	60–100	100–120

TABLE 11.3   Elements of the Primary Survey

Airway: Assess for obstruction because of direct injury, foreign bodies, or edema as well as identify patients at risk due to their inability to protect the airway secondary to a depressed level of consciousness. Establish a definitive airway.

Breathing: Assess for the absence of breath sounds or presence of diminished breath sounds (consistent with either pneumothorax or hemothorax), gross chest wall injuries (flail chest, sucking chest wound), dyspnea, hyperresonance or dullness to chest percussion (suggesting tension pneumothorax or hemothorax). Perform thoracentesis for hemothorax and nontension pneumothoraces and needle decompression for tension pneumothorax.

Circulation: Assess for the presence of hypovolemia, sources of hemorrhage, and cardiac dysfunction. Evaluate the jugular veins for distention and distant heart sounds to evaluate for cardiac tamponade requiring pericardiocentesis. Control hemorrhage with packing, clotting products, pressure, and temporary sutures. Ensure adequate access for volume resuscitation (e.g., bilateral upper extremity large-bore intravenous catheters).

Disability: Determine gross mental status and assess for neurologic dysfunction including motor examinations. Identify the presence of head or spinal cord injury. Utilize the Glasgow Coma Scale (Table 11.1).

Exposure: Complete removal of patients' clothing to perform a brief physical examination while controlling for hypothermia.

are unlikely to require emergent reoperative intervention. Although intraoperative resuscitation may have been adequate, vigilance is of the utmost importance because patients may have missed injuries or further decompensate owing to the physiologic response to traumatic and operative insults.

1. Changing trends in the management of trauma, including **damage control surgery** and hemostatic resuscitation, have shifted the priorities of initial efforts away from vigorous resuscitation to permissive hypotension until hemostasis can be achieved. Accordingly, patients may be relatively underresuscitated at the conclusion of surgery. These patients are often unsuitable for admission to the PACU.

2. Sufficient **expertise** and **personnel** must be available given the often unpredictable postoperative course of trauma patients and high incidence of shock, respiratory failure, and other complications as outlined below.

3. Heightened **physical security** may be required in certain circumstances, and the receiving PACU must be able to accommodate such needs.

B. Admission to an **intensive care unit** (ICU) should be pursued for patients who require ongoing resuscitation, mechanical ventilation, or who have suffered multisystem injuries. When limited physical space within an ICU precludes admission, involvement of the **ICU team** while the patient remains in the PACU should be advocated.

IV. MANAGEMENT OF COMMON PACU PROBLEMS

A. Circulatory **shock**, a low-perfusion state marked by inadequate tissue oxygenation, is commonly encountered in trauma patients. **Resuscitation** is the process by which shock is treated, perfusion is restored, and tissue oxygenation is normalized. Intraoperatively, resuscitation may be purposefully delayed or slowed until hemostasis is obtained because robust systemic perfusion may worsen hemorrhage and preclude clot formation. However, the **goal** of resuscitation shifts postoperatively following the accomplishment of hemostasis and then focuses on normotension and normovolemia.

1. An approach to the **differential diagnosis** of shock is presented in Table 11.4. Although there are numerous potential etiologies, **hemorrhagic** shock is the most common in this patient population. (Please refer to Chapter 21 for a detailed discussion.) As such, hypotension in trauma patients is typically synonymous with hypovolemia. However, **obstructive** shock should always be considered in the differential because it can be rapidly progressive and fatal.

Bedside **ultrasonography**, including transthoracic ultrasound, can help to quickly assess the etiology of shock as demonstrated through experience with FAST and the growing utilization of ultrasound in critical care environments.

2. The **systemic inflammatory response syndrome** (SIRS) describes a cytokine response to surgical stress or antecedent trauma, which is marked by tachycardia, tachypnea, fever, and leukocytosis. When coupled with hypovolemia or a sufficiently robust inflammatory response, SIRS can progress to include hypotension and resultant

TABLE 11.4	Differential Diagnosis of Shock in the Immediately Postoperative Trauma Patient	
Shock Etiology		**Specific Considerations**
Hypovolemic		Hemorrhage, burns, underresuscitation, gastrointestinal losses
Obstructive		Tamponade, tension pneumothorax, pulmonary embolism, aortic disruption, abdominal compartment syndrome
Cardiogenic		Myocardial infarction, cardiac contusion, dysrhythmia, heart failure
Distributive	Septic	Bacteremia, pneumonia, pancreatitis, surgical site infection, catheter-related infection
	Neurogenic	Spinal cord injury
	Anaphylactic	Antibiotics, latex
Endocrine		Acute and relative adrenal insufficiency, thyrotoxicosis
Toxic		Group A *Streptococcus*, necrotizing soft tissue infection

distributive shock. Even when faced with likely SIRS, other etiologies of shock should be carefully considered and excluded.

3. The **treatment** of shock relies on accurate diagnosis, and correction, of the underlying cause. As a general principle, hypovolemia should be convincingly corrected prior to the use of vasopressors so as not to mask inadequate hemostasis. **Refractory hypovolemia** may represent inadequate or failed hemostasis, and the surgical team should be immediately notified if such a suspicion develops. Multiple laboratory markers have been used to judge the adequacy of resuscitation following trauma, including pH, lactate, base excess, and central or mixed venous oxygen saturation. Although base excess is easy to measure and of clear prognostic value, lactate appears to be a more accurate biomarker.

   a. Aggressive resuscitation during hemorrhage requires **coordination** of multiple considerations: adequate intravascular access, supply of blood products, equipment (warmers and/or rapid infusers), and personnel. A plan to quickly address all of these needs must be in place for all PACUs that admit trauma patients.

   b. **Intravenous fluids** should be used judiciously and only when faced with clinical evidence of severe hypovolemia. Reflexive infusion of fluid to rectify all causes of hypotension can quickly lead to pulmonary edema, abdominal compartment syndrome (ACS), dilutional coagulopathy, and other consequences of overt fluid overload. Available evidence does not support the use of colloids, compared to crystalloids, in trauma patients. Furthermore, albumin has been associated with higher mortality rates in the setting of traumatic brain injury (TBI).

B. **Hypothermia** is a frequent complication of general anesthesia, and trauma patients are particularly susceptible following transport and evaluation, hemorrhage, resuscitation, and often extensive surgical exposure. Even a mild degree of hypothermia has been associated with **numerous adverse outcomes** and contributes heavily toward the development of coagulopathy, acidosis, and death in trauma patients. **Core temperature** should be measured no less often than every 15 minutes until a definitive trend has been established. Values less than 36.0°C must prompt immediate intervention. **Forced air warming** devices are a mainstay of treatment given both their safety and efficacy, and fluids should be warmed during ongoing resuscitation. The vasodilatation that accompanies **rewarming** may precipitously unmask hypovolemia; as such, close attention should be paid to hemodynamics during this period. Please refer to Chapter 22 for a detailed discussion.

C. **Neurologic considerations**, while seemingly routine, are pivotal to the prompt and successful postoperative recovery of trauma patients.

   1. **Pain management** is often a challenge owing to the combination of pain from the initial injury and subsequent surgical insult. Pulmonary function can be easily compromised following injury to the chest or abdomen because splinting impairs respiratory efforts leading to hypoventilation, gradual alveolar derecruitment, and poor oxygenation. Furthermore, it has been argued that aggressive pain control, in blunting the sympathetic response to pain, may ameliorate microcirculatory vasoconstriction, improve tissue perfusion, halt fibrinolysis, and protect against disruption of the endothelial glycocalyx. Please refer to Chapter 14 for a detailed discussion of pain management in the PACU.

      a. **Opioids** are a mainstay of postoperative pain control. Compared to interval dosing, patient-controlled analgesia (PCA) is often thought to be the most appropriate way to facilitate adequate and timely pain control postoperatively because this patient population may require heightened doses owing to tolerance and extensive injury.

b. **Pharmacologic adjuncts** should be used with caution. **Nonsteroidal anti-inflammatory drugs** (NSAIDs) impair platelet function through their inhibition of cyclooxygenase-1. Although this concern often precludes their use following trauma, large retrospective studies and meta-analyses have failed to demonstrate a significant impact of ketorolac on the incidence of surgical bleeding. **Acetaminophen** should be limited to 3,000 mg/24 hours and avoided in patients subjected to prolonged hypotension because they may develop concomitant ischemic hepatitis.

c. **Ketamine** is a useful adjunct to opioids when administered in low doses by either infusion or intermittent dosing. Concerns that ketamine may contribute to posttraumatic stress disorder have dissipated because contemporary experience with its use has grown. Although some practitioners avoid the use of ketamine over concerns about its effects on intracranial and intraocular pressure, these effects have been greatly exaggerated and are no longer relevant in current practice.

d. **Regional anesthesia** is often overlooked as a viable option for postoperative pain control in the trauma population because the emergent nature of surgery often necessitates rapid intervention and complicates the informed consent process. However, postoperative peripheral nerve blockade should be considered in amenable cases of orthopedic trauma. Attention should be paid to the patient's coagulation status, the possibility of preexisting nerve injury, and the likelihood of compartment syndrome. Pain associated with compartment syndrome is often poorly masked by regional anesthesia in the absence of dense motor blockade, and some have argued that the recognition of compartment syndrome may not necessarily be delayed.

e. **Neuraxial anesthesia** is frequently not a viable option for postoperative pain control following trauma owing to the high incidence of hypovolemia and coagulopathy. However, patients with blunt chest injury and three or more rib fractures may benefit from the utilization of an epidural catheter in the absence of contraindications.

2. Postoperative **delirium** is not uncommon following emergency surgery for trauma. Although the underlying etiology is unclear, evidence from elective surgery suggests that preoperative benzodiazepines, abdominal surgery, and a long operative course are all contributing factors. With regard to trauma patients, drug and/or alcohol intoxication, disorientation, inadequate analgesia, fear, and sympathetic overstimulation are additional considerations.

a. Postoperative delirium not only poses a **serious risk** to patients and their caretakers but may be the first sign of an underlying physiologic derangement.

b. The **evaluation** and **treatment** of postoperative delirium is covered in Chapter 19. Trauma patients should be quickly evaluated for respiratory and metabolic causes of delirium because these are not only correctable but potentially life-threatening. Thereafter, inadequate analgesia and either intoxication or withdrawal may be likely culprits. When supportive interventions fail, haloperidol or other antipsychotic medications should be considered when symptoms are severe and patient safety is at risk. Indiscriminate

TABLE 11.5	Approach to Delayed Awakening Following Emergency Surgery for Trauma	
Underlying Etiology	**Specific Causes**	**Evaluation**
Drug effects	Intoxication	Serum ethanol, toxicology screening
	Residual neuromuscular blockade	Peripheral nerve stimulation
	Residual anesthetic	Chart review, cranial nerve examination, clinical evaluation
Metabolic	Hypoglycemia	Capillary glucose
	Hypothermia	Core thermometry
	Acidosis	Arterial blood gas
Neurologic	Traumatic brain injury	Computed tomography, review mechanism of injury
	Cerebral ischemia	Computed tomography, complete neurologic examination
	Intracranial pathology	Computed tomography, cranial nerve examination
	Seizure	Electroencephalography
Respiratory	Hypercarbia	Arterial blood gas
	Hypoxemia	Pulse oximetry, arterial blood gas
	Dyshemoglobinemia	Pulse or arterial CO oximetry

benzodiazepine use may only precipitate worsened delirium and often proves to be counterproductive.

3. **Delayed awakening**, either in the operative suite or PACU, has a broad differential following trauma owing to multiple possible contributors. Table 11.5 presents a basic approach to the diagnosis and evaluation of this problem in trauma patients. **Treatment** is directed toward correction of the underlying contributing factors, where possible, and is otherwise supportive. Airway protection is always of the utmost importance. As such, extubated patients who fail to awaken after approximately 90 minutes, or those with a continued decline in consciousness, may require endotracheal intubation until symptoms resolve. **Naloxone** and **flumazenil** should be used with extreme caution in this population because administration in the setting of chronic abuse may precipitate symptoms of acute withdrawal.

D. **Respiratory failure** represents a major contributor to morbidity and mortality, especially among the elderly and following blunt thoracic trauma. Although often multifactorial, common peritraumatic considerations are outlined below.

1. **Rib fractures** are remarkably painful, and suboptimal analgesia leads to the inevitable development of respiratory splinting and atelectasis. Thoracic epidural analgesia or paravertebral nerve block should be considered for patients with evidence of respiratory compromise secondary to pain. **Noninvasive positive pressure ventilation** is a well-proven option to manage respiratory insufficiency secondary to rib fractures and flail chest syndrome.

2. **Pulmonary contusion** often accompanies blunt thoracic injury and leads to progressive shunting and hypoxemia. Initial chest radiographs can be deceptively reassuring; however, ongoing resuscitation, intraoperative positive pressure ventilation, and the systemic inflammatory response to trauma can all contribute to progressive pulmonary dysfunction.

   a. Even minor lung injury can blossom into the **acute respiratory distress syndrome**, which portends a poor prognosis. Care is largely supportive and centers on avoidance of overzealous volume expansion and lung-protective ventilation strategies. Positive pressure ventilation is often required and should be titrated to deliver tidal volumes of 4 to 6 mL/kg of ideal body weight, with plateau airway pressures less than 30 cm H_2O. These patients require prompt transfer to an ICU. In the setting of severe ARDS, transfer to an ECMO-capable center should be considered.

E. **Cardiac** complications may manifest as a direct result of traumatic injury or indirectly if the physiologic stress response outpaces physiologic reserves.

   1. **Blunt cardiac injury** (BCI) following thoracic trauma can range in severity from minor electrocardiographic abnormalities to overt myocardial rupture. In the population of trauma patients likely to be encountered in the PACU, **arrhythmia** and **cardiac dysfunction** are the two most likely sequelae.

      a. The **diagnostic** approach to BCI is controversial. An **EKG** demonstrating malignant arrhythmias, new conduction abnormalities, or ST or T wave changes is suggestive of BCI in patients with thoracic trauma. However, a normal EKG cannot definitively exclude BCI; as such, current guidelines recommend the use of cardiac **biomarkers** as a confirmatory test. However, biomarkers may be elevated even in the absence of thoracic trauma or overt myocardial injury owing to the stress response to polytraumatic injury. Regardless, **echocardiography** should be pursued in patients with refractory shock when BCI is clinically suspected because the culprit may be structural damage and not simply cardiac dysfunction secondary to myocardial contusion.

      b. **Management** of BCI is mostly supportive. Contused myocardium is arrhythmogenic, which can be problematic because arrhythmia is poorly tolerated in this population. Treatment should proceed per ACLS algorithms with heightened attention to the prompt **correction of metabolic abnormalities**, which further contribute to the genesis and perpetuation of arrhythmia. After discharge from the PACU, patients with suspected BCI should be admitted to either a **telemetry** or ICU setting for at least 24 hours. **Cardiology** consultation may be helpful to establish ongoing follow-up.

   2. **Myocardial ischemia** and **infarction** (MI) are ultimately the result of mismatching between myocardial oxygen demand and supply. The physiologic stress response to both trauma and surgical intervention can easily precipitate acute cardiac events in patients with underlying heart disease. As is the case with most perioperative MI, **symptomatic angina is rare**. Distracting injuries may further reduce its detection among trauma patients. As such, arrhythmia and hypotension may be the only presenting symptoms. MI has been found to be a rare consequence of BCI that typically presents shortly following the inciting injury. Patients in the PACU with a suspected MI are likely to respond to the typical interventions aimed at restoring a favorable supply to demand ratio: pharmacologic intervention,

analgesia, supplemental oxygen, and avoidance of anemia. β-Block-ade and preload reduction are often poorly tolerated in postacute trauma patients and must be titrated judiciously.

Interestingly, retrospective data suggest that **pulmonary artery catheterization** is associated with better outcomes in elderly trauma patients with moderate shock. This finding highlights the likely importance of careful and judicious resuscitation in avoiding deleterious cardiac outcomes among frail patients.

F. Immediate postoperative **infection** and **sepsis** are extremely uncommon following elective surgery and only rarely manifest themselves in the PACU. However, trauma patients are at an increased risk for immediate infectious complications postoperatively in the setting of penetrating trauma, contaminated wounds, emergent procedures, aspiration, and invasive devices. Although postoperative **fever** often represents a normal cytokine response to trauma or surgery, persistent or high-degree fever should prompt immediate clinical examination of the patient, attention to the surgical site, and consideration of other etiologies as outlined in Chapter 22.

G. The prevention and treatment of **coagulopathy** is a critical element in the care of trauma patients. With an estimated incidence of approximately 30%, coagulopathy has been consistently associated with increased transfusion requirements, longer hospital and ICU stays, prolonged duration of mechanical ventilation, organ system dysfunction, and death. Although the subgroup of trauma patients selected for admission to the PACU are unlikely to demonstrate fulminant coagulopathy, the inflammatory response to trauma may unexpectedly precipitate abnormal coagulation and impaired hemostasis.

1. The **etiology** of coagulopathy relates to a disruption in the homeostatic balance between clotting and fibrinolysis. **Hypothermia**, **acidosis**, and **hemodilution** are three classic causes of enzymatic dysfunction. However, increasing attention has been drawn to the importance of **consumptive coagulopathy** and pathologic **fibrinolysis** associated with acute traumatic coagulopathy (ATC) as contributing factors.

2. **Diagnostic** studies are often impractical intraoperatively given the time needed for result turnaround and the dynamic nature of coagulation. As such, plasma-rich transfusion strategies during massive transfusion with a 1:1:2 ratio of plasma and platelets to red blood cells are often employed. Postoperatively, **coagulation studies** including partial thromboplastin time (PTT), prothrombin time, international normalized ratio (INR), fibrinogen, and complete blood counts (CBC) can be used to gauge the severity of coagulopathy and guide treatment efforts. Notably, **fibrinogen** is typically the first factor to become depleted during ATC. If available, thromboelastography (TEG) and related viscoelastic assays can be utilized to generate a graphic representation of clotting function.

3. The **treatment** of ATC should be aimed at interrupting the **lethal triad** of hypothermia, acidosis, and coagulopathy. Initial supportive measures must aim to restore normothermia, bolster systemic perfusion to correct tissue hypoxia, and achieve normovolemia without diluting clotting factors. Empiric plasma-rich resuscitation strategies have been associated with improved perioperative hemostasis during massive resuscitation; however, the optimal duration of this strategy once hemostasis has been achieved remains unclear. Postoperatively, the transfusion of blood product components can be guided by diagnostic studies.

a. **Antifibrinolytics** are lysine analogs that interrupt the degradation of fibrin by plasmin and thus work to prevent ATC. **Tranexamic acid** (TXA) is one such drug and the only pharmaceutical agent with robust prospective evidence demonstrating a reduction in mortality following traumatic hemorrhage. TXA is effective when given **within 3 hours** of injury, but may be deleterious if treatment is initiated thereafter. Unfortunately, TXA remains unavailable at many centers in the United States despite its relatively low cost. **Aminocaproic acid** is often used in its absence despite uncertainty about the optimal timing, dosage, and duration of treatment.

b. **Recombinant factor VIIa** garnered initial anecdotal evidence for its efficacy when faced with diffuse microvascular bleeding associated with ATC. However, subsequent randomized prospective trials failed to demonstrate any impact of this expensive treatment on mortality. As such, its current role is largely as a salvage therapy.

c. More recently, **prothrombin complex concentrates** (PCCs) have been developed by processing pooled human plasma into a preserved and easily reconstitutable solution containing factors II, VII, IX, and X in addition to proteins C and S. Compared to fresh frozen plasma, the ability to immediately administer PCC coupled with reduced fluid volume, infectious complications, and immune risks makes PCC an attractive alternative. Experience with PCCs to correct coagulopathy following both cardiac surgery and trauma is growing, largely among providers in Europe. The high cost of treatment has limited their widespread adoption in the United States thus far. At this time, the only well-defined role of PCCs is in the emergent reversal of vitamin K antagonist anticoagulants.

d. Similarly, **fibrinogen concentrate** is also being considered for its potential role in the correction of ATC in combination with antifibrinolytic agents, given that fibrinogen is rapidly depleted.

V. SPECIFIC CONSIDERATIONS

A. **Airway injury** poses a serious risk to patients and is typically identified during the primary survey. Penetrating trauma is the most common culprit. Subcutaneous emphysema, decreased breath sounds (because of pneumothorax), hemoptysis, and dyspnea are all physical examination findings suggestive of an airway injury. Should any of these findings present postoperatively, an occult injury should be suspected and immediate consideration given to the establishment of a definitive airway.

B. **Head trauma** represents a growing subsegment of traumatic injury. From 2001 to 2010, the rates of TBI-related ED visits increased across all age groups by at least 50%, except the 25- to 44-year-old group, where there was a 40% increase. TBI is responsible for about 33% of all deaths caused by injury of any kind, and there are approximately 5.3 million people with permanent disabilities as a result of head injury.

1. Seizures, weakness, cognitive dysfunction, reduced alertness, and changes in airway reflexes are common **presenting symptoms** in patients with neurotrauma. Underlying causes include subarachnoid hemorrhage, subdural hemorrhage, intracerebral hemorrhage, and diffuse axonal injury. Importance is placed on ensuring that intracranial and extracranial hemodynamics are optimized to allow adequate cerebral perfusion pressure and cerebral blood flow in an effort to avoid secondary brain injury because of ischemia and hypoxia. Additionally, emphasis should be placed on the maintenance of **normocapnia**.

2. Patients with known **intracranial hypertension** are often most appropriately managed in an ICU. However, all PACU providers should be familiar with the principles of management as outlined in Chapter 7.

C. **Penetrating neck injury** requires prompt attention to airway management and the control of hemorrhage during the primary survey because the neck is rich in neurologic, vascular, alimentary, and endocrine structures.

1. To facilitate injury classification, the neck is divided into **three anatomic zones**: Zone 1 from the sternal notch to cricoid cartilage, Zone 2 from the cricoid cartilage to the angle of the mandible, and Zone 3 from the angle of the mandible to the skull base. The majority of injuries occur in Zone 2, which is in part because of its lack of nearby osseous structures.

2. **Hard signs** of neck injury include dysphagia, dysphonia, an obvious air leak, hemorrhage, expanding hematoma, subcutaneous emphysema, auscultatory bruit, and palpable thrill. Identification of these findings during the primary survey warrants immediate surgical intervention.

3. In the absence of obvious injury, the **classical approach** calls for surgical exploration of all injuries to Zone II in which the platysma was violated. However, the availability of high-quality helical computed tomography (CT) scans and CT angiography (CTA) has changed the management of penetrating neck injury such that **CTA** is now commonly obtained to evaluate all injuries regardless of anatomic zone in the absence of obvious operative indications. These patients require **heightened scrutiny** postoperatively.

D. **Thoracic trauma** varies in severity from benign contusion to injuries resulting in immediate and unavoidable death. PACU providers should be proficient in the detection and management of tension pneumothorax, hemothorax, and cardiac tamponade because these can be rapidly fatal in the absence of intervention.

1. **Hemothorax** can be evidenced by large effusions on a radiograph, decreased breath sounds, hemodynamic instability, and worsening hypoxemia. Although a large hemothorax is typically uncovered during the primary survey, injury of smaller vasculature can delay its detection until well into the postoperative period. Thoracocentesis is both diagnostic and therapeutic.

2. Similarly, **pneumothorax** may not be detected during the primary survey because findings can be subtle. Furthermore, supine radiographs can appear deceptively normal. The intraoperative provisioning of positive pressure ventilation can worsen a small pneumothorax and delay its recognition. Absent or diminished breath sounds with respiratory distress are suggestive findings. Symptoms may progress to include elevated airway pressures, hemodynamic instability, and tracheal deviation in the case of a tension pneumothorax. Needle decompression and/or tube thoracostomy should be pursued. Postoperatively, **upright** chest radiographs and **ultrasonography** can be useful adjuncts if a pneumothorax is suspected.

3. Distant heart sounds, jugular venous distention (JVD), and hemodynamic instability are indicative of **cardiac tamponade** and necessitate pericardiocentesis. JVD may not be present with concomitant hypotension.

E. **Abdominal trauma** is classified by the mechanism of injury to ascertain the likely pattern of injury. Blunt abdominal trauma from motor vehicle crashes, falls, and assault may result in crush injury, shearing injury to organs and vasculature, or increased intraabdominal pressure resulting in a ruptured viscous. Penetrating injury, typically the result of gunshot or stab wounds, commonly involves the small bowel, liver, stomach, colon, and vascular structures. Initial ultrasound examination has largely replaced diagnostic peritoneal lavage, because it allows the provider to assess for operative indications in the unstable patient and permits nonoperative management with serial examinations.

1. In both penetrating and blunt abdominal trauma, the **liver** is the most commonly injured solid organ. In greater than 95% of cases managed nonoperatively, rebleeding does not occur. Transfusion requirements are typically higher in operative cases versus nonoperative cases, potentially related to the severity of injury requiring operative management. Complications following hepatic injury include liver abscesses and biliary tract injuries with biloma and hemobilia.

2. Injury to the **spleen** may cause massive hemorrhage with hemodynamic instability. The failure rate of nonoperative management approaches 5% to 10% and increases with more severe grades of injury. Rebleeding following hemostasis may occur days to weeks after injury. It is imperative for providers to closely follow hematocrit values, and an ongoing transfusion requirement may indicate the need for either operative management or angiography with embolization. Operative management for massive hemorrhage often requires splenectomy.

    a. Patients who undergo splenectomy may have a transient **thrombocytosis**, and current guidelines recommend the administration of aspirin should the platelet count exceed 1,000,000. Additionally, patients typically develop a **leukocytosis** following splenectomy. As such, evaluation of alternative markers of infection is necessary.

    b. In patients who are deemed compliant, **vaccination** against *Haemophilus influenza*, *Pneumococcus*, and *Meningococcus* may be administered at follow-up 2 weeks following surgery. For all others, vaccination upon hospital discharge is indicated.

3. Traumatic **pancreatic** injuries are associated with significant morbidity and mortality and are typically seen in the setting of duodenal injury and upper lumbar trauma. Because the pancreas is a retroperitoneal organ, patients may not present with peritoneal signs. Elevated **amylase** and **lipase** postoperatively may point to a pancreatic injury.

    a. Patients who undergo an emergent **pancreaticoduodenectomy for trauma** should be admitted to an ICU postoperatively because they typically have a higher injury burden and more complicated postoperative course compared to other patients who sustained blunt trauma.

4. In penetrating trauma, the small bowel is the most commonly injured **hollow viscous organ**. Injury to both the small bowel and colon may also result from blunt trauma, especially with improperly worn seatbelts. Indications for operative intervention include intraperitoneal free air and fluid, peritonitis, and hemodynamic instability. Although free fluid may be bowel contents, it is typically blood from solid organ injury. Serial abdominal examinations and close monitoring of arterial blood gases (base deficit), lactate, and white blood cell (WBC) count are indicated in patients who are hemodynamically stable without gross evidence of injury on CT scan.

5. **Abdominal compartment syndrome (ACS)** is caused by intraabdominal hypertension that results in decreased end-organ perfusion leading

to ischemia and tissue death. ACS is fatal if left untreated because ischemia develops in the hypoperfused gut and kidneys, and multiple organ dysfunction syndrome ensues. Because of the increased abdominal pressure, ventilation in these patients proves difficult owing to impaired diaphragmatic excursion and decreased abdominal compliance. Additionally, because of compression of the inferior vena cava, venous return to the heart is impaired, which can lead to a mixed shock state and exacerbation of tissue hypoperfusion.

a. ACS is **subdivided** into primary, secondary, and recurrent types. Primary ACS is associated with injury of the abdominopelvic space requiring operative or interventional radiologic intervention. Visceral edema from third space losses and progressive bleeding from surgery or coagulopathy are important factors in the development of primary ACS. Secondary ACS is caused by conditions not originating in the abdominopelvic space. Sepsis and the resultant capillary leak that occurs contribute to this condition. However, the most commonly encountered cause of secondary ACS in trauma is **massive resuscitation** (greater than 10 L of crystalloid or 10 units red blood cells). Recurrent ACS occurs following surgical treatment of primary or secondary ACS.

b. **Clinical signs** of ACS include elevated airway pressures, elevated central venous pressure (CVP), worsening markers of resuscitation despite clinical euvolemia, oliguria, and refractory shock. Its onset can be insidious, and providers must maintain a **high degree of suspicion** in patients with risk factors for ACS. Measurement of intraabdominal pressure by a Foley catheter can aid in the diagnosis: pressures over 12 mm Hg are abnormal and readings greater than 20 mm Hg are more worrisome. Ultimately, however, ACS is a **clinical diagnosis** that mandates prompt decompressive laparotomy.

F. Although a majority of **orthopedic trauma** is managed electively, pelvic trauma with concomitant vascular, genitourinary, or colorectal injury often necessitates emergent intervention. Significant pelvic fractures may lead to vascular injury requiring surgical repair and/or interventional radiology for angiography and embolization. A **baseline examination** of the affected region or limb following intervention is important, because changes to the examination whether acutely or over a period of hours may necessitate further intervention.

G. **Compartment syndrome** results from injury to fascial components and is most often the result of orthopedic or vascular trauma. Subsequent edema can lead to compromised perfusion and resultant tissue necrosis, infection, loss of function, and need for surgical intervention.

1. Several **causes** of compartment syndrome should be considered following trauma.

a. **Crush injury**, with significant musculoskeletal and vascular injury, is most often associated with compartment syndrome. Increasing compartment pressure secondary to bleeding (from vascular injury or orthopedic injury) and/or tissue swelling within the fascial compartment leads to venous obstruction; however, continued arterial inflow promotes further engorgement, ischemia, and tissue necrosis.

b. **Reperfusion injury**, which occurs commonly following repair of vascular injury, is caused by the release of various neurohormonal inflammatory mediators accumulated during antecedent tissue ischemia. Along with oxygen radicals, they promote increased capillary permeability and tissue edema. Typically resulting in

SIRS or circulatory shock, the syndrome is worsened by associated hemodynamic instability.

  c. Long bone **fracture** and muscular trauma are other possible causes.

2. **Recognition** of compartment syndrome is important for PACU providers because the findings are often **subtle** and easily overlooked in a postoperative trauma patient. Classic **signs and symptoms** include swelling, pain on passive stretching, pain out of proportion to exam, paresthesia, abnormal skin color, motor deficits, and loss of peripheral pulses.

  a. Notably, pulselessness is a **late finding**, and the presence of distal pulses does not exclude compartment syndrome.

  b. The measurement of compartment pressures is an important diagnostic modality, particularly in patients with impaired consciousness. Commercially available needle and catheter manometry sets can quickly assess compartment pressures when clinical concern is raised. Pressures typically are considered normal if less than 20 mm Hg. In patients who are symptomatic, pressures between 20 and 30 mm Hg warrant further investigation and possible operative intervention. Any compartment with a pressure >30 mm Hg should undergo fasciotomy.

3. Clinical suspicion of compartment syndrome in the PACU warrants careful evaluation of the patient in consultation with the surgical team. Definitive **treatment** involves prompt fasciotomy.

Suggested Readings

Centers for Disease Control and Prevention, National Center for Injury Prevention and Control. Web-based injury statistics query and reporting system (WISQARS). Available at: http://www.cdc.gov/injury/wisqars/. Accessed March 1, 2015.

Clancy K, Velopulos C, Bilaniuk JW, et al. Screening for blunt cardiac injury: an Eastern Association for the Surgery of Trauma practice management guideline. *J Trauma Acute Care Surg* 2012;73:S301–S306.

Friese RS, Shafi S, Gentilello LM. Pulmonary artery catheter use is associated with reduced mortality in severely injured patients: a National Trauma Data Bank analysis of 53,312 patients. *Crit Care Med* 2006;34:1597–1601.

Gage A, Rivara F, Wang J, et al. The effect of epidural placement in patients after blunt thoracic trauma. *J Trauma Acute Care Surg* 2014;76:39–45.

Grossman MD, Born C. Tertiary survey of the trauma patient in the intensive care unit. *Surg Clin North Am* 2000;80:805–824.

Holcomb JB, Tilley BC, Baraniuk S, et al. Transfusion of plasma, platelets, and red blood cells in a 1:1:1 vs a 1:1:2 ratio and mortality in patients with severe trauma: the PROPPR randomized clinical trial. *JAMA* 2015;313:471–482.

Kirkpatrick AW, Roberts DJ, De Waele J, et al. Intra-abdominal hypertension and the abdominal compartment syndrome: updated consensus definitions and clinical practice guidelines from the World Society of the Abdominal Compartment Syndrome. *Intensive Care Med* 2013;39:1190–1206.

McNicol ED, Schumann R, Haroutounian S. A systematic review and meta-analysis of ketamine for the prevention of persistent post-surgical pain. *Acta Anaesthesiol Scand* 2014;58:1199–1213.

Morrison CA, Carrick MM, Norman MA, et al. Hypotensive resuscitation strategy reduces transfusion requirements and severe postoperative coagulopathy in trauma patients with hemorrhagic shock: preliminary results of a randomized controlled trial. *J Trauma* 2011;70:652–663.

Murthi SB, Hess JR, Hess A, et al. Focused rapid echocardiographic evaluation versus vascular catheter-based assessment of cardiac output and function in critically ill trauma patients. *J Trauma Acute Care Surg* 2012;72:1158–1164.

Myburgh J, Cooper DJ, Finfer S, et al. Saline or albumin for fluid resuscitation in patients with traumatic brain injury. *N Engl J Med* 2007;357:874–884.

Peitzman AB, Fabian TC, Rhodes M, et al. *The Trauma Manual: Trauma and Acute Care Surgery*. Philadelphia, PA: Wolters Kluwer Health; 2012.

Shakur H, Roberts I, Bautista R, et al. Effects of tranexamic acid on death, vascular occlusive events, and blood transfusion in trauma patients with significant haemorrhage (CRASH-2): a randomised, placebo-controlled trial. *Lancet* 2010;376:23–32.

Spahn DR, Bouillon B, Cerny V, et al. Management of bleeding and coagulopathy following major trauma: an updated European guideline. *Crit Care* 2013;17:R76.

Strom BL, Berlin JA, Kinman JL, et al. Parenteral ketorolac and risk of gastrointestinal and operative site bleeding. A postmarketing surveillance study. *JAMA* 1996;275:376–382.

Postoperative Care for the Burn Patient

Andrew Vardanian and Jeremy Goverman

INTRODUCTION

Burn injuries cause significant morbidity and mortality, often requiring operative intervention. The most common causes of burn injury are fire/flames (43%) and scald injuries (33%). Other causes include contact with hot objects, electrical and chemical burns. The most prevalent age group with burn injuries are those 20 to 60 years of age, accounting for more than 50% of all burn injuries. Advances in burn care have allowed the overall mortality rate to decrease from 3.4% to 2.7% in men and 4.6% to 3.3% over the 10-year period from 2004 to 2013.

Burn patients undergo various operations in three phases of care—acute, subacute, and long term or reconstructive. The most common procedures are debridement (excision) of burn wounds, skin grafting, placement of wound dressings, and venous catheter placement. The specific type of grafting varies from use of autografts, allografts (cadaveric), and xenografts (porcine) depending on depth of burn and institutional protocols. The location of excision and grafting is dependent on the location of the burn injury, and may entail simple application of grafts on large surface areas such as the back or torso, or more detailed insetting as often required with grafting to the hand.

Each phase of burn surgery has important postoperative considerations. Common postoperative complications are reviewed as well as special circumstances in burn care such as chemical burns, electrical injuries, and frostbite.

PHASES OF BURN SURGERY

Burn surgery can be divided into acute, subacute, and long term or reconstructive (see Table 12.1). In the acute setting, the primary goal is survival. Patient survival is paramount, but other important considerations in the acute phase are limb and digit preservation. Border-zone (zone of stasis) tissue that may survive with appropriate resuscitation and burn care reduces the overall amount of burn wound requiring further treatment. The different types of operations that are usually required are decompressive procedures such as escharotomy and fasciotomy, early excision of burn wounds to remove dead tissue (eschar), and skin grafting to restore the integrity of the skin. Other common procedures are central and arterial line placement, enteral feeding tube placement, and bronchoscopy.

In the subacute phase, the initial resuscitation period has ended and primary wound excision and grafting has occurred. The burn surgeon tailors care for ongoing patient and wound care needs. Incompletely debrided wounds and/or areas of graft loss are reexcised. New skin graft donor sites or healed donor sites from prior graft harvests are used to regraft open surfaces. Adjustments are made to joint surfaces and digits that commonly have graft loss in large total body surface area (TBSA) burns. In massive burns (>90% TBSA), cultured epidermal autografts may be utilized in the subacute phase of burn surgery. Other commonly performed procedures include tracheostomy

		Postoperative Care
Phase of Burn Surgery	**Types of Operations**	**Considerations**
Early/acute	Decompressive procedures (escharotomy, fasciotomy)	Patient positioning
		Temperature regulation
		Monitoring
		Goal-directed therapy
	Excision	Wound care
	Skin grafting	Nutrition
		Pharmacologic support
		Pain control and sedation
		PT/OT
Subacute	Excision	Wound care
	Skin grafting	Pain control
	Use of CEA	Prevention of infection
		Nutrition
		PT/OT
Long-term/ reconstructive	Skin resurfacing/laser treatments	Patient positioning and splinting
	Local tissue rearrangements (Z-plasty)	Postoperative pain and nausea
	Contracture release	Wound care
		Nutrition
		PT/OT

TABLE 12.1 Phases of Burn Surgery

PT/OT, physical therapy/occupational therapy; CEA, cultured epidermal autografts.

(percutaneous or open), typically for prolonged intubation, and central line changes as indicated.

The long-term or burn reconstructive phase has great diversity in the types of operations and may range from contracture release, split-thickness or full thickness skin grafting, and local tissue rearrangements, to more complex tissue transfer including free-tissue transfer. Because life-threatening injuries have been previously addressed, the purpose of surgery during this phase is to improve functional and aesthetic outcomes.

POSTOPERATIVE CARE: THE ACUTE AND SUBACUTE PHASES OF BURN SURGERY

Decompressive procedures (escharotomy, fasciotomy), burn wound excision (escharectomy), and skin grafting (autografting or allografting) are the main procedures done for the acute burn patient. Escharotomies may be performed at the bedside in the intensive care unit (ICU) with electrocautery, but may also be performed in the operating room. The purpose is to release overlying burned tissue, often in circumferential and large TBSA burns requiring massive fluid resuscitation, to allow tissue decompression and to improve perfusion. The chest and abdomen may be released in this manner to allow improved respiratory dynamics and to decrease abdominal compartment syndrome. Abdominal compartment syndrome may require urgent decompressive laparotomy. Ocular compartment pressure is released with lateral canthotomy. Deep thermal injuries, ischemia-reperfusion injury, edema related to resuscitation, or electrical injuries may also cause fascial compartment syndrome of the extremities. Fasciotomies are commonly performed to release compartments of the hand, forearm, or lower extremity.

Patient Positioning

Burn wound debridement and grafting require proper patient positioning in the operating room in order to maximize surgeon access to the sites of injury. The arms or legs are frequently elevated to allow proper wound debridement or graft harvesting. The patient may need to be placed in prone, lateral, or supine positions at various times during the operation.

Temperature Regulation

Maintenance of core body temperature is important in the postoperative period to prevent worsening coagulopathy and to regulate hypermetabolism, both of which may result in worsening tissue perfusion and metabolic acidosis. Loss of body heat occurs quickly in the burn patient. With loss of the epidermis, the burn patient is unable to properly thermoregulate using cutaneous vasoconstriction. Heat dissipates from the body core to superficial tissues. It is highly important to use warmed fluids and to heat postoperative care rooms to maintain normothermia in the burn patient. Covering the head and extremities may be useful as well as the use of radiant heaters and forced-air warming blankets.

Monitoring and Goal-Directed Therapy

Postoperative care necessitates goal-directed therapy and must be tailored to the specific needs of the individual burn patient. ICU level of care is often necessary with appropriate resuscitation and monitoring of heart rate, blood pressure, mean arterial pressure, body temperature, oxygen saturation, and volumes of fluid input and output. Burn TBSA of 20% causes maximal stimulation of inflammatory mediators, which impairs vascular tone and cardiac function, and results in an exaggerated systemic inflammatory and hypermetabolic response. Vasoactive medications such as α agonists, α/β agonists, and ADH agonists may be necessary to maintain adequate mean arterial pressure. Care must be taken to avoid overresuscitation, which can result in compartment syndrome, progression of burn wound depth, loss of skin grafts, and increased infectious complications.

Postoperative care involves monitoring lab values such as the hemoglobin level, platelet count, INR, and PTT. Bleeding may occur after excision and skin grafting, and blood transfusions may be necessary. An estimate of blood loss within the first 3 days of burn surgery ranges from 0.45 to 0.75 mL/cm^2 burn area excised. With large raw, open surface areas, ongoing blood loss may occur in the postoperative period. Hemoglobin levels must be checked to prevent critical anemia. Dressings must be monitored for excessive saturation, which can herald ongoing bleeding.

Electrolyte abnormalities, renal function, and hepatic function must be assessed. Arterial pH, base deficit, and lactate levels are used to assess global perfusion and thus to manage ongoing resuscitation with fluid administration and/or titration of vasoactive medication. Arterial blood gas values assist with ventilator management.

Ventilator management is patient and institution dependent. Low-pressure, low tidal volume protocols are typically followed to prevent barotrauma. The decision to extubate is multifactorial and depends on hemodynamic stability, mental status, and resolution of significant airway edema or inhalation injury.

Wound Care

Wound care is paramount to graft survival and donor site outcomes. Skin grafts are fragile on initial transfer to the recipient sites. Loss can occur through shear, hematoma/seroma under the skin graft, infection, or poor nutrition. Strategies in the postoperative period must target each of these potential causes of graft loss.

Dressings are applied to prevent shear. Various types of dressings (bolsters, stents) may be used; however, the principle of the burn dressing is to stabilize and protect the graft in the postoperative period. A veil-like dressing is first applied to the wound bed over the skin graft, and stabilized with a large roll of dry sterile dressing that may be secured with a kerlix wrap on an extremity or with large sheets of thick gauze that are sutured in place over the abdomen, chest, flanks, or back. Care must be taken to prevent removal of the burn dressing during patient transfer from the operating room to the recovery suites or ICUs. Negative pressure wound therapy (NPWT) can also be used to bolster a skin graft to the wound bed. A veil-like dressing or xeroform can be placed over the skin graft and a sponge is applied and secured with occlusive clear tape to create a vacuum seal. Care must be taken in the postoperative period to ensure the NPWT is functional. Pitfalls include occlusion of the tubing, a break in the occlusive seal, or malfunction of the device, though the latter may occur if batteries are not recharged during patient transfer. Early identification of a leak or malfunction is important to prevent dislodgement of the sponge or build-up of fluid (hematoma/seroma) that can cause graft loss.

Hematoma is prevented by meticulous hemostasis in the operating room. Identification of significant bleeding or saturation of dressings in the postoperative period may allow early identification of hemorrhage or hematoma that may cause graft loss. Seroma is less likely with meshed grafts and more common in sheet grafts. Graft loss from seroma is prevented intraoperatively with use of pie crusting, though monitoring the function of NPWT may help minimize seroma formation postoperatively. Infection may be prevented with adequate excision of burn wounds and the use of topical antimicrobial agents, such as silvadene, sulfamylon, or silver nitrate soaks applied to the graft or over the burn dressing, as preferred by the individual burn center. Dressings are typically removed on postoperative days 5 to 7, at which time skin graft integration has taken place.

Donor Site Wound Care

Donor site care in the postoperative period is important to maximize wound healing and to prevent a partial thickness injury from converting to a full thickness or chronic wound that requires future debridement and skin grafting. Foam dressings, often containing silver (i.e., Mepilex Ag), are commonly used for donor sites. These dressings combine soft silicone adhesive technology with the sustained antimicrobial action of ionic silver. The dressing is applied directly over the donor site and secured with staples, sutures, or kerlix wrap. The dressing is removed 5 to 7 days postoperatively. Data suggest that Mepilex Ag decreases pain with dressing changes. Other donor site options include xeroform, telfa, adaptec, tegaderm, and dry sterile dressings. Postoperatively, telfa, adaptec, and dry sterile dressings are removed and changed as necessary. Xeroform and tegaderm typically remain in place until wound epithelialization has completed. In large TBSA burns, donor sites can be managed with similar dressings to the recipient sites to allow wound care with sulfamylon or silver nitrate soaks. Donor site care is highly dependent on burn surgeon/burn center preference.

Nutrition and Pharmacologic Agents

Nutrition in the postoperative period is highly important for graft and patient survival given the hypermetabolic state of acute burn patients. Early enteral nutrition is necessary to promote caloric goals and to provide adequate amino acids, carbohydrates, and lipids. Two medications used to modulate the hypermetabolic response in burn patients are testosterone analogues (oxandrolone) and β-blockers. Multiple randomized controlled trials have shown that oxandrolone improves donor site healing, net nitrogen balance, and protein synthesis, decreases weight loss, and shortens hospital length of stay. Propranolol also improves skeletal muscle protein metabolism, especially in the pediatric burn population. In addition, modulation of hypermetabolism and reduction in resting energy expenditure can be achieved by elevating the ambient room temperature.

Pain Control and Sedation

Adequate analgesia and sedation is highly important in the postoperative period. Various regimens are used for postoperative pain control. Examples include fentanyl, hydromorphone, or morphine drips often with the addition of NSAIDs and/or acetaminophen. Sedation regimens include midazolam, dexmedetomidine, or propofol. Quetiapine and haldol are also used in regimens tailored for patient-specific postoperative goals.

POSTOPERATIVE CARE: THE RECONSTRUCTIVE PHASE OF BURN SURGERY

The reconstructive phase of burn surgery may begin as early as 3 to 4 weeks postinjury and may last for an entire lifetime. The initial life-threatening events have been resolved and the focus is on the optimization of functional and aesthetic outcomes. Common issues are release of contractures that limit joint range of motion, for example, use of the digits or movement of the elbow or arm. In the head and neck region, ear deformities, ectropion, lower lip, and neck contractures are common problems that affect the burn patient. Operative planning and techniques are tailored to patient-specific needs. Standard postoperative care applies to most reconstructive phase burn patients.

In particular, patients with significant neck contractures or microstomia from burn injury may have difficult airways, which must be monitored in the postoperative period. For neck contractures, treatment includes contracture release and split-thickness skin grafting. This allows release of tight scars and replacement of missing tissue with donor skin. Recurrent contracture is high; however, improved neck mobility and range of motion result.

Temperature Regulation

The reconstructive burn patient typically has minimal or no open wounds, and therefore does not have the same risk for hypothermia as the acutely burned patient. These patients more closely resemble other elective surgical patients in the postoperative period. However, because of altered cutaneous vasoconstriction/vasodilation in grafted skin sites, these patients may be at higher risk for hyperthermia in warm environments. Core body temperature must be monitored during the postoperative period.

Wound Care

Basic principles of postoperative wound care have been discussed (please see Chapter 13). Dressings must remain clean and without saturation. Dressings must be secure but not overly constrictive as to cause ischemia. They should allow for inspection of the wound to evaluate for wound infection.

Bolsters may be applied over skin graft sites to prevent shear and to reduce hematoma/seroma. The ear, for example, requires bolster placement given its three-dimensional contour. Other recipient sites may be managed with NPWT. Bolsters and VAC dressings are typically removed 5 to 7 days postoperatively. Splinting or K-wire placement may also be used in the hand to prevent shear and to improve outcomes of grafting over joints. Specific types of splints are tailored to the individual reconstructive needs of the patient. Standard dressings are also applied to donor sites as aforementioned such as Mepilex Ag, xeroform, or Tegaderm dressings.

Postoperative Pain and Nausea

Pain and nausea control are similar to management of other postoperative patients (please see Chapter 15).

POSTOPERATIVE COMPLICATIONS IN THE BURN PATIENT

Postoperative care for the burn patient requires familiarity with potential postoperative complications. Most are similar to complications in other trauma and acute care surgery patients. Table 12.2 lists important postoperative complications in the burn patient. They include pneumonia, cellulitis, urinary tract infection, respiratory failure, septicemia, wound infection, renal failure, cardiac complications (arrhythmia), bacteremia, and central line–associated bloodstream infection.

Sepsis is difficult to identify and diagnose in postoperative burn patients. Because of hypermetabolism, burn patients are tachycardic. They may have fever and leukocytosis, further confounding the diagnosis. Overall, a high index of suspicion and low threshold for empiric antibiotics and cultures is warranted. The American Burn Association defines sepsis as a change in the clinical state of the burn patient that triggers the concern for infection. The trigger must include at least three of the following of temperature ($>39°C$ or $<36.5°C$), progressive tachycardia, progressive tachypnea, thrombocytopenia, hyperglycemia, or the inability to continue enteral feedings for more than 24 hours. Additional documentation of positive cultures, pathologic tissue source, or clinical response to antimicrobials is necessary. These data may be useful to correctly diagnose sepsis in the postoperative burn patient.

SPECIAL CONSIDERATIONS FOR POSTOPERATIVE CARE IN THE BURN PATIENT

Chemical

Initial care of chemical burns involves decontamination with irrigation or with specific agents such as calcium gluconate gel in the case of hydrofluoric acid burns. Once stabilized, patients undergo necessary debridement as with other acute burn patients. Postoperative care must adhere to the principles aforementioned regarding wound care, pain control, and observation for postoperative complications.

TABLE 12.2	Major Complications After Burn Injury

Pneumonia
Cellulitis
Urinary tract infection
Respiratory failure
Sepsis
Wound infection
Renal failure
Arrhythmia
Bacteremia
Catheter-related bloodstream infection
ARDS
Other blood/systemic infection
Other hematologic infections

Note: Pneumonia is the most common complication (5.8% of fire/flame injured patients), followed by cellulitis and urinary tract infection.
ARDS, acute respiratory distress syndrome.

Electrical

The principles of postoperative care after electrical injury are similar to those of other burn patients. Four types of injury occur with high-voltage electrical injuries: flash, flame, arc, and current-invoked injury. The arc and electrical current may produce a burn on clothing, which creates a flame injury or a flash burn. The arc is usually limited and is from rapid ionization of current. The true electrical burn produces extensive soft tissue injury that extends beyond areas visible at initial examination. The severity depends on the type of current, voltage, and duration of contact. Operative management typically consists of serial debridement, which ensues after patients are adequately resuscitated and other issues such as current-induced arrhythmias have been addressed. Postoperative care must emphasize adequate resuscitation and optimal wound care to identify infection that may be the result of evolving wound necrosis.

Frostbite Injury

Patients with frostbite injury usually do not undergo urgent surgical debridement of wounds but may undergo catheter-directed thrombolysis in the first 24 to 48 hours after initial injury. Initial treatment includes immediate rewarming and fluid resuscitation as needed. Vascular assessment is made for capillary refill, skin color, and palpable versus Doppler positive inflow. If there is presence of circulatory compromise, angiography is done. Tissue plasminogen activator (TPA) may be used to treat vascular compromise. An intra-arterial catheter is placed into the necessary vessel, and TPA is administered per institutional protocols. Heparin is infused to goal PTT levels of 50 to 70. Repeat angiographs are done every 12 hours for a maximum of 48 hours. Indications for discontinuation include reperfusion, drop in fibrinogen level (<150 mg/dL), and duration greater than 48 hours. Heparin is continued for 96 hours after TPA is discontinued.

Postoperative care requires careful assessment of catheter sites to monitor for signs of bleeding or hematoma. Local wound care continues until the wounds are healed or amputation is needed. Small intact blisters are left in place, whereas ruptured blisters are debrided to evaluate underlying tissue perfusion. Topical antimicrobials are typically applied and wounds are covered with dry sterile dressings.

Suggested Readings

American Burn Association, National Burn Repository 2014. Version 10.0. Available at: http://www.ameriburn.org/2014NBRAnnualReport.pdf.

Bittner EA, Shank E, Woodson L, et al. Acute and perioperative care of the burn-injured patient. *Anesthesiology* 2015;122:448–464

Gee Kee EL, Kimble RM, Cuttle L, et al. Randomized controlled trial of three burns dressings for partial thickness burns in children. *Burns* 2015;41(5):946–955.

Greenhalgh DG, Saffle JR, Holmes JH 4th, et al, American Burn Association Consensus Conference on Burn Sepsis and Infection Group. American Burn Association consensus conference to define sepsis and infection in burns. *J Burn Care Res* 2007;28(6):776–790.

Herndon DN, ed. *Total Burn Care.* 4th ed. Philadelphia, PA: Saunders Elsevier; 2012.

Ibrahim AE, Goverman J, Sarhane KA, et al. The emerging role of tissue plasminogen activator in the management of severe frostbite. *J Burn Care Res* 2015;36(2): e62–e66.

Jeschke MG, Pinto R, Kraft R, et al; Inflammation and the Host Response to Injury Collaborative Research Program. Morbidity and survival probability in burn patients in modern burn care. *Crit Care Med* 2015;43(4):808–815.

Sheridan RL, Martin RF, eds. Management of burns. *Surg Clin North Am* 2014;94(4): 721–944.

Tompkins RG. Survival from burns in the new millennium: 70 years' experience from a single institution. *Ann Surg* 2015;261(2):263–268.

Postoperative Care for the Plastic Surgical Patient

Andrew Vardanian and William (Jay) Gerald Austen

INTRODUCTION

This chapter provides a general reference for common postoperative issues in the plastic surgery patient (Table 13.1). Special considerations for the craniofacial, breast, hand, and cosmetic surgery are also discussed.

Postoperative Monitoring

As with other surgical patients in the postoperative period, the plastic surgery patient requires close monitoring of vital signs including temperature, heart rate, blood pressure, and oxygen saturation. Although postoperative fever is common, persistent or progressive temperature elevation may indicate infection that requires further evaluation and treatment. Heart rate should be monitored, because tachycardia may result from uncontrolled pain, hypovolemia, arrhythmia, or anemia. Blood pressure must remain normotensive. Elevations in blood pressure may result in bleeding that requires exploration and reoperation. Postoperative hematoma caused by hypertension is well-described after rhytidectomy, especially in male patients, but may also occur after breast surgery or abdominoplasty. Monitoring both oxygen

TABLE 13.1	Postoperative Care for the Plastic Surgery Patient: General Considerations		
General Considerations	**Postoperative Strategy**
Vital signs	Monitor hemodynamics and oxygen saturation
Pain control	Monitor for adequacy
	Adjunctive medications
Nausea/vomiting	Antiemetics
	Minimize opiates
Antibiotics	Perioperative
	Operative case/patient-specific indications
Wound care	Monitor for infection
	Monitor NPWT device function
	Optimize graft take and reduce donor site morbidity
Drain care	Monitor for bleeding or infection
	Improve tissue adhesion and prevent seroma
Patient positioning	Avoid compression of vascular pedicle
	Optimize wound healing
	Reduce edema (craniofacial, extremity)
Bowel regimen	Stool softeners
	Hydration
VTE prophylaxis	Mechanical, chemical prophylaxis
	Early ambulation

NPWT, negative pressure wound therapy; VTE, venous thromboembolism.

saturation and respiratory rate is important for those on patient-controlled analgesia (PCA) or high levels of opiates. Unexplained tachypnea, decreased oxygen saturation, with tachycardia merit workup for pulmonary embolism.

Pain Control

As many plastic surgery operations are elective in nature, adequate pain control is of high importance. Various institutional regimens exist with regard to pain control. A common protocol uses PCA with morphine or hydromorphone in those who must remain NPO during the postoperative period. When oral intake is tolerated by the patient, a PO regimen is used, commonly oxycodone at 5 mg for mild pain, 10 mg for moderate pain, and 15 mg for severe pain in standard intervals of 4 hours. These values may be increased in the opiate-tolerant patient, typically with 5-mg increments. Intravenous morphine or hydromorphone is used for breakthrough pain. In addition, adjunctive medications such as acetaminophen, intravenous or PO, are dosed separately and given at 6-hour intervals. Staggered dosing of these medications (given 2 to 3 hours between administration of opiate medication) improves patient pain management. Of note, oxycodone and acetaminophen are given separately, rather than through a combination pill (such as Percocet). This allows uptitration of oxycodone, should pain control necessitate higher dosing, while avoiding higher doses of acetaminophen.

Nausea

Postoperative nausea, although common, can affect a patient's entire perception of the operative experience. Most nausea is a direct consequence of general anesthesia or postoperative pain control with opiates. Patients are treated with ondansetron, metoclopramide, or prochlorperazine and other medications such as scopolamine patch or corticosteroids. Though the specific postoperative regimen varies, the awareness of nausea as a significant factor in the postoperative quality of care merits its timely attention and treatment by the health care team. Retching and vomiting associated with nausea, though less common, may obviously cause significant discomfort. Such forced and spasmodic abdominothoracic movement against a closed glottis raises intrathoracic pressure and has untoward results after facial, cosmetic, and reconstructive surgery.

Antibiotics

Standard prophylactic antibiotics are used in plastic surgery to prevent surgical site infections (SSIs). These include the first-generation cephalosporin cefazolin in coverage of *Staphylococcus* and *Streptococcus* species, with some coverage against Gram-negative bacteria. In patients with cephalosporin allergy or contraindication, clindamycin is used for its effectiveness against *Staphylococcus* and *Streptococcus* species. Clindamycin has additional coverage for anaerobic Gram-negative rods. In patients with known methicillin-resistant *Staphylococcus aureus*, vancomycin is often used.

Postoperative guidelines for antibiotic use (antibiotic choice and duration) are not established and practices vary by surgeon preference. In the majority of cases, breast surgery using tissue expander or implant-based reconstruction has continued antibiotic therapy in the postoperative period. The duration varies, with some surgeons discontinuing antibiotics after 24 hours and others continuing antibiotics for 1 to 2 weeks while drains are in place. Because of the heterogeneity of published results, definitive evidence-based recommendations cannot be made, and antibiotic treatment in the postoperative period remains surgeon-dependent.

Wound Management and Skin Grafting

Wound management after plastic surgery ranges from simple inspection to negative pressure wound therapy (NPWT) that requires complex dressing changes. General principles are to leave operative dressings intact until 48 hours postoperatively, at which time wound edges have epithelialized. Dressings are applied to be secure but not overly constrictive to cause pressure necrosis of skin flaps. Dressings should allow the surgeon to examine the wound/surgical site for postoperative hematoma or tissue ischemia that requires immediate attention.

The timing and frequency for postoperative wound care and dressing changes is surgeon dependent. Dressings should remain clean and without saturation with blood or drain fluid. The majority of surgical dressings are changed or removed at 48 hours. Some surgeons use minimal or no dressings. This is often the case when an adhesive is applied along the surgical incision at the end of the operation, to create an impermeable seal. Adhesives commonly used include dermabond topical (2-octyl cyanoacrylate), dermabond prineo, and histoacryl (*n*-butyl-2 cyanoacrylate).

Binders or ACE wraps may be used to add compression to large surface areas, such as after abdominoplasty or liposuction. They must not be too tight to compromise blood flow. Hand surgery patients have splints that immobilize and protect the operative site after fracture or tendon repair. Cosmetic face and neck lift patients often have elastic or ACE wraps that provide gentle compression in an appropriate vector to prevent seroma/hematoma.

Various dressings may be used after skin grafting. Options for recipient sites include bolsters that are applied intraoperatively and are left in place without manipulation to avoid shear force on the graft. Bolsters are typically fastened with silk sutures, which are removed on postoperative days 5 to 7. Other common dressings for skin graft recipient sites are NPWT using the wound VAC. They are typically removed on postoperative days 5 to 7.

Donor sites have various options for management. Tegaderm, a nonocclusive transparent dressing, is commonly used as a donor site dressing. As fluid accumulates below the dressing, a small incision can be made postoperatively to allow egress of fluid with application of a smaller Tegaderm over the incision site. Xeroform can be applied on donor sites and allowed to stay in place until the skin surface reepithelializes. Other dressings for donor sites include use of Mepilex Ag foam dressings that may be removed in 5 to 7 days postoperatively.

Drain Care

Drains are used to allow removal of serous fluid and blood from tissue spaces, promoting tissue adherence and wound healing. Postoperative drain care depends on the type of drain used. Two general categories of drains are closed suction and passive systems.

Closed suction drains may be TLS (test tube–type device), Hemovac type, or bulb-suction types such as Blake and Jackson–Pratt. TLS drains are used in small enclosed spaces, such as an auricular pocket created during microtia repair or other similar spaces created with craniofacial procedures. TLS drains require frequent change of the collecting test tube, which has negative pressure to allow suction of small quantities of fluid. Drain care requires attention to the proper functioning of the drainage system. A plastic clamp is used to close the tubing system, while the old test tube is removed and a new test tube is secured in place. The plastic clamp is then removed to allow proper drainage. The quantity of fluid in the old test tube may be measured and recorded.

Bulb-suction-type drains have an array of sizes, with smaller ones used for drainage of the scalp or a tissue flap on the face after rhytidectomy. Larger bulb-suction drains are used to evacuate fluid from larger potential spaces. Examples include the abdominal wall after abdominoplasty or deep inferior epigastric artery perforator (DIEP) breast reconstruction or drainage of the posterior back after use of the latissimus dorsi muscle for free tissue or pedicle-based reconstructions. Bulb-suction drains are also used in recipient sites such as the breast or upper or lower extremity after free tissue transfer. The quality and quantity of fluid must be examined postoperatively. High-output sanguineous drainage or the presence of clotted blood in the drain tubing or collecting bulb may indicate hemorrhage, which may necessitate exploration. High serous output often indicates the need for continued drainage. An increase in drain output after expander/implant-based breast reconstruction may indicate a latent infection that requires further evaluation. A change in the quality of drained fluid, such as odor or purulence, may indicate infection and warrants evaluation.

Passive drains are Penrose-type drains or catheters that allow egress of fluid from the wound bed onto dressings. These are typically used in areas of the body where there is concern for any trauma, such as local tissue injury that can occur through a closed-suction system. An example is use of a Penrose drain to allow drainage of fluid near a vascular anastomosis in the head and neck region after free tissue transfer.

Patient Positioning

Plastic surgery patients require careful attention to postoperative positioning. Patients who have undergone cosmetic abdominoplasty or breast reconstruction using DIEP flaps may have high tension on the abdominal closure. Optimal positioning is achieved by using the semi-Fowler position with the head of bed at 30 to 45 degrees and the hips flexed, often with use of a pillow for support behind the knees. Proper positioning prevents excessive stretch of the abdominal tissue flaps and promotes maximal delivery of blood from the lateral intercostal perforators to optimize wound healing. When walking, patients must maintain a semi-flexed, or skiers position, in the first 1 to 2 weeks postoperatively. Duration depends on the tightness of closure and surgeon preference.

Patients that have undergone pedicle latissimus dorsi breast or chest wall reconstruction must have the ipsilateral arm elevated and abducted 30 degrees on a pillow to prevent compression of the vascular pedicle. Patients that have undergone breast reconstruction using tissue expanders/implants or autologous reconstruction require avoidance of pressure on the reconstructed breast mound. Postcraniofacial surgery patients must sit with the head of bed at 30 to 45 degrees to facilitate drainage and reduce edema. Patients after cosmetic face and neck lifts have a pillow placed behind the neck for the first 12 to 24 hours postoperatively to prevent neck flexion that interferes with adhesion of the skin and subcutaneous tissues after appropriate skin draping. Patients after hand surgery are required to maintain elevation of the hand above the level of the heart to prevent excessive swelling, which can occur if the extremity is held in the dependent position. Similarly, patients with free flap reconstruction of the lower extremity are required to keep the limb at a neutral position on level with the heart to avoid excessive edema and to optimize venous drainage, which may compromise the flap if the limb is held in a dependent position.

Free Flap Care and Monitoring

Patients who have undergone free tissue transfer require careful postoperative care and monitoring to identify early signs of flap compromise and to optimize reconstructive success. Patient positioning is paramount to prevent pressure on the newly transferred free flap and to promote wound healing of the donor site. Examples include the use of the semi-Fowler position after use of free transverse rectus abdominis myocutaneous (TRAM) or DIEP breast reconstruction to optimize the integrity of the abdominal closure. As aforementioned, drains are used to remove excess fluid from both donor and reconstruction sites. Closed suction–type drains are commonly used for the abdominal donor site with use of the TRAM or DIEP free flap and also for the large dissected surface area created on the back with use of the latissimus dorsi free flap for head and neck or lower extremity reconstruction. Passive drains, such as a Penrose, are carefully placed within recipient sites along the head and neck and extremities to allow drainage of fluid without the risk of suction near a vascular anastomosis.

Postoperatively, free flap care and monitoring protocols include maintaining normal vital signs with strict avoidance of hypotension or hypertension. IV hydration is highly important to ensure adequate tissue perfusion as well as avoidance of potential vasoconstrictors such as pressors or caffeine. Most centers initiate active flap warming for the first 48 hours to maximize vasodilation of the perforators. Warming may be done by placing the patient in a warm room or with use of an isolated forced-air warming blanket such as the Bair Hugger that is placed over the free flap itself to promote local tissue vasodilation.

Basic principles for flap monitoring are inspection and assessment of vascular patency. Inspection of the flap is of paramount importance. With inspection, the observer evaluates the flap color. The flap should appear pink with normal temperature. The presence of a blue, cyanotic, or mottled appearance or a cool temperature indicates flap compromise and heralds the need for urgent intervention. Surgeons may utilize temperature probes on the flaps with controls placed on normal tissue. A temperature discrepancy of greater than 3°C signifies concern for flap compromise. With palpation, the tissue turgor is evaluated to ensure a soft, normal feel. A firm, hard, or swollen flap indicates flap compromise and seroma or hematoma that requires further evaluation.

The patency of the vascular anastomoses, both arterial and venous, is highly important and must be closely monitored. Capillary refill is assessed. Normal capillary refill is 2 to 3 seconds. If capillary refill is brisk, with filling less than 1 second, there is concern for venous congestion and further evaluation is needed to avoid flap loss. Venous congestion may be caused by a thrombus in the vein. If capillary refill is greater than 3 seconds, there may be an arterial inflow problem, which also requires urgent evaluation.

A handheld Doppler is used to check the arterial anastomosis by evaluating a fasciocutaneous or musculocutaneous perforator that is marked intraoperatively by the surgical team. The Doppler signal is checked hourly for the first 48 hours and then every 2 hours for the next 24 hours, and then every 4 hours until the patient is discharged from the hospital. A triphasic Doppler signal indicates excellent arterial blood flow. A venous signal may also be identified and monitored by the surgical staff. Other methods of flap monitoring to assess tissue perfusion include tissue oximetry such as ViOptix, which allows noninvasive real-time measurement of local tissue oxygen saturation in a free flap. A drop in signal heralds flap compromise and necessitates further evaluation.

Bowel Regimen

Though common in the surgical population after gastrointestinal surgery, the use of a bowel regimen is often overlooked in the postoperative care of the plastic surgery patients. Proper bowel regimen, however, is important in plastic surgery, especially after body contouring, abdominoplasty, or free tissue transfer using the TRAM or DIEP flap reconstruction. These operations have longer procedure time, necessitate opiate pain control, and are associated with greater immobility, which contribute to constipation. A standard regimen includes docusate, senna, bisacodyl, and suppositories as necessary to promote normal postoperative bowel function.

Venous Thromboembolism Prophylaxis

Plastic surgery patients have high risk for postoperative venous thromboembolism (VTE), with symptomatic VTE cited at 2.2% after flap-based breast reconstruction after mastectomy, 7.7% after circumferential abdominoplasty, 5.0% after abdominoplasty, and 2.9% after breast or upper body contouring. Heparin or enoxaparin is recommended for prevention of VTE in the postoperative plastic surgery patient. The Caprini risk assessment model has been used to identify patients with greater risk for VTE, especially those that undergo major surgery with longer duration, increasing age, presence of malignancy, and confinement to the bed greater than 72 hours in the postoperative period. Given the current data, it is prudent to utilize chemoprophylaxis to reduce postoperative VTE, especially in patients that undergo body contouring, abdominoplasty, and free tissue reconstruction. Moreover, the use of early ambulation in all patients is advised and must be emphasized by all members of the health care team.

SPECIAL CONSIDERATIONS

Plastic surgery patients that undergo craniofacial, breast, hand, and cosmetic surgery require special postoperative considerations. Key management issues are briefly described for common procedures, and are summarized in Table 13.2. There are myriad types of operations that necessitate specialty care within these categories, and further information can be obtained in the selected references.

The Craniofacial Patient

Craniofacial surgery is an extensive topic but can be divided into intracranial or extracranial operations with important postoperative considerations. Intracranial operations involve both neurosurgery and plastic surgery teams and have exposure of the meninges. Examples include facial bipartition,

TABLE 13.2	Postoperative Care for the Plastic Surgery Patient: Special Considerations		
Category	**Monitoring**	**Complications**	**Preventive Strategy**
Craniofacial			
• Intracranial surgery (i.e., monobloc, cranial vault remodeling)	• Evaluate drain output • Monitor for CSF drainage	• Hematoma • Seroma • Edema • Infection • Rare events: Meningitis Hemorrhage	• Elevation of head of bed • Wound and drain care • Correction of anemia and coagulopathy
• Extracranial bone related (i.e., ORIF facial fractures orthognathic surgery, distraction)	• Mandible: Integrity of MMF or guiding elastics • Facial fractures: ZMC, orbital floor/wall, extraocular movements, vision	• Hematoma • Infection • Hardware malfunction	• Elevation of head of bed • Wound and drain care; • Peridex mouthwash and oral care • Wire cutters/ scissors at bedside
• Extracranial soft tissue (i.e., cleft lip/cleft palate)	• Integrity of soft tissues and incisions	• Wound dehiscence • Tissue flap ischemia	• Use of elbow splints • Dental packing or palatal splint • Oral care

| | Postoperative Care for the Plastic Surgery Patient: Special Considerations (*continued*) | | |

Category	Monitoring	Complications	Preventive Strategy
Breast			
• Reduction/ mastopexy • Augmentation • Reconstruction (expander/ implant based or combination latissimus dorsi with implant) • Free flap DIEP/ TRAM (see below)	• Evaluate skin flap integrity, incision, nipple • Examine drain output (quantity/ quality)	• Infection (cellulitis) • Skin flap or nipple ischemia/ necrosis • Wound dehiscence • Expander/ implant exposure • Seroma/ hematoma	• Drain care • Noncompressive dressings • Proper positioning • Antibiotics (implant-based reconstruction)
Hand			
• Tendon repair • Soft tissue • Bone	• Evaluate edema, pain, integrity of splint and repair	• Infection • Skin flap ischemia • Rupture of repair (tendon) • Hardware problems	• Elevation of hand • K-wire/pin-site care • Splint care
Cosmetic			
• Face • Body contouring	• Evaluate edema, soft tissues, and incisions	• Infection • Wound problems • Hematoma • Seroma	• Elevation and proper positioning • Drain and wound care • No nose blowing (after rhinoplasty) • Cool compresses • Compressive garments (after brachioplasty)
Microvascular free tissue transfer	• Evaluate flap color, temperature, capillary refill and Doppler (vascular anastomosis)	• Arterial or venous problems • Wound dehiscence • Flap ischemia • Fat necrosis	• Hemodynamic monitoring, flap warming, hydration, avoidance of vasoconstrictors, proper positioning

ORIF, open reduction internal fixation; MMF, maxillomandibular fixation; ZMC, zygomaticomaxillary complex; DIEP, deep inferior epigastric artery perforator flap; TRAM, transverse rectus abdominis myocutaneous flap.

fronto-orbital advancement, or cranial vault remodeling for craniosynostosis. Postoperative management requires intensive care unit admission, strict hemodynamic monitoring, and hourly neurologic examinations. Postoperative complications actively examined for include hemorrhage (strict monitoring of drain output), elevated intracranial pressure from cerebral edema (evaluation for papilledema), cerebrospinal leak from unrecognized dural tear (evaluation for rhinorrhea or increased drain output), or infection (meningitis being uncommon but severe). Facial and periorbital/eyelid swelling are common and can last from 4 to 5 days, often worse 36 to 48 hours postoperatively.

Extracranial operations include a broad spectrum of procedures from ORIF of facial fractures, orthognathic surgery, mandibular or midface distraction, and cleft lip and palate surgery.

Facial fractures are managed in the postoperative period with elevation of the head of bed and placement of iced gauze on the face to decrease swelling. Oral and dental care is initiated with Peridex (chlorhexidine gluconate 0.12%) mouthwash. Occlusion is monitored after orthognathic surgery. If the jaw is wired in occlusion, wire cutters are placed at the bedside for use in case of vomiting or airway emergency. Similarly, scissors are placed at the bedside if guiding elastics are used. Turning arms of distraction devices are checked regularly to ensure their proper function. Device entrance sites are cared for with twice-daily application of bacitracin ointment.

Cleft lip and palate patients require placement of elbow splints before leaving the operating rooms to prevent manual disruption of the repair. A tongue stitch is placed through the distal tongue and loosely secured to the cheek to allow tongue retraction to facilitate intubation in case of an airway emergency. The child is admitted overnight for monitoring and IV hydration with transition to oral intake by 24 hours postoperatively. The repair is monitored for wound dehiscence, ischemia to the tissue flaps, excessive swelling, or bleeding. Palatal splints or dental putty may be used to protect a palatal repair or alveolar bone graft site.

The Breast Patient

Postoperative care for the plastic surgery breast patient includes many of the principles already discussed with pain and nausea control of paramount importance. Drain output and quality is observed to monitor for signs of bleeding that would necessitate urgent reoperation. A variety of dressings are used postoperatively. Some patients do not have dressings, with simple application of a sports bra or use of Steri-Strips over the incision lines. Others have secure but nonconstricting dressings to allow evaluation for cellulitis, the viability of skin flaps, or postoperative hematomas.

Breast reconstruction includes tissue expander/implant-based reconstructions or free tissue reconstruction. Reconstruction is done in an immediate or delayed fashion. Tissue expander/implant-based reconstructions have postoperative drains, and perioperative antibiotics are commonly used. When a tissue expander or implant is placed in the subpectoral pocket, significant muscle spasms may occur postoperatively. Treatment with baclofen or other muscle relaxers is warranted. Implant-based reconstruction may be used in combination with pedicle flaps such as the latissimus dorsi flap. As aforementioned, patient positioning is important in this scenario, with elevation and abduction of the arm at 30 degrees to prevent compression of the vascular pedicle.

Patients that undergo mastopexy or reduction mammaplasty must have evaluation of the nipple for viability and the skin flaps for evidence of ischemia or necrosis. Nipple ischemia in the immediate postoperative period necessitates release of sutures and return to the operating room for decompression.

The Hand Surgery Patient

Splints should be secured with the hand elevated to reduce swelling. The choice of splint used depends on the specific procedure done such as extensor or flexor tendon repair or ORIF of a distal radius, carpal, or metacarpal fracture. Dressings are secure, but allow monitoring of capillary refill or the presence of a hematoma. If there are K-wires or external fixator pins in position, entrance site care can be done with half-strength hydrogen peroxide with normal saline or betadine and normal saline. Bacitracin and/or xeroform is applied to the entrance sites in an effort to prevent infection. After drainage or surgery for hand infections, passive drains such as the Penrose drain may be used to allow drainage of fluid. Frequent packing and dressing changes must be done as indicated by the context of the procedure.

The Cosmetic Surgery Patient

Postoperative practices after cosmetic surgery are surgeon dependent. Compression garments are used after body contouring, such as brachioplasty, to reduce postoperative edema and seroma formation. Ace-wraps and abdominal binders are used to apply gentle pressure after liposuction of the torso, abdomen, or flanks. Compressive, band-like dressings are used for face and neck lift patients to optimize contour of the cervicomental angle and to prevent edema. The head of bed is elevated to help decrease facial swelling and edema. Iced gauze and other types of cool compresses are used after blepharoplasty to reduce eyelid swelling.

Nasal splints may be used after rhinoplasty to open the nares or to contour the nasal dorsum and supratip region to reduce postoperative swelling. Medrol dose packs may also be used to reduce postoperative edema. Cool compresses are placed below the eyes for 48 hours and the patient is instructed to sit and sleep with the head of bed elevated at 45 degrees to decrease edema. Drainage from the nose is common, and the patient is instructed to change gauze pads below the nose as needed until the drainage stops, typically 48 hours postoperatively. The patient is instructed not to sneeze or blow through the nose, but rather through the mouth for the first 3 weeks postoperatively. Nasal congestion is common and can be treated for the first 2 weeks with over-the-counter normal saline or a short course of oxymetazoline. Nasal splints are removed at the surgeon's discretion, often 5 to 7 days postoperatively. Contact sports or strenuous activity must be avoided for 4 to 6 weeks postoperatively.

Suggested Readings

Ariyan S, Martin J, Lal A, et al. Antibiotic prophylaxis for preventing surgical site infection in plastic surgery: an evidence based consensus conference statement from the American Association of Plastic Surgeons. *Plast Reconstr Surg* 2015;135(6):1723–1739.

Guyuron B, Eriksson E, Persing JA, et al, eds. *Plastic Surgery Indications and Practice*. 1st ed. Philadelphia, PA: Saunders; 2008.

Pannucci CJ, Bailey SH, Dreszer G, et al. Validation of the Caprini risk assessment model in plastic and reconstructive surgery patients. *J Am Coll Surg* 2011;212(1):105–112.

Thaller SR, Bradley JP, Garri JI, eds. *Craniofacial Surgery*. New York, NY: Informa-Healthcare; 2007.

Thorne CH, Chung KC, Gosain AK, et al, eds. *Grabb & Smith's Plastic Surgery*. 7th ed. Philadelphia, PA: Lippincott, Williams & Wilkins; 2014.

Wolfe SW, Hotchkiss RN, Pederson WC, et al, eds. *Green's Operative Hand Surgery*. 6th ed. Philadelphia, PA: Elsevier; 2011.

Postoperative Complications

14 Postoperative Pain Management

Mark Hoeft

INTRODUCTION

Pain, as defined by the International Association for the Study of Pain, is "an unpleasant sensory and emotional experience associated with actual or potential tissue damage, or described in terms of such damage." Pain management is important to the care of the postoperative patient for early return of function, comfort, and patient satisfaction. Currently, pain management is a quality measure for the Joint Commission and for reimbursement through the Centers for Medicare and Medicaid Services' Hospital Consumer Assessment of Healthcare Providers and Systems (HCAHPS). Pain is a difficult measure because there are no truly objective signs and is impacted by various psychosocial factors. The utilization of nonopioid- or opioid-sparing techniques such as regional blocks, neuraxial techniques, and nonopioid adjuncts has become tantamount given the rise in opioid abuse in the United States. It is estimated that 25 million people initiated pain relievers for nonmedical uses between 2002 and 2011, and the number of deaths per year attributed to prescription opioid medications reached 16,651 in 2010.

EPIDEMIOLOGY

Although multiple modalities to treat postoperative pain exist including opioid and nonopioid pain medications, and regional and neuraxial anesthesia techniques, pain worldwide continues to be a major issue postoperatively, with an estimated 50% of patients experiencing severe to intolerable pain after surgery and trauma. Many risk factors contribute to poor postoperative pain control following surgery. Patients at risk for poorly controlled pain include those with baseline young age, female sex, preoperative chronic pain intensity, chronic opioid use, preexisting psychiatric diagnoses, preexisting addiction issues, anesthetic technique (e.g., remifentanil-induced hyperalgesia), incision size, and the specific surgical procedure performed (total knee replacements, thoracotomy, etc.).

KEY PATHOPHYSIOLOGY

Basic Pain Sensation in the Normal Individual

Sensation of pain can be divided into four steps: transduction, transmission, modulation, and perception. In transduction, the ability of the body to sense noxious stimuli (nociception) depends on the activation of nociceptors (pain receptors). These receptors are divided into thermal, mechanical, and polymodal nociceptors. Thermal receptors are excited by extremes of temperature; mechanical receptors respond to sharp objects that penetrate, squeeze, or pinch; whereas polymodal receptors respond to the destructive mediators of thermal, mechanical, and chemical stimuli such as potassium, serotonin, bradykinin, histamine, prostaglandins, leukotrienes, or substance P. Following transduction, the nociceptor signal is translated into an electrical signal that allows for transmission of the stimuli via the peripheral nerves. Pain pathways are typically mediated through A delta and C fibers via the dorsal root ganglion and then transmitted through one of three major ascending nociceptive pathways (spinothalamic, spinoreticular, or spinomesence-phalic). Modulation of pain (suppression or worsening of a painful stimulus) occurs either peripherally at the receptor, at the level of the spinal cord, or in supraspinal structures (i.e., the brain stem, thalamus, or cortex). Finally, the perception of pain takes place at the level of the thalamus, somatosensory cortex, anterior cingulate gyrus, insula, cerebellum, and frontal cortex. The thalamus and somatosensory cortex are thought to allow for the localization of pain, whereas the anterior cingulate gyrus is involved in the emotional response to the stimulus. The insula, cerebellum, and frontal cortex allow for one to remember and to learn from a painful experience and to develop avoidance behavior.

Acute versus Chronic Pain

The clinical definition of acute versus chronic pain is determined in a temporal fashion with an arbitrary timeframe of 3 to 6 months defining the cutoff point between acute and chronic.

Acute pain can be defined as a noxious stimulus caused by injury or abnormal functioning of viscera or musculature. It is usually noted following posttraumatic, postoperative, obstetrical, and acute medical illnesses (i.e., myocardial infarction or nephrolithiasis). It is typically classified as somatic or visceral in nature. Somatic pain is caused by the activation of nociceptors in the skin, subcutaneous tissues, and mucous membranes. This pain is typically well localized and is described as a sharp, throbbing, or burning sensation. Visceral pain arises from injury of the organs and is typically described as dull, distention, achy, and is poorly localized. Acute pain follows the pathways listed above and may resolve within seconds to weeks following resolution of the insult.

Chronic pain can be secondary to lesions of peripheral nerves, the spinal cord, or supraspinal structures. Chronic pain can be complicated by many psychological factors such as attention-seeking behavior, and emotional stresses that can precipitate pain (cluster headaches), and pure psychogenic mechanisms.

The types of acute and chronic pain are subdivided into four categories: nociceptive, inflammatory, neuropathic, and dysfunctional. Nociceptive pain occurs through suprathreshold stimulation of pain receptors and typically serves as a protective mechanism. Typically, no injury or changes to the nervous system are seen in nociceptive pain. This type of pain is typically seen in the acute setting of trauma or following surgery. The pain type works as an adaptive mechanism to allow for protection of the injured body part. Nociceptive pain can be chronic in nature, as is seen in certain pathologic states such as osteoarthritis where destruction of the joint can lead to stimulation of the nociceptors with movement.

Inflammatory pain is secondary to mediators (e.g., bradykinin, serotonin) released by injured tissues and inflammatory cells. These mediators lead to a decreased threshold for the perception of pain secondary to changes in the peripheral and central nervous system.

This pain can be either acute following trauma or surgery or chronic in the setting of cancer or osteoarthritis and as nociceptive pain. Upon the removal of inflammation, the hypersensitivity will typically resolve.

Neuropathic pain is secondary to a lesion of the peripheral or central nervous system.

These pathologic states can include diabetic neuropathy, thalamic strokes, and postherpetic neuralgia. All neuropathic pain syndromes have positive signs and symptoms (e.g., allodynia, hyperalgesia) and negative symptoms (i.e., weakness, sensory loss, and decreased reflexes). As opposed to inflammatory pain, neuropathic pain will remain long after the resolution of the inciting insult. Dysfunctional pain is a diagnosis of exclusion where no noxious stimuli, inflammation, or pathologic lesion can be elucidated. Common diseases included under this heading include fibromyalgia and irritable bowel syndrome.

CLINICAL SIGNIFICANCE

Undertreated pain has been linked with increased morbidity and mortality, postoperative pneumonia, deep vein thrombosis, myocardial ischemia and infarction, depression, and readmissions, whereas improved pain control is associated with early mobilization, improved patient satisfaction, and reduced cost of care. Although surgery is performed to correct pathology or aid in resolving pain as a symptom of the pathology, it can contribute to 22.5% and 17.5% of the chronic pain seen in surgical and trauma patients, respectively.

WORKUP

Evaluation and Assessment of Pain

Effective postoperative pain management starts with a preoperative assessment and plan, especially in opioid-tolerant patients or patients with preexisting chronic pain. Opioid-induced hyperalgesia and/or opioid tolerance may result in higher doses of opioids and the addition of nonopioid analgesics for adequate pain control. A preoperative assessment prior to surgery may be warranted to allow for an opioid wean prior to surgery to reduce the patient's tolerance and hyperalgesia. A preoperative assessment may also be utilized to discuss other pain management options including regional and neuraxial analgesia, along with postoperative expectations for pain management with the patient. A thorough evaluation and assessment of the patient's pain is necessary to elucidate prior chronic pain history, baseline (preoperative) pain scores, prior medication trials, addiction history, aberrant behavior, and worsening pain suggestive of an acute process that may require intervention. Many states now have prescription monitoring programs available to allow clinicians to review patients' opioid and benzodiazepine prescriptions from other providers to assess for compliance and/or aberrant, drug-seeking behavior.

Laboratory results including renal function (opioid and NSAID use), liver function tests (acetaminophen), urine or blood toxicology (opioids), coagulation studies (neuraxial and regional anesthesia), and white blood cell and platelet counts (neuraxial and regional anesthesia) may be helpful in formulating a plan for the management of postoperative pain. A thorough review of the patient's medications is necessary prior to regional or neuraxial anesthesia to rule out anticoagulant use.

Pain Assessment Tools

When assessing postoperative pain, a verbal numeric scale is typically used. The scale ranges from 0 to 10, with 0 representing no pain and 10 representing the worst pain imaginable. Important qualitative descriptors of pain to assess are the location, radiation, and the quality (sharp or dull) of the pain. Multiple pain assessment tools include the numerical rating scale, visual analog scale, and Wong–Baker FACES Pain Rating Scale.

WHAT FACTORS TRIGGER INCREASED MONITORING, AND HOW IS THIS ACCOMPLISHED?

Opioids

Increased monitoring may be required in certain subsets of postsurgical patients at risk for adverse events from pain medications such as the opioids.

Those patients with obstructive sleep apnea, chronic obstructive pulmonary disease, renal failure, liver failure, and altered mental status and the elderly may experience unwanted side effects from utilization of the opioids such as mental status changes and respiratory depression. An understanding of the metabolism and elimination of these medications along with dose adjustment or avoidance is of utmost importance. Utilization of the opioids in these populations, especially in combination with other psychotropic medications, can have devastating results, including hypoxemia and death. For those patients of concern, continuous pulse oximetry and capnography may be utilized to more quickly notify clinicians of potential adverse events.

Risk Factors for Opioid Abuse

It is important to screen all patients for the risks for addiction and aberrant pain behaviors in the perioperative periods to determine a cogent plan for pain management. Multiple risk factors are associated with opioid addiction and aberrant behavior including personal or family history of substance abuse, concurrent smoking, prior illicit drug abuse, and mental health issues. Multiple screening tools exist for the determination of risk for opioid addiction and aberrant behavior for patients with chronic pain including Opioid Risk Tool (ORT) and the Screener and Opioid Assessment for Patients with Pain (SOAPP) to assess the risk of long-term opioid therapy.

Some of the major challenges surrounding opioids include those of tolerance, physical dependence, withdrawal, and addiction. Tolerance is defined as a fixed dose of an opioid providing less analgesia over time that may lead to escalating doses of narcotics to achieve the same pain relief. Physical dependence is a physiologic state that is manifest by abruptly stopping opioid medications, which then results in a withdrawal state. Opioid withdrawal presents with irritability, anxiety, insomnia, diaphoresis, yawning, rhinorrhea, and lacrimation. As time progresses, the symptoms may include fevers, chills, myalgia, abdominal cramping, diarrhea, and tachycardia. Opioid withdrawal is self-limiting and can typically last 3 to 7 days. As opposed to physical dependence, addiction is defined by opioid use, resulting in physical, psychological, or social dysfunction and continued use of the opioid despite the overlying issues. Behaviors that are most indicative of addictive behaviors are buying street drugs, stealing money to obtain drugs, attempting to obtain opioids from multiple sources, acts of prostitution to obtain drugs, forging prescriptions, and selling prescription drugs.

Communication

For those patients at high risk of opioid abuse, addiction, dependence, or diversion, communication with the patient's primary care physician, surgeon, pain physician, psychiatrists, substance abuse provider, or other opioid prescribers is important for determination/suspicion of the patient's substance abuse history and risk factors to aid in the development of a perioperative plan to minimize medications with high addiction potential. For those patients requiring medications with high addiction potential, close follow-up with their primary care physician, surgeon, or pain physician is recommended along with a short course of opioid. Utilization of an opioid contract, designation of a single provider to write for opioids, random drug screens, and opioid risk stratification may be necessary.

MANAGEMENT OPTIONS

Pain is often treated utilizing a multimodal approach, meaning multiple treatment methods may be combined to provide analgesia, with the hope of decreasing pain and opioid usage. The treatment of acute pain can often begin prior to the initial surgical insult. In the preoperative period, preemptive analgesia is often utilized to decrease or stop nociceptive input. Nonsteroidal anti-inflammatory drugs (NSAIDs) such as celecoxib (PO), ketorolac (IV), and ibuprofen (PO) or acetaminophen can be used preoperatively in combination with other medications such as gabapentin to prevent central sensitization. The main advantage of celecoxib and other cyclooxygenase-2 (COX-2) inhibitors over other NSAIDs include the decreased risk of gastrointestinal bleeding, but other adverse events such as myocardial infarction, stroke, allergic reaction to sulfonamide drugs, and renal issues may be seen with the use of COX-2 inhibitors.

Preemptive analgesia can also be obtained through neuraxial and regional techniques, such as peripheral nerve blocks of the femoral nerve, and brachial plexus. In those patients with moderate to severe pain, opioid analgesics such as hydromorphone or morphine may be used in combination with acetaminophen or NSAIDs for analgesia. Surgeons may aid in providing pain relief through infiltration of local anesthetics such as lidocaine or bupivacaine at the surgical site.

In those patients not able to take oral medications postoperatively, patient-controlled analgesia (PCA) devices allow patients to deliver pain medication through the pressing of a button that allows the medication to be delivered via an intravenous route or an epidural catheter. These devices typically allow patients to deliver a predetermined amount of pain medicine at specific time intervals. There is a lockout period in which the patient can attempt to deliver pain medication; however, none will be given to prevent overdosing on opioid pain medication. A continuous (basal) rate may also be added to provide a baseline level of analgesia without the patient needing to administer the medication.

Below are listed common procedures and medication classes utilized in the postoperative management of pain.

Neuraxial and Regional Analgesia
Continuous Epidural Analgesia

   Indications: postoperative pain relief following lower extremity, pelvic, abdominal, and thoracic surgery, rib fractures

   Medications: local anesthetics, opioids, clonidine

   Adverse effects: local anesthetic toxicity, hypotension, somnolence, pruritus, motor blockade, nausea

   Contraindications: patient refusal, bacteremia, hypotension, coagulopathy, increased intracranial pressure

   Complications: epidural hematoma, epidural abscess, neurologic injuries, high spinal, postdural puncture headache, intravascular injection

Regional Blocks
Patient-Controlled Analgesia

   Indications: blockade of peripheral nerves of the upper (interscalene, supraclavicular, infraclavicular, axillary) and lower (femoral, popliteal, saphenous, and ankle) extremities for primary anesthetic for surgery and/or postoperative pain control, transversus abdominis plane block, paravertebral block

   Medications: local anesthetics (bupivacaine, ropivacaine, mepivacaine)

   Adverse effects: hoarseness (blocking of recurrent laryngeal nerve), shortness of breath (blocking of phrenic nerve), Horner syndrome (blocking of stellate ganglion)

   Complications: pneumothorax, hematoma, abscess, neurologic injuries, intravascular injection, hematoma

Pain Medication

Indications: postoperative pain control

Route of administration: intravenous or subcutaneous systemic administration of opioid pain medications by patient

Mechanism of action: μ-receptor agonist

Medications: morphine, hydromorphone, fentanyl, methadone, meperidine

Adverse effects: oversedation, respiratory depression, itching, ileus, nausea, vomiting, addiction, physical dependence

Other consideration: best used in patients unable to tolerate oral pain medications. Dependent on patient's ability to comprehend the PCA device. Higher baseline anxiety levels and less social support is associated with higher PCA use and opioid consumption.

Nonsteroidal Anti-Inflammatory Drugs

Indications: mild to severe inflammatory pain

Mechanism of action: inhibition of COX enzyme

Adverse effects: gastrointestinal upset/ulcer, renal failure, bleeding, allergic reaction

Opioids

Indications: moderate to severe postoperative pain

Route of administration: intravenous, oral, transdermal, buccal, intranasal, intrathecal, subcutaneous (See Table 14.1 for common opioid dosing)

Mechanism of action: μ-, δ-, and κ-opioid receptors. The receptors are most abundant in the dorsal horn of the spinal cord and also in the dorsal root ganglion and peripheral nerves

Adverse effects: oversedation, respiratory depression, itching, constipation, ileus, nausea, vomiting, addiction, physical dependence

Anticonvulsants (Gabapentin, Carbamazepine, and Oxcarbazepine, Pregabalin)

The anticonvulsants work through very diverse mechanisms of action, including modulation of voltage-gated calcium channels, sodium channels, GABA, and glutamine receptors. FDA-approved pain indications include trigeminal neuralgia (carbamazepine), postherpetic neuralgia (gabapentin, pregabalin), diabetic neuropathy (pregabalin), fibromyalgia (pregabalin), and migraine

 TABLE 14.1 Common Oral Opioid Pharmacodynamics and Dosing

Opioids	Half-Life	Duration (h)	Equianalgesic Oral Doses (mg)	Initial Dose (mg)	Dosing Interval (h)
Codeine	3	3–4	80	30–60	4
Hydromorphone	2–3	2–3	2	2–4	4
Hydrocodone	1–3	3–6	10	5–7.5	4–6
Oxycodone	2–3	3–6	7	5–10	6
Methadone	15–30	4–6	10–20	20	6–8
Morphine	2–3.5	3–4	10	10–30	3–4
Propoxyphene	6–12	3–6	43–45	100	6
Tramadol	6–7	3–6	40	50	4–6

prophylaxis (divalproex, topiramate). Common adverse effects include somnolence, fatigue, and withdrawal (abrupt cessation of gabapentin).

Serotonin–Norepinephrine Reuptake Inhibitors (Venlafaxine, Duloxetine)

Serotonin–norepinephrine reuptake inhibitors (SNRIs), as their class implies, block the reuptake of norepinephrine and serotonin. Duloxetine is the first antidepressant to have a specific pain indication (diabetic neuropathy) in the United States. These medications have also been demonstrated to be useful in the treatment of fibromyalgia. The side-effect profile tends to be lower in SNRIs than in the tricyclic antidepressants (TCAs).

Tricyclic Antidepressants (Nortriptyline, Amitriptyline)

Indications: These agents are used for the treatment of neuropathic pain syndromes such as postherpetic neuralgia, diabetic neuropathy, pain secondary to spinal cord injury, cancer-related neuropathic pain, and other pain syndromes such as low back pain, osteoarthritis, and fibromyalgia.

Mechanism of action: TCAs contribute to the improvement in pain symptoms through their actions on multiple sites, including serotonergic, noradrenergic, opioidergic, NMDA receptors, adenosine receptors, sodium channels, and calcium channels. The effects of TCAs can include elevation of mood, normalization of sleep patterns, and muscle relaxation.

Adverse effects: somnolence, urinary retention, dry mouth, increased fall risk in elderly, drowsiness, dizziness, weight gain, orthostatic hypotension, and lethargy

Tizanidine

Indications: Tizanidine is commonly used in pain medicine as a muscle relaxant and/or sleep aid.

Mechanism of action: α_2-agonist

Adverse effects: hypotension, dry mouth, and somnolence

Low-Dose Ketamine Infusion

Indications: severe postoperative pain

Mechanism of action: NMDA antagonist

Adverse effects: hallucinations, salivation, tachycardia, hypertension

Lidocaine Infusion

Indications: postoperative pain (trauma, intraabdominal surgery), central pain, cancer pain, diabetic neuropathy

Mechanism of action: sodium channel blockade, inhibition of G-coupled proteins, and NMDA receptors

Adverse effects: nausea, vomiting, abdominal pain, diarrhea, dizziness, perioral numbness, tremor, dry mouth, metallic taste, insomnia, and tachycardia

Suggested Readings

Gerbershagen HJ, Pogatzki-Zahn E, Aduckathil S, et al. Procedure-specific risk factor analysis for the development of severe postoperative pain. *Anesthesiology* 2014;120:1237–1245.

Gil KM, Ginsberg B, Muir M, et al. Patient-controlled analgesia in postoperative pain: the relation of psychological factors to pain and analgesic use. *Clin J Pain* 1990;6:137–142.

Guignard B, Bossard AE, Coste C, et al. Acute opioid tolerance: intraoperative remifentanil increases postoperative pain and morphine requirement. *Anesthesiology* 2000;93:409–417.

International Association for the Study of Pain. Unrelieved pain is a major global healthcare problem. *International Association for the Study of Pain* 2004–2005. Available at: http://www.iasp-pain.org/files/Content/ContentFolders/GlobalYear AgainstPain2/20042005RighttoPainRelief/factsheet.pdf. Accessed June 14, 2015.

Kalkman CJ, Visser K, Moen J, et al. Preoperative prediction of severe postoperative pain. *Pain* 2003;105:415–423.

Macintyre PE, Walker S, Power I, et al. Editorial I: Acute pain management: scientific evidence revisited. *Br J Anaesth* 2006;96:1–4.

Overdyk FJ, Carter R, Maddox RR, et al. Continuous oximetry/capnometry monitoring reveals frequent desaturation and bradypnea during patient-controlled analgesia. *Anesth Analg* 2007;105:412–418.

15 Postoperative Nausea and Vomiting

Ryan J. Horvath and William Benedetto

I. INTRODUCTION

Postoperative nausea and vomiting (PONV) continues to be a common occurrence in the postanesthesia care unit (PACU) setting, affecting at least 30% of patients after general anesthesia and greater than 80% in populations with multiple risk factors without prophylaxis. The sequelae of PONV range from the relatively benign (patient discomfort and poor patient satisfaction) to the more severe (electrolyte abnormalities, dehydration, pain especially with abdominal and thoracic surgery, wound or anastomotic dehiscence, hypertension, increased intracranial pressure, pneumothorax, and aspiration). PONV is also a major contributor to PACU length of stay, limiting discharge for ambulatory surgery and increasing hospital admission rates, costing hundreds of millions of dollars per year in the United States alone. Therefore, prevention and treatment of PONV is of paramount importance. The focus of this chapter is to describe the risk factors related to PONV, discuss PONV prophylaxis and rescue, and summarize the therapies for PONV.

II. RISK FACTORS: PATIENT

Several studies have been undertaken to assess patient risk factors related to PONV, and several predictive models have been developed to help determine which patients would benefit most from PONV prophylaxis. Recent evidence-based analysis has shown that the following risk factors are most closely associated with PONV: **female gender, history of PONV, nonsmoking status, history of motion sickness, and age.**

A. **Female gender** is highly correlated with PONV, with a risk greater than 2.5 times that of males. The mechanism for this effect is, however, not well understood. Smaller trials have shown that females are more sensitive to emetogenic stimuli and 2 to 3 times more likely to suffer from PONV than men. This susceptibility is thought to be hormonally mediated because these studies suggest that females are 4 times more likely to suffer from PONV during menses and 4 times less likely to suffer from PONV after menopause compared with baseline. However, large randomized controlled trials have failed to support these variations in PONV susceptibility with hormonal cycles.

B. Patients who have a **history of PONV** after prior surgeries are approximately 2 times more likely to suffer from PONV from subsequent surgeries than the general population. In addition, a **history of motion sickness** is thought to indicate a susceptibility to PONV that may be genetically mediated because sufferers of motion sickness and PONV are more likely to have first-degree relatives with their own history of PONV compared with controls.

C. **Nonsmokers** are approximately 2 times more likely to suffer from PONV than smokers. The protective action of smoking on PONV is currently unknown; however, many diverse hypotheses have been generated and await testing. Induction of cytochrome P450 by cigarette smoke contaminants has been shown to lead to increased anesthetic gas metabolism, although the small change in metabolism is unlikely to account for the marked differences in PONV susceptibility between smokers and nonsmokers. Another hypothesis is that smoking and nicotine alter the neurotransmitter milieu responsible for PONV.

D. **Age** has been shown to be protective for PONV, with approximately a 20% risk reduction with each decade of life. PONV, however, is relatively uncommon in children aged less than 3, but is more prevalent in adolescence and early adulthood before decreasing with increasing age. The mechanism of this trend is unknown; however, several hypotheses have been proposed, including hormonal variations in adolescence and puberty and reduced autonomic reflexes in the aged adult.

III. **RISK FACTORS: SURGERY**

Evidence for the impact of surgical type on PONV is limited by publication bias; however, there is a strong historical consensus on high-risk surgeries that are associated with PONV.

A. **Ophthalmic** surgeries, especially strabismus surgeries, are well known to cause dizziness and PONV.

B. **ENT** middle ear surgeries can lead to profound PONV, and ENT procedures with bleeding down the GI track can lead to emesis.

C. **Gynecologic**, **urologic**, and **abdominal** procedures can lead to visceral stimulation that is highly emetogenic. In addition, **laparoscopic procedures** with insufflation can cause visceral pressure and retained abdominal CO_2, causing PONV.

D. Other surgical factors that are less well studied but may still have a role in PONV include incisional pain, hypotension, hypoxia, ileus, and the presence of a nasogastric tube.

E. In addition, special care should be given to patients undergoing surgeries following which retching or vomiting would be highly detrimental, especially laryngeal/tracheal surgery, surgeries with vulnerable vascular anastomoses, or those during which intracranial hypertension is present.

IV. **RISK FACTORS: ANESTHESIA**

The type of anesthesia delivered has long been known to affect PONV, especially in susceptible populations. Recent meta-analysis suggests that the most strongly associated anesthesia risk factors for PONV are the **use of volatile anesthetics, duration of anesthesia, use of nitrous oxide**, and **postoperative opioids**.

A. **Volatile anesthetics** have been shown to be the strongest predictor of early PONV, and it is unsurprising that prolonged exposure to volatile anesthetics further increases the risk of PONV.

B. **Nitrous oxide** has been shown to be associated with PONV, especially when the duration exceeds 45 minutes to 1 hour. Proposed mechanisms of nitrous oxide–induced PONV include bowel distention, middle ear pressure changes, and direct effects on receptors in emetogenic centers in the brain.

C. **Postoperative opioids** are thought to cause PONV through peripheral μ-opioid receptor activation, leading to reduced peristaltic activity and to decreased gastric and colonic emptying and visceral distention.

V. **PONV RISK SCORES AND PROPHYLAXIS**

Medications used to treat PONV are not without side effects; therefore, many risk scores have been developed to stratify patients' likelihood of developing PONV to help guide the choice of prophylaxis. Most of these assign points to known patient, surgical, and anesthesia risk factors (such as those listed above) and give approximate PONV risk

| | TABLE 15.1 | Modified Apfel Score for Adults Used to Assess Properative Risk of PONV | | |

Risk Factor	Points	Total Points	Risk of PONV (%)
Female gender	1	0	10
Nonsmoker	1	1	20
History of PONV	1	2	40
Postoperative opioids	1	3	60
Total	1–4	4	80

and suggestions for prophylaxis. There is continued debate as to the benefits of routine PONV prophylaxis given cost-effectiveness of treatment and possible medication side effects; however, in certain patient populations, it is warranted.

A. The **Modified Apfel risk score for adults** (Table 15.1) is one of the most studied and validated risk scores. It assigns points for several risk factors and estimates the risk of PONV.

B. Many other PONV risk scores have been created on the basis of the Apfel score and often include a small number of additional risk factors in their tabulation; however, they all aim to stratify patients into low-, moderate-, and high-risk groups.

C. Patients with a **low risk of PONV** (10% to 20%) require no routine prophylaxis. However, if there are surgical- or anesthesia-related risk factors, then administration of PONV prophylaxis from one pharmacologic class (see below) is reasonable.

D. Patients with a **moderate risk of PONV** (20% to 40%) require prophylaxis from one to two pharmacologic classes (see below).

E. Patients with a **high risk of PONV** (60% to 80%) require prophylaxis from two to three pharmacologic classes (see below) and would benefit from avoidance of nitrous oxide, volatile anesthetics, and postoperative opioids.

F. **Total intravenous anesthesia** (TIVA), involving a propofol infusion and analgesics, and **regional anesthesia,** are both effective methods of limiting PONV, especially in high-risk patients.

VI. **PONV RESCUE**

PONV rescue is necessary when no prophylaxis was given or when prophylaxis fails.

A. If **no PONV prophylaxis was given**, then treatment should begin with a medication from one pharmacologic class.

B. If **PONV prophylaxis failed**, then treatment should continue with an antiemetic from a different class than previously administered.

C. Most antiemetic medications have been shown to **reduce PONV** by approximately **25%.**

D. Antiemetics elicit **synergism** (combined effect greater than the additive effect of individual therapies) when administered from different pharmacologic classes. Therefore, it is more effective to administer antiemetics from several different classes than from a single pharmacologic class. The most investigated and common combination therapy used clinically includes ondansetron, dexamethasone, and haloperidol/droperidol.

E. If **PONV** becomes **refractory** to standard rescue therapy, then occasionally a sedating infusion of propofol is necessary in the PACU. This will, however, require the patient to remain in a PACU or intensive care setting for the duration of therapy.

VII. AGENTS: BY PHARMACOLOGIC CLASS

A. Serotonin (5-HT$_3$) Receptor Antagonists

Serotonin (5-HT$_3$) receptor antagonists are the most commonly administered and investigated medications for both prophylaxis against and treatment of PONV. Basic and clinical research suggests that 5-HT$_3$ antagonists block 5-HT$_3$ receptors centrally in the medullary chemoreceptor trigger zone in the floor of the fourth ventricle and peripherally on vagal nerve terminals.

1. **Ondansetron** (Zofran, 4 to 8 mg IV at the end of surgery), the "gold standard" antiemetic and prototypical 5-HT$_3$ receptor antagonist, has shown efficacy as both prophylaxis against and rescue from PONV.

2. Second-generation 5-HT$_3$ antagonists include: **Palonosetron** (0.075 mg IV at the end of surgery, 40 hour half-life), **Granisetron** (0.35 to 3 mg IV at the end of surgery), **Tropisetron** (2 mg IV at the end of surgery, not approved in the United States), **Dolasetron** (12.5 mg IV at the end of surgery, caution given increased risk of torsades de pointes arrhythmias, no longer available in the United States), and **Ramosetron** (0.3 mg IV at the end of surgery, not approved in the United States). Research into the efficacy of these newer agents is ongoing.

3. Common **side effects** for the class of 5-HT$_3$ receptor antagonists include headache, drowsiness/sedation, and constipation. Less common, but of great clinical importance, is the propensity of these medications to increase QTc interval. Although the amount of QTc prolongation (approximately 5 to 20 ms in clinically relevant doses for most agents) in isolation does not usually limit its use or redosing, it can become significant when 5-HT$_3$ receptor antagonists are administered in conjunction with other medication with similar propensity to prolong the QTc interval.

B. Tranquilizers

Members of the tranquilizer group are a diverse collection of antiemetic medications that include butyrophenones, antipsychotics, and sedatives. In addition to their ability to treat nausea and vomiting, they all share a propensity for sedation at higher doses.

1. **Haloperidol** (Haldol, 0.5 to 2 mg IV or IM at the end of surgery) has been found to be effective on both the prophylaxis against and rescue from PONV. It should be noted, however, that it has antipsychotic and sedative activity at higher doses (5 mg or greater with repeated dosing). Side effects of haloperidol dosed for antipsychosis include extrapyramidal effects and QTc prolongation. Although extrapyramidal side effects are rare following lower PONV dosing, QTc prolongation can still occur. Caution should be used in patients with prolonged QTc (>450 ms) and when haloperidol is used in conjunction with other QTc prolonging agents.

2. **Droperidol** (Inapsine, 0.625 to 1.25 mg IV at the end of surgery) now carries an FDA black box warning concerning QTc prolongation and torsades de pointes arrhythmias at doses similar to those used for PONV. This action has caused many institutions to severely limit its clinical use.

3. Other members of this class of PONV agents include **Prochlorperazine** (Compazine, 5 to 10 mg IV), **Hydroxyzine** (Vistaril, 25 to 100 mg IM), **Perphenazine** (5 mg IV), and **Dixyrazine** (10 mg IV). Dixyrazine has been shown to be effective in preventing PONV; however, newer data are inconclusive regarding the effectiveness of Prochlorperazine, Hydroxyzine, or Perphenazine for the prevention or treatment of PONV.

C. **Dopamine Receptor Antagonists**

Dopamine receptor antagonists are thought to prevent PONV through inhibition of both central and peripheral dopamine receptors. Antagonism of central D_2 receptors in the medullary chemoreceptor trigger zone reduces nausea and in the area postrema reduces vomiting. In addition, antagonism of peripheral dopamine receptors along the gastrointestinal tract increases motility without increasing secretions, leading to enhanced gastric emptying.

1. **Metoclopramide** (Reglan, 10 to 20 mg IV) is the prototypical dopamine receptor antagonist, which has weak efficacy when used as a rescue medication in the first 24 hours after surgery for treatment of PONV.

2. Side effects of dopamine receptor antagonists include dyskinesia or extrapyramidal side effects.

D. **Cholinergic Receptor Antagonists**

Cholinergic receptor antagonists, including scopolamine, have been shown to have efficacy in preventing both motion sickness and PONV.

1. **Scopolamine** (1.5 mg transdermal patch, applied >2 hours prior to surgery) is best used prophylactically in conjunction with other antiemetic agents. Of note, it should not be redosed.

2. Side effects of cholinergic receptor antagonists include visual disturbances, dry mouth, and dizziness.

E. **Corticosteroids**

Corticosteroids, especially dexamethasone, are known to be effective in the prevention of PONV. Studies support that PONV is inhibited centrally; however, the exact mechanism of action is currently unknown.

1. **Dexamethasone** (4 to 8 mg IV, administered at the start of surgery) has been shown to be effective in preventing PONV. Of note, it should not be redosed.

2. **Methylprednisolone** (40 mg IV, administered at the start of surgery) has been shown to be effective in preventing PONV.

3. Side effects of corticosteroid use for prevention of PONV include significant increases in blood glucose 6 to 12 hours after administration; therefore, caution should be used in diabetic patients. There is currently insufficient evidence to support an increased risk of wound infection after single-dose administration of corticosteroids for PONV; however, it is prudent to use caution in patients with increased concern for postoperative infection.

F. **Neurokinin-1 Antagonists**

Neurokinin-1 (NK-1) antagonists are a new class of antiemetics that competitively inhibit Substance P binding to the NK-1 receptor in the CNS.

1. **Aprepitant** (Emend capsule, 40 or 80 mg PO) has been found to be highly effective as a rescue antiemetic; however, its use for prophylaxis has yet to be established. Oral formulation and expense have so far limited its clinical use.

2. **Fosaprepitant** (Emend injection, 150 mg IV) is an IV formulation of the prodrug of Aprepitant. Clinical use has been similarly limited by expense.

3. **Cosapitant** (150 mg PO) has yet to be approved for use in the United States.

4. **Rolapitant** (200 mg PO) has a 180-hour half-life, but has yet to be approved in the United States.

G. **Antihistamines**

1. **Dimenhydrinate** (1 mg/kg) has been shown to have antiemetic efficacy similar to ondansetron and dexamethasone; however, optimal timing and dosing are currently unknown.

2. **Meclizine** (50 mg PO) is another antihistamine that has been shown to have some efficacy for the prevention of PONV.

H. Other Antiemetics

1. **Propofol** is a sedative-hypnotic medication, which, acting through γ-aminobutyric acid receptors, is commonly used for induction or maintenance of anesthesia. Its use as part of a TIVA can significantly reduce PONV, especially in patients with multiple risk factors. At subhypnotic doses (1 mg/kg bolus and 20 µg/kg/min infusion), propofol has been shown to be effective for rescue of PONV.

2. α_2-**agonists** clonidine and dexmedetomidine have shown weak antiemetic efficacy. Possible mechanisms for this effect include their propensity for opioid sparing, sedation, or direct central antiemetic activity.

I. Nonpharmacologic Therapies

There are many nonpharmacologic therapies for the prevention and treatment of PONV; however, few have been rigorously studied.

1. Acupuncture/acupressure and IV fluid hydration have shown some limited efficacy in treating PONV.

2. The following therapies have **not** been found to be effective in the treatment of PONV: music therapy, isopropyl alcohol inhalation, intraoperative supplemental oxygen, intraoperative gastric decompression, proton pump inhibition, ginger root, nicotine path, cannabinoids, and hypnosis.

J. Pediatric

Studies show that PONV in children is up to twice as prevalent as in adult populations. Similar to adults, children at moderate to high risk should receive combination therapy from multiple pharmacologic classes.

1. **Ondansetron** (0.05 to 0.1 mg/kg) is the most studied antiemetic in pediatric populations, and its use as PONV prophylaxis and safety has been supported even in 1-month-old children.

2. **Dexamethasone** (0.5 mg/kg) is commonly used in pediatric populations, often in combination with ondansetron.

VIII. CONCLUSIONS

PONV is a common and costly occurrence in the perioperative setting. Prophylaxis is warranted in patients with risk factors for PONV or undergoing high-risk surgical procedures and is best achieved through administration of antiemetics from multiple pharmacologic classes. PONV rescue is similarly best achieved through multimodal approaches.

Suggested Readings

Apfel CC, Heidrich FM, Jukar-Rao S, et al. Evidence-based analysis of risk factors for postoperative nausea and vomiting. *Br J Anesth* 2012;109:742–753.

Apfel CC, Läärä E, Koivuranta M, et al. A simplified risk score for predicting postoperative nausea and vomiting. *Anesthesiology* 1999;91:693–699.

Apfelbaum JL, Silverstein JH, Chung FF, et al. Practice guidelines for postanesthetic care: an updated report by the American Society of Anesthesiologists Task Force on Postanesthetic Care. *Anesthesiology* 2013;118:291–307.

Gan TJ, Diemunsch P, Habib AS, et al. Consensus guideline for the management of postoperative nausea and vomiting. *Anesth Analg* 2014;118:85–113.

Jokinen J, Smith AF, Roewer N, et al. Management of postoperative nausea and vomiting: how to deal with refractory PONV. *Anesthesiol Clin* 2012;30:481–493.

Silverstein JH, Apfelbaum JL, Barlow JC, et al. Practice guidelines for postanesthetic care: a report by the American Society of Anesthesiologists Task Force on Postanesthetic Care. *Anesthesiology* 2002;96:742–752.

Skolnik A, Gan TJ. Update on the management of postoperative nausea and vomiting. *Curr Opin Anaesthesiol* 2014;27:605–609.

Postoperative Airway Complications

Tara Kelly and Mazen Maktabi

Although anesthesiologists are well informed on optimization for safe intubation and intraoperative ventilation, less focus has been placed on postoperative airway complications. It has been reported that postoperative airway complications are relatively common (1.3% to 19%), almost 30% of all adverse events associated with anesthesia occur at the end of anesthesia or during recovery, and further emphasis and attention on this phase of anesthesia is needed. This chapter focuses on risk factors, diagnosis, and management of airway complications occurring in the early postoperative period.

As anesthesiologists, our first interaction with the postoperative patient is actually in the operating room, around emergence and the time of extubation. As stated by Popat et al, extubation "is not simply a reversal of the process of intubation because conditions are less favourable than at the start of anesthesia." Adequate planning for tracheal extubation involves preoperative identification of patients with difficult airways. The Difficult Airway Society has created four steps for anesthesiologists to follow in the "Basic Algorithm": planning for extubation, preparing for extubation, performing extubation, and providing postextubation care. This airway algorithm is further divided into "Low-Risk Algorithm" and an "At-Risk Algorithm" to optimize extubation based on patient and surgical specific factors.

PATIENT-SPECIFIC FACTORS

Because of the lack of consistency of research definitions regarding postoperative airway complications, limitations in identifying patient-specific factors exist. Specific factors that have been demonstrated to increase the risk of postoperative airway complications include male sex, age >60 years, diabetes, obesity, and obstructive sleep apnea (OSA).

Obstructive Sleep Apnea and Noninvasive Ventilation

Two types of noninvasive ventilation (NIV) are commonly used in the postoperative period: noninvasive continuous positive pressure ventilation and noninvasive positive pressure ventilation. Both types of NIV support and decrease the work of breathing, improve atelectasis to allow for better gas exchange, and reduce left ventricular afterload to improve cardiac output. The use of NIV postoperatively should be strongly considered in high-risk patient populations, including the elderly, obese, patients with a history of chronic obstructive lung disease, postabdominal and thoracic surgery patients, or those who use NIV at home. In high-risk populations, postoperative NIV reduces reintubation rates after surgery, decreases postsurgical risk of pneumonia, and increases hospital survival.

Obesity

Obese (body mass index [BMI] ≥30 kg/m^2) and morbidly obese (BMI ≥ 35 kg/m^2) patients present many challenges to the anesthesiologist, including the risk of postoperative airway complications. Anesthesiologists must consider the high rate of OSA in obese populations because OSA is often associated with decreased pharyngeal tone that can be sensitive to anesthetics and opioids (Popat et al., 2012). In the postanesthetic care unit (PACU), obese patients should, if possible, be placed in a head and back up position at a minimum of 25 degrees to decrease the reduction of functional residual capacity, reduce atelectasis, and improve gas exchange. Obese patients have a susceptibility to obesity hypoventilation syndrome (OHS), which is defined as the combination of obesity (BMI $\geq 30 \, kg/m^2$), daytime awake hypercapnia (partial pressure of arterial carbon dioxide $\geq 45 \, mm \, Hg$), and hypoxemia (partial pressure of oxygen $\leq 70 \, mm \, Hg$) (Chau et al., 2012). Patients with OHS are at an increased risk for postoperative ventilatory decline in the PACU often secondary to opioids owing to their propensity for upper airway obstruction, impaired pulmonary mechanics, and depressed central respiratory drive. Often, these patients require and improve with NIV, as described earlier.

SURGICAL FACTORS

Surgical procedures lasting more than 4 hours and those performed on an emergent basis appear to increase the risk for postoperative airway complications. Patients undergoing surgical procedures of the tonsils, adenoids, vocal cords, and trachea are at increased risk of postoperative airway events. In addition, surgical procedures that are in the prone position increase the risk of postoperative airway events, given the increased edema of the airway during the procedure. Similarly, thoracic procedures and abdominal procedures that involve the diaphragm also increase the risk of postoperative airway and pulmonary complications.

Thyroid Surgery

Greater than 90,000 thyroid surgeries are performed per year in the United States. Thyroid surgery presents a number of causes for postoperative airway compromises. Transient and permanent recurrent laryngeal nerve (RLN) paralysis, hypocalcemia, tracheomalacia, and postoperative hematoma are potential life-threatening complications of the airways because they impact airway patency postoperatively.

Hematoma

The incidence of postoperative hematoma has been reported to range from 0.19% to 4%, with the greatest risk during the first 6 hours following thyroid surgery; however, this serious risk can persist throughout the first postoperative 24 hours. The concern of airway obstruction following hematoma formation is the rationale for postoperative hospitalization following central neck surgery. Risk is attributed to surgical technique, patient predisposition, and thyroid pathology. It has been found that patients who develop postthyroid surgery hematoma are 3 times more likely to die than patients who did not experience postoperative hematoma. Patient discharge within 24 hours is safe and recommended in specific patient groups. A "thyroid kit" should always be kept at the bedside of postoperative thyroid surgery patients. It should contain sterile basic surgical equipment (blades, scissors, surgical clamps, and gauzes) that facilitates opening and decompressing a postoperative thyroid hematoma. A high index of suspicion for a threatening hematoma should exist when patients complain of new onset of difficulty in breathing or developing hoarseness in the PACU. Management of acute hematoma causing respiratory compromise involves promptly alerting the surgical and PACU teams and, if needed, removing sutures and opening the wound to relieve airway compression. Emergent surgical exploration may then be indicated. It should be emphasized that early intervention in cases of developing postoperative thyroid hematoma is important because delay in management of airway compression will lead to impairment of lymphatic

TABLE 16.1	Clinical Findings Associated with Postoperative Wound Hematoma		
	Respiratory	**Neck**	**General**
Early	Change in voice quality	Elevated drain output	Restlessness
	Difficulty breathing	Suture line bleeding	Agitation
To	Inspiratory stridor	Anterior neck swelling	Panic
	Cyanosis	Facial edema/plethora	Somnolence
Late	Respiratory arrest	Tracheal deviation	Unresponsiveness

From Palumbo MA, Aidlen JP, Daniels AH, et al. Airway compromise due to wound hematoma following anterior cervical spine surgery. *Open Orthop* 2012;6:108–113.

and venous drainage with consequent increasing edema and swelling of the airway, in which case evacuation of the hematoma may not resolve airway compression. In such situations, a surgical airway can be lifesaving (Table 16.1).

Hypocalcemia

Up to 83% of postthyroidectomy patients experience some degree of hypocalcemia postoperatively; however, a smaller subgroup requires treatment for symptomatic hypocalcemia. Patient populations with a higher rate of symptomatic hypocalcemia include patients with advanced thyroid cancers, Graves' disease, or symptomatic hyperparathyroidism prior to surgery. Of note, although autotransplantation of at least one parathyroid gland during surgery minimizes the risk of permanent hypoparathyroidism, it is associated with an increased rate of acute hypocalcemia in the postoperative period. Airway compromise from hypocalcemia generally manifests 12 to 48 hours postprocedure as stridor and poor air movement, and may be associated with tingling in the lips.

Recurrent Laryngeal Nerve Paralysis/Palsy

Bilateral RLN paralysis following thyroidectomy has been reported to be as low as 0.58%; however, unilateral RLN damage is more common (3.5% to 6.6%). Although improvements in intraoperative nerve monitoring and even direct visualization by a flexible endoscope at the end of surgery are reassuring, the consequences of unpreparedness in the PACU can be life threatening.

Carotid Endarterectomy

Airway compromise from postoperative neck hematoma and postoperative neck edema is a feared consequence of carotid endarterectomies (CEAs).

Neck Hematoma

With an incidence of 5.5%, neck hematoma is a serious complication of CEA. On average, neck hematomas present about 6 hours postoperatively, and 50% will need surgical exploration. The distortion of the airway occurs by both hematoma formation and edema formation. The need for urgent or emergent reintubation in a patient with an expanding neck hematoma can be challenging even for the experienced anesthesiologist. In a patient with respiratory compromise, decompression of the hematoma by removing sutures at the surgical incision may improve intubating conditions and therefore should occur before or concurrently with attempts to secure the airway (Shakespeare et al., 2010).

Airway Edema

Edema, secondary to either mucosal trauma or lymphatic and venous congestion, is thought to complicate CEA. There have been numerous reports of hematoma evacuation not improving airway compromise, leading to the theory of airway edema as the causal agent for airway compromise. In the setting of persistent airway edema, postoperative intubation and mechanical ventilation provide a secured airway and time for the edema to resolve (Munro et al., 1996) Administration of corticosteroids may also facilitate the resolution of airway edema (Hughs et al., 1997) (Table 16.2).

Anterior Cervical Spine Surgery

Airway obstruction occurring after anterior cervical surgery has a reported incidence of 1.2% to 6.1% and can be because of pharyngeal swelling, hematoma formation, cerebrospinal fluid leak, angioedema, and graft dislodgement. The incidence of postoperative neck hematoma following anterior cervical discectomies and/or fusion ranges between 0.2% and 1.9%. Risk factors associated with airway obstruction include surgical duration greater than 5 hours, surgical exposure of more than three vertebral bodies, blood loss greater than 300 mL, and exposure involving C2, C3, or C4. An important clinical point is that many of these patients will have a neck collar in place postoperatively, which will mask and therefore delay early diagnosis and visualization of neck swelling. This underscores the importance of early detection of signs of periairway swelling such as voice changes, mild stridor, difficulty talking, and agitation. Other airway complications of anterior cervical spine surgery in the PACU are unilateral or bilateral RLN palsy, respiratory failure due to cervical neural compression (because of a dislodged graft or direct compression by

	Additional Risk Factors for Postoperative Airway Compromise		
Surgical	**Patient**	**Anesthetic**	**Institutional**
Exposure of >3 vertebral bodies	Morbid obesity	Suboptimal airway visualization	No 24-h in-house anesthesia care
Exposure of C2–C4 levels	Obstructive sleep apnea	Multiple intubation attempts	No 24-h in-house surgical staff
Blood loss >300 mL	Pulmonary disease		
Operative time >5 h	Cervical myelopathy		
Dual approach operations	Prior anterior cervical surgery		

From Palumbo MA, Aidlen JP, Daniels AH, et al. Airway compromise due to wound hematoma following anterior cervical spine surgery. *Open Orthop* 2012;6:108–113.

TABLE 16.3	Probable Etiology of Airway Compromise After Anterior Cervical Spine Surgery	
Postoperative Period	**Time Elapsed from Surgery**	**Probable Causative Factor**
Immediately	<12 h	Wound hematoma
Early	12–72 h	Pharyngeal/prevertebral edema
Late	>72 h	Abscess, CSF accumulation, construct failure

From Bertalanffy H, Eggert HR. Complications of anterior cervical discectomy without fusion in 450 consecutive patients. *Acta Neurochir (Wien)* 1989;99(1/2):41–50.

a hematoma). Table 16.3 lists the likely causes of airway problems following cervical spine surgery in relation to timing of occurrence of the complications.

ANESTHESIA SPECIFIC FACTORS

Studies have identified that specific anesthetic practices may increase the rate of postoperative airway complications. These practices include premedication with opioids alone or opioids and benzodiazepines, induction with thiopental (when compared with propofol), intraoperative fentanyl at doses >2 µg/kg/hour, the use of a combination of fentanyl and morphine, and misuse and inadequate reversal of neuromuscular blocking drugs.

Residual Neuromuscular Blockade

The incomplete recovery from neuromuscular blocking drugs, both intermediate-acting and long-acting agents, increases a patient's risk of developing postoperative respiratory complications. In lightly anesthetized healthy volunteers, residual neuromuscular blockade leads to attenuation of hypoxic ventilation response, upper airway obstruction, pharyngeal dysfunction, and decreased respiratory motor strength. In addition, it has been found that the use of excessive doses of neostigmine to reverse neuromuscular blockade also increases a patient's risk for respiratory complications.

Laryngeal Mask Airway

Use of a laryngeal mask airway (LMA) is common practice among anesthesiologists in the United States. Postoperative complications associated with LMA use include damage to the RLN and hypoglossal nerve, referred to as Tapia syndrome. Clinically, Tapia syndrome often presents as dysarthria, dysphagia, dyspnea, inability to elevate the soft palate on the affected side, and the deviation of the tongue to the affected side (Wadelek et al., 2012; Shah et al., 2015) Possible risk factors include use of nitrous oxide, inappropriately sized LMAs, lateral positioning, difficult LMA insertion, and prolonged operative time. Conservative treatment, including speech therapy, often may provide full recovery for this neurapraxic injury (Wadelek et al., 2012; Shah et al., 2015)

Wire-Reinforced Tubes

Wire-reinforced tubes (WRTs) have a stainless steel wire that runs in a helical fashion within their wall along the entire length of the tube. They can be deformed in an irreversible fashion if they are bitten by the patient, resulting in airway obstruction. The primary indication for use of a WRT intraoperatively is in surgeries where kinking and obstruction of the endotracheal tube is a possibility, such as in severe flexion of the neck in upper cervical spine surgery, posterior fossa surgery, neck surgery, otolaryngology, and oral surgery. If a WRT is used as part of intraoperative anesthesia care and if the decision is made to keep the patient intubated postoperatively, every effort should be made to exchange this tube for a regular endotracheal tube before exiting the operating rooms in order to prevent the possibility of permanently kinking this tube by biting. If the patient's airway is swollen or presents a risk making changing the tube difficult or risky, effective bite blocks should be securely placed to prevent biting on the tube. In addition, clearly visible warning reminders in the patient postoperative orders and signs on the WRT and by the patient's bed should be placed to remind the nursing, respiratory therapy, and ICU medical staff of the presence of the WRT so that utmost vigilance is exercised in preventing the patient from biting the tube in the postoperative period.

In providing postoperative care, it is important to recognize and anticipate risk factors associated with postoperative airway compromise, intervene early to prevent worsening of the airway status, and ensure the early availability of assistance and equipment to reintubate a patient in the PACU if necessary.

Suggested Readings

Abboud B, Sleilaty G, Rizk H, et al. Safety of thyroidectomy and cervical neck dissection without drains. *Can J Surg* 2012;55:199–203.

Campbell MJ, McCoy KL, Shen WT, et al. A multi-institutional international study of risk factors for hematoma after thyroidectomy. *Surgery* 2013;156(6):1283–1291.

Canet J, Gallart L, Gomar C, et al. Prediction of postoperative pulmonary complications in a population-based surgical cohort. *Anesthesiology* 2010;113:1338–1350.

Cavallone LF, Vannucci A. Extubation of the difficult airway and extubation failure. *Anesth Analg* 2013;116(2):368–383.

Chau EH, Lam D, Wong J, et al. Obesity hypoventilation syndrome: a review of epidemiology, pathophysiology, and perioperative considerations. *Anesthesiology* 2012;117:188–205.

Cook TM, Woodhall N, Frerk C, on behalf of the Fourth National Audit Project. Major complications of airway management in the UK: results of the Fourth National Audit Project of the College of Anaesthetists and the Difficult Airway Society. Part 1: Anaesthesia. *Br J Anesth* 2011;106:617–631.

Dixon BJ, Dixon JB, Carden JR, et al. Preoxygenation is more effective in the 25 degrees head up position than in the supine position in severely obese patients: a randomized controlled study. *Anesthesiology* 2005;102:1110–1115.

Glossop AJ, Shepard N, Brydon DC, et al. Non-invasive ventilation for weaning, avoiding reintubation after extubation and in the postoperative period: a meta analysis. *Br J Anaesth* 2012;109:305–314.

Hazem MZ, Naif AA, Ahmed AS. Recurrent laryngeal nerve injury in thyroid surgery. *Oman Med J* 2011;2:34–38.

Hughs R, McGuire G, Montanera W, et al. Upper airway edema after carotid endarterectomy: the effect of steroid administration. *Anesth Analg* 1997;84(3):475–478.

Isono S. Obstructive sleep apnea of obese adults: pathophysiology and perioperative airway management. *Anesthesiology* 2009;110(4):908–921.

Jaber S, Pierre M, Chanques G. Role of non-invasive ventilation (NIV) in the perioperative period. *Best Pract Res Clin Anaesthesiol* 2010;24:253–265.

Lo CY, Kwok KF, Yuen PW. A prospective evaluation of recurrent laryngeal nerve paralysis during thyroidectomy. *Arch Surg* 2000;135:204–207.

Munro FJ, Makin AP, Reid J. Airway problems after carotid endarterectomy. *Br J Anesth* 1996;76:156–159.

Murphy GS, Szokol JW, Marymont JH, et al. Residual neuromuscular blockade and critical respiratory events in the postanesthesia care unit. *Int Anesth Res Soc* 2008;107(1):130–137.

Palumbo MA, Aidlen JP, Daniels AH, et al. Airway compromise due to laryngeal edema after anterior cervical spine surgery. *J Clin Anesth* 2013;25(1):66–72.

Palumbo MA, Aidlen JP, Daniels AH, et al. Airway compromise due to wound hematoma following anterior cervical spine surgery. *Open Orthop J* 2012;6:108–113.

Pompei L, Della Rocca G. The postoperative airway: unique challenges? *Curr Opin Crit Care* 2013;19:359–363.

Popat M, Mitchell V, Dravid R, et al. Difficult Airway Society Guidelines for the management of tracheal extubation. *Anaesthesia* 2012;67:318–340.

Rose DK, Cohen MM, Wigglesworth DF, et al. Critical respiratory events in the postanesthesia care unit: patient, surgical and anesthetic factors. *Anesthesiology* 1994;81(2):410–418.

Sagi HC, Beutler W, Carroll E, et al. Airway complications associated with surgery on the anterior cervical spine. *Spine* 2002;27(9):949–953.

Shah AC, Barnes C, Spiekerman CF, et al. Hypoglossal nerve palsy after airway management for general anesthesia: an analysis of 69 patients. *Anesth Analg* 2015;120(1):105–120.

Shakespeare WA, Lanier WL, Perkins WJ, et al. Airway management in patients who develop neck hematomas after carotid endarterectomy. *Anesth Analg* 2010;110(2):588–593.

Takahoko K, Iwasaki H, Sasakawa T, et al. Unilateral hypoglossal nerve palsy after use of the laryngeal mask airway supreme. *Case Rep Anesthesiol* 2014;2014:369563.

Wadelek J, Kolbusz J, Orlicz P, et al. Tapia's syndrome after arthroscopic shoulder stabilization under general anesthesia and LMA. *Anesthesiol Intensive Ther* 2012;44:31–34.

Weiss A, Lee KC, Brumund KT, et al. Risk factors for hematoma after thyroidectomy: results from the nationwide inpatient sample. *Surgery* 2014;156(2):399–404.

Wingert DJ, Friesen SR, Iliopoulos IJ, et al. Post thyroidectomy hypocalcemia: incidence and risk factors. *Am J Surg* 1986;152:606–610.

Postoperative Respiratory Complications

Tao Shen and Richard M. Pino

I. INTRODUCTION

Postoperative respiratory complications occur commonly and are a significant source of morbidity and mortality. A large Australian review showed respiratory and airway complications occurring in 2.2% of 8,372 postanesthetic care unit (PACU) admissions. Notable complications were inadequate oxygenation and ventilation, upper airway obstruction, and aspiration. Because most respiratory events culminate in hypoxemia as the common pathway, routine use of pulse oximetry in the PACU can lead to timely detection of these complications. However, because most patients receive supplemental oxygen therapy, desaturation may not occur until late in the course of respiratory events, and PACU providers must use other parameters and clinical signs to assist in their assessments of pulmonary status. In the evaluation of the patient with postoperative pulmonary issues, the anesthesiologist in the PACU must decide which issues can continue to be treated in the PACU with the extension of care on the hospital floor or which patients will require triaging to an ICU either for more definitive care or for extensive observation.

II. CONTRIBUTING FACTORS

A. The development of postoperative respiratory complications is a synergy between a patient's medical condition and the effects of general anesthesia (GA) and surgery on the respiratory system.

1. **Patient factors**

    Age > 70 years, ASA classification $\geq$ 2, cigarette smoking, malnutrition (serum albumin < 30 g/L), functional dependence, and comorbidities such as underlying chronic respiratory disease, congestive heart failure, and neuromuscular weakness all decrease pulmonary reserve and increase susceptibility to effects of surgery and anesthesia.

    a. Patients with **asthma** have increased risk of bronchospasm, pneumonia, and respiratory failure if history of frequent exacerbations, recent hospitalization, or tracheal intubation for asthma. Complication rates for general versus regional anesthesia were similar in a study of over 1,500 asthmatic patients.

    b. **Chronic obstructive pulmonary disease (COPD)** is associated with high risk of developing postoperative pulmonary complications. Patients can have chronically fatigued respiratory muscles, unrecognized cor pulmonale, and bronchospasm in addition to their fixed obstructive disease.

    c. **Obstructive sleep apnea (OSA)** is greatly affected by anesthesia and surgery, and patients are at risk for more frequent and severe episodes of postoperative hypoxemia. Sedatives and analgesics decrease pharyngeal tone and attenuate responses to hypoxia and hypercarbia. GA alone results in transient alterations in sleep architecture, which combined with use of opioids may be important factors in the development of postoperative sleep disturbance and propensity for obstruction.

d. **Smoking cessation** should be emphasized in all patients. Carbon monoxide and nicotine normalize after 12 to 48 hours of abstinence. Airway reactivity is reduced after 1 week, and sputum volume is halved at 2 weeks. Stopping smoking 4 to 6 weeks prior to surgery is shown to reduce the overall incidence of perioperative respiratory complications.

2. **Surgical factors**

   a. Thoracic and abdominal surgery (including major vascular surgeries) results in dysfunction **of the diaphragm.** This occurs via functional disruption of respiratory muscles from surgical incisions and retracting, irritation, or injury of the phrenic and intercostal nerves, and effects of postoperative pain limiting deep breathing. These factors produce a restrictive respiratory pattern in the acute postoperative period. In patients undergoing laparotomy, functional residual capacity (FRC) decreases to approximately 50% of baseline, returning to normal over 1 to 2 weeks. **Neurosurgery** can affect control of respiration, and surgeries involving the **head and neck** increase the risk for airway complications postoperatively.

   b. The **degree of surgical insult** such as level of aggressiveness, procedure duration (>3 hours), and amount of blood lost is associated with postoperative pulmonary complications, likely as part of the systemic inflammatory response syndrome, large fluid shifts during resuscitation, and amplification of local factors described earlier. The need for intraoperative **blood transfusion** is an independent risk factor, as is **emergency surgery**.

3. **Anesthetic factors**

   a. **GA reduces FRC** with an immediate and universal development of atelectasis in the dependent parts of the lung. FRC is reduced by approximately 20% under GA with greater reduction in patients with obesity and COPD. This occurs from loss of chest wall muscle tone and upward displacement of the diaphragm causing compression atelectasis. The reduced FRC, in part, also decreases lung compliance and increases airway resistance. The relative reduction in FRC to closing volume produces intrapulmonary shunting and ventilation–perfusion mismatches. Anesthesia is also associated with **inhibition of hypoxic and hypercapnic ventilatory drive**, which persists for a variable period of time postoperatively and predisposes to hypoventilation and hypoxemia.

   b. **Epidural anesthesia** without GA creates little to no atelectasis formation. Neuraxial techniques may therefore be preferred in high-risk patients.

   c. **Residual anesthetics, sedatives, and analgesics** blunt hypoxic and hypercapnic ventilator drives, predisposing to hypoventilation and hypoxemia.

B. **Risk Stratification**

Although patients at increased risk for developing postoperative respiratory complications can be identified, it is difficult to quantify their risk with more precision.

1. Laboratory studies, baseline arterial blood gases, pulmonary function testing, and preoperative chest radiograph have not been shown to be helpful, unless there is a question of diagnosis or presence of unexplained symptoms.

2. Predictive **pulmonary risk indices** for postoperative respiratory failure or pneumonia (Table 17.1) have been developed. The major contributors to patients' risk remain clinical factors. These results were based on the analysis of Veteran Affairs patient database, which,

TABLE 17.1	Respiratory Failure Risk Index	
Preoperative Predictor		**Point Value**
Type of surgery		
• Abdominal aortic aneurysm		27
• Thoracic		21
• Neurosurgery, upper abdominal, peripheral vascular		14
• Neck		11
• Emergency surgery		11
Albumin < 30 g/L		9
Blood urea nitrogen (>30 mg/dL)		8
Partially or fully dependent functional status		7
History of chronic obstructive pulmonary disease		6
Age (y)		
• ≥70		6
• 60–69		4
Respiratory failure risk: ≤10 points, 0.5%; 11–19, 2.2%; 20–27, 5%; 28–40, 11.6%; >40, 30.5%		

From Arozullah AM, Daley J, Henderson WG, et al. Multifactorial risk index for predicting postoperative respiratory failure in men after major noncardiac surgery. The National Veterans Administration Surgical Quality Improvement Program. *Ann Surg* 2000;232:242–253.

although encompassing a high number of patients, was skewed to include mostly male veterans.

III. UPPER AIRWAY OBSTRUCTION

A. Upper airway obstruction is most often caused by inadequate recovery of airway reflexes and muscle tone.

B. **Clinical signs** typically include poor chest excursion, discoordinate abdominal and chest wall motion during inspiration, and intercostal and suprasternal retraction. Inspiratory stridor and snoring may be present if the obstruction is partial; complete obstruction is silent.

C. At-risk groups are patients with history of OSA, craniofacial abnormalities, redundant soft tissues (obesity), acromegaly, and tonsillar and adenoidal hypertrophy

D. **Differential Diagnoses**

1. **Pharyngeal obstruction** from a sagging tongue and poor pharyngeal tone in the semiconscious patient is the most common cause of postoperative airway obstruction. The most studied upper airway dilator muscles are the genioglossus and tensor palatini muscles, both of which are involved in stabilizing airway patency in response to negative pharyngeal pressure during inspiration. Residual anesthetic and neuromuscular blockade can cause dilator muscle dysfunction and airway collapse in the postoperative patient.

    a. Pharyngeal obstruction usually responds to simple airway maneuvers including chin tilt and jaw thrust (anteriorly displacing mandible), lateral decubitus positioning, and use of oral- or nasopharyngeal airways. Nasal airways are typically better tolerated, because they do not stimulate the gag reflex.

    b. Patients with OSA can benefit from continuous positive airway pressure (CPAP), ideally from the time of extubation onward. It is advantageous for the patient to bring his/her own CPAP machine to the hospital.

2. **Laryngeal obstruction**

   a. **Laryngospasm** is caused by intense tonic contraction of the laryngeal muscles and descent of the epiglottis over the laryngeal inlet. Laryngospasm in the PACU is generally precipitated by an airway irritant (e.g., secretions, blood) in a patient still emerging from anesthesia. Partial laryngospasm can be difficult to discern from other causes of airway obstruction because some air movement still occurs. **Vocal cord paresis** can result from recurrent laryngeal nerve (RLN) injury or mechanical injury to the vocal cords. Injury to the RLN prevents abduction of the ipsilateral vocal cord, which fixes in a paramedian position because of unopposed action of the cricothyroid muscle (supplied by the superior laryngeal nerve). The RLN and vocal cords can be injured during thyroid, parathyroid, laryngeal, and thoracic surgery as well as from trauma sustained during rigid bronchoscopy and intubation. Unilateral RNL injury presents typically with hoarseness, with the primary concern being risk of gastric aspiration. Both laryngospasm and vocal cord paresis can be clinically manifested by stridor and extremely high-pitched vocalization. Paradoxical respiration (chest retraction during inspiration while the abdomen is distended) may also be noticed. A brief application of positive pressure ventilation will be efficacious to "break open" the vocal cords if laryngospasm is the problem. If this treatment is not effective, there should be no delay in securing the airway with tracheal intubation especially if bilateral vocal cord abduction from nerve injury is likely. Most vocal cord paralysis is transient, and recovery occurs over the course of weeks to months. Permanent paralysis occurs. Complete laryngospasm and vocal cord paralysis can cause **negative pressure pulmonary edema**.

   b. **Laryngeal edema** more frequently occurs in children (who have smaller airway diameter), after prolonged surgeries with large fluid administration, and surgeries involving head-down or prone positioning. Intraoperative difficult intubation and airway instrumentation alert to possible airway edema from direct injury. The cuff leak test is neither sensitive nor specific and should not be relied upon as the sole test in deciding whether to extubate a patient with suspected airway edema who arrives in the PACU intubated. In most cases, treatment involves supplemental oxygen, sitting the patient **upright** to facilitate venous drainage, **fluid restriction**, possible **diuresis**, and administration of **nebulized epinephrine** (2.25% solution, 0.5 to 1.0 mL in normal saline). Intravenous **dexamethasone** 4 to 8 mg IV every 6 hours for 24 hours can also help reduce swelling. **Heliox** (80% helium, 20% oxygen), which improves airflow by reducing gas density, can be used while waiting for other medical treatments to take effect. In severe cases, reintubation is required.

3. **External airway compression**, most commonly by hematomas, can develop after thyroidectomy, parathyroid surgery, carotid endarterectomy, and radical neck dissections. The pressure from the expanding hematoma within the neck tissue disrupts venous and lymphatic drainage, which further escalates edema. Patients may present with local pain and pressure, dysphagia, and respiratory distress. Tracheal deviation and biphasic stridor may be seen. Tracheal intubation should be rapidly established, which may be extremely challenging because of altered neck anatomy. Treatment involves emergent reexploration in the OR. Subcutaneous clot can be evacuated at the bedside by removing surgical sutures.

IV. **HYPOVENTILATION**
  A. Hypoventilation occurs from **inappropriately low alveolar ventilation**, resulting in hypercapnia ($PaCO_2 > 45$ mm Hg) and respiratory acidosis. It is common after GA, and is mild and temporary in most instances. When severe, hypoventilation can cause hypoxemia, CO_2 narcosis ($PaCO_2$ 90 to 120 mm Hg), and eventually apnea.
  B. **Signs of hypoventilation** may vary from somnolence, low respiratory rate, signs of airway obstruction, rapid and shallow breathing, to labored breathing. Tachycardia, hypertension, and cardiac irritability can result from sympathetic stimulation. Severe respiratory acidosis can cause myocardial depression and hypotension. Mild hypercapnia may not be tolerated in patients with preexisting cardiopulmonary disease, such as pulmonary hypertension.
  C. In patients with spontaneous ventilation, supplemental oxygen often masks the ability to detect abnormalities in ventilation in the PACU. **Pulse oximetry** can only reliably detect hypoventilation if the patient is breathing room air.
  D. **Differential Diagnoses**
    1. **Decreased ventilatory drive**
       Hypoventilation in the PACU is most commonly because of the residual depressant effects of anesthetics on the respiratory drive.
       a. **Opioids** produce respiratory depression by shifting the CO_2 response curve downward and to the right, characteristically producing a slow respiratory rate with large tidal volumes. Excessive sedation is usually present and the patient may become apneic without stimulation. Indeed, the ventilatory depression from opioids becomes significantly worse when the patient falls asleep. The effect of opioids acts **synergistically**, with residual **volatile anesthetics** and **benzodiazepines** often administered as a combination to the patient intraoperatively.
       b. The safest method to treat anesthetic-related hypoventilation is continuation of **assisted ventilation** until the drugs are cleared. Otherwise, **pharmacologic reversal** can be considered.
          1. Treatment of excessive narcotization includes incremental doses of **naloxone** (0.04 to 0.08 mg in adults), the effect of which is seen within 1 to 2 minutes. Large doses of naloxone can result in unwanted reversal of analgesia as well as sympathetic surge precipitating hypertensive crisis, pulmonary edema, and myocardial ischemia. Notably, the duration of action of naloxone is 30 to 60 minutes, which is shorter than most opioids, and patients should be monitored closely for relapse into hypoventilation.
          2. **Flumazenil** (increments of 0.2 to 1 mg IV every 5 minutes, maximum 5 mg) can be given to reverse the sedative effects of benzodiazepines. The onset of flumazenil is 1 to 2 minutes, peaking at 5 to 10 minutes. Its redistribution half-life is only 5 to 15 minutes, and patients may relapse into sedation. In patients on chronic benzodiazepines, flumazenil may precipitate withdrawal seizures.
       c. **Central nervous system disorders** are rare de novo causes of hypoventilation in the postoperative period. They, of course, must be considered after intracranial surgeries and surgeries involving the carotid and vertebral arteries. These include intracranial strokes and bleeding (particularly in the brain stem), cerebral embolic events, and mass effect from tumor and abscesses.
    2. **Ventilatory insufficiency** in the PACU can be because of inadequate chest movements from respiratory muscle weakness, incisional

pain, and diaphragmatic dysfunction. Marked hypoventilation and respiratory acidosis can occur when these factors are superimposed on an impaired ventilatory reserve because of preexisting pulmonary, neuromuscular, or neurologic disease. Patients often present with tachypnea, low tidal volumes, discoordinated chest movements, and generalized weakness.

a. **Residual neuromuscular blockade** in the PACU usually results from **inadequate reversal. Altered pharmacokinetics** (e.g., with hypothermia, renal and hepatic dysfunction), **drug–drug interactions,** and **metabolic derangements** (e.g., hypokalemia, hypophosphatemia, hypocalcaemia, hypermagnesemia) can affect the predictability of reversal of muscle relaxants. Evidence of neuromuscular recovery should include a train-of-four ratio >0.9, maintenance of a patent airway, adequate ventilation and oxygenation, and a sustained head lift of >5 seconds (most sensitive). If muscle weakness persists after adequate pharmacologic reversal, it may be best to restart or continue mechanical ventilation, administer anxiolytics, and wait for recovery of muscle strength. **Overdosing neostigmine** in an attempt to reverse paralysis may in itself cause weakness in a fashion similar to a depolarizing muscle relaxant. At this point, special situations such as pseudocholinesterase deficiency and succinylcholine-induced phase II block should be considered. Table 17.2 lists the factors that can prolong the effect of muscle relaxants.

b. There are some **conditions that influence the response to neuromuscular blocking agents,** which require extra attention in the PACU.

1. **Myasthenia gravis** and **myasthenic syndrome**—produce extreme sensitivity to nondepolarizing muscle relaxants and profound postoperative weakness. The use of acetylcholinesterase

TABLE 17.2	Factors Causing Prolonged Neuromuscular Blockade

Drugs
- Antibiotics
  - Aminoglycosides, e.g., gentamicin, tobramycin
  - Tetracyclines
  - Polymyxins
- Volatile anesthetic agents
- Local anesthetics (especially if given IV)
- Anticholinesterase inhibitors
- Antiarrhythmics, e.g., quinidine
- Calcium channel blockers
- Magnesium
- Dantrolene
- Lithium

Altered Physiology and Metabolism
- Hypothermia
- Acidosis and acidosis
- Hepatic and renal dysfunction

Electrolyte Abnormalities
- Hypocalcemia
- Hypokalemia
- Hypermagnesemia
- Hypernatremia

inhibitors for treatment in myasthenia gravis may prolong the action of depolarizing muscle relaxants through inhibition of pseudocholinesterases.

2. **Myotonic syndromes** (e.g., myotonic dystrophy)—characterized by impaired muscle relaxation and persistent contraction after stimulation (myotonia) and progressive muscle wasting because of abnormal calcium metabolism. Myotonic triggers include hypothermia, shivering, etomidate, propofol, methohexital, succinylcholine, and neostigmine. These patients have a weakened respiratory effort and extreme sensitivity to the respiratory depressant effects of opioids, benzodiazepines, and inhalational agents.

c. The diaphragm accounts for 70% of lung volume change during normal respiration. **Diaphragmatic dysfunction** following upper abdominal and thoracic surgeries can significantly reduce ventilation and cause hypercarbia. **Phrenic nerve** irritation or injury can result from surgical trauma as well as ipsilateral brachial plexus blocks (interscalene > supraclavicular > infraclavicular). **Restrictive factors** such as obesity, gastric distension, high intraabdominal pressures, tight dressings, and body casts also inhibit respiratory muscle and cause CO_2 retention.

d. Patients with **preexisting airflow limitations** (e.g., from **COPD**) have a high ventilatory workload at baseline, worsened by surgical trauma, airway reactivity, and secretions, which further reduce ventilation and gas exchange.

e. **Splinting because of incisional pain** decreases alveolar ventilation (rapid, shallow breathing), causing atelectasis, hypercapnia, and hypoxemia. Deep breathing and pulmonary toilet can be facilitated with early and effective pain relief (e.g., epidural analgesia, intercostal nerve blocks), which is especially important in patients with underlying respiratory and neuromuscular diseases.

V. HYPOXEMIA

A. Hypoxemia is common in the postoperative period. Observational studies in the PACU found 30% to 55% of patients had at least one episode whereby O_2 saturations (SpO_2) < 90% and 10% to 13% had SpO_2 <80%. In patients who arrive in the PACU without supplemental oxygen, 30% had SpO_2 <90%.

B. Mild hypoxemia is well tolerated in young healthy patients. With progressive duration and severity, acidosis and circulatory depression occur, which are poorly tolerated in patients with preexisting heart and lung disease (e.g., pulmonary hypertension).

C. Hypoxemia is usually promptly detected by pulse oximetry. One of the first **clinical manifestations** of hypoxemia is restlessness and confusion. Other signs may include dyspnea, tachycardia from sympathetic stimulation, and cardiac irritability (e.g., premature atrial and ventricular complexes). Bradycardia and hypotension are late signs. **Cyanosis** is classically described when more than 5 g/dL of deoxyhemoglobin is present, and thus may be absent in patients with severe anemia.

D. **Differential Diagnoses**

The most common cause of hypoxemia in the recovering patient is a combination of hypoventilation and intrapulmonary shunting. Systematically, evaluation of the hypoxemic postoperative patient should include consideration of each of these causes of hypoxemia:

1. **Atelectasis**

A decrease in FRC begins with induction of GA and persists for many days postoperatively. A reduction in FRC can move the end-expiratory point into the closing capacity, promoting airway closure during tidal breaths in the dependent lung, initiating shunting or reducing ventilation/perfusion ratios. Any situation that results in either increased closing capacity (e.g., advanced age) or reduced FRC (e.g., obesity, infection, aspiration, pulmonary edema, thoracic and upper abdominal surgery) places the patient at increased risk for hypoxemia. Nevertheless, the FRC/closing capacity relationship is not the sole determinant of impaired gas exchange during the perioperative period; other important factors include a reduction in chest wall muscle tone and changes in bronchomotor and vascular tone that persist into the postoperative period.

a. **Treatment** involves maneuvers to increase vital capacity such as deep breathing, incentive spirometry, and sitting upright. Adequate analgesia is important to prevent splinting. Noninvasive ventilation is shown to be effective in treating more severe hypoxemia in some patient groups and decrease the incidence of reintubation.

b. **Severe intrapulmonary shunting** occurs when the shunt fraction is >15% and is commonly associated with radiographic findings of atelectasis and pulmonary infiltrates. In these patients, causative factors such as endobronchial intubation, bronchial obstruction with secretion or blood, aspiration pneumonia and pneumonitis, pulmonary edema, and pneumothorax should be suspected and treated accordingly.

2. **Hypoventilation**

Hypoxemia exclusively because of hypoventilation is uncommon, especially in patients receiving supplemental oxygen. Hypoventilation promotes alveolar collapse and increases the partial pressure of CO_2, which in turn decreases the alveolar oxygen tension.

3. **Diffusion hypoxia**

This can occur during rapid washout of nitrous oxide on emergence from GA. Because nitrous oxide is 32 times more soluble than nitrogen, it dilutes the inspired air and thus alveolar oxygen concentration. Diffusion hypoxia is rarely seen clinically because it is easily prevented by oxygen administration after extubation.

4. **Pulmonary edema**

Commonly detected by the presence of wheezing, the most common time of appearance of pulmonary edema is observed within 60 minutes of completion of surgery. Causes of pulmonary edema can be divided into:

a. **Increased vascular hydrostatic pressure** (cardiogenic pulmonary edema) usually occurs in patients with preexisting cardiac disease and can be precipitated by large fluid administration, dysrhythmias, and myocardial ischemia. Evaluation by a cardiologist may be prudent, especially for the management of acute coronary events that require catheterization and intervention. Diuretics, vasodilators, and inotropes remain the mainstay of treatment.

b. **Increased pulmonary capillary permeability**—seen following a variety of clinical situations such as sepsis, trauma, burn, aspiration, blood product transfusion, and disseminated intravascular coagulation. It can progress to adult respiratory distress syndrome. Treatment is mainly supportive and involves addressing the underlying condition.

c. **Sustained reduction in interstitial hydrostatic pressure**—also known as negative pressure pulmonary edema, this results when the patient attempts forceful inspirations against a closed glottis, usually with laryngospasm on emergence. Treatment may involve noninvasive ventilation. The use of diuretics is controversial. The condition usually resolves within 24 hours when recognized early and respiratory support is provided promptly.

5. **Pulmonary aspiration**

Gastric contents can enter the trachea during induction, emergence, or PACU admission because of depressed airway reflexes. Topical local anesthetic to facilitate fiberoptic bronchoscopy can leave the airway unprotected for several hours postoperatively. Signs of significant aspiration include bronchospasm, hypoxemia, atelectasis, and cardiovascular instability. Initial treatment consists of oropharyngeal suctioning, bronchodilators for bronchospasm, and oxygen therapy. Mechanical ventilation may be required if hypoxemia is severe. Antibiotics may be indicated if the aspiration is suspected to contain a high bacterial load (e.g., with small bowel obstruction). Steroids are of no benefit. Patients who remain asymptomatic after 2 hours of their aspiration event are unlikely to develop pulmonary complications.

6. **Pneumothorax** should be considered following central line placement, supraclavicular and intercostal blocks, chest trauma (including rib fractures), neck surgery, and intraabdominal and retroperitoneal surgeries (which may have injured the diaphragm). Patients with subpleural blebs and bullae may have developed pneumothorax during positive pressure ventilation. Chest tube insertion is generally indicated for all symptomatic pneumothorax or one that is greater than 15% to 20% of the volume of the lung.

7. **Pulmonary embolism** is an uncommon cause of postoperative hypoxemia, but should be considered in patients with malignancy, deep venous thrombosis, multiple trauma, orthopedic surgery (fat embolism), and intracranial surgery (air embolism).

E. **Approach to the Hypoxemic Patient in the PACU**

1. **Immediate actions**
   a. Assess airway patency
   b. Assess for hemodynamic stability
   c. Administer or increase supplemental oxygen.
   d. Consider immediate treatments such as endotracheal intubation for acute airway compromise, decompression of tension pneumothorax, and cardioversion of unstable rhythms.

2. **Clinical features**
   a. Bedside examination for associated symptoms (such as chest pain, palpitations), respiratory rate, mental status and auscultation for equal air movements, and presence of stridor, wheezing, and crackles.
   b. Observe trend of vital signs, telemetry, and oxygen requirement. Note administration of medications such as opioids, anxiolytics, sedating antiemetics (e.g., promethazine).
   c. Consider common clinical patterns:
      1. Low respiratory rate and sedation with slow downward drift in SpO_2: residual anesthetics, opioids, and sedatives
      2. Tachypnea and restlessness: inadequate analgesia, muscle weakness, diaphragmatic dysfunction, metabolic acidosis
      3. Tachypnea and wheeze: segmental bronchial obstruction, bronchospasm, pulmonary edema
      4. Acute onset of hypoxemia: pneumothorax, airway obstruction, large pulmonary embolism, acute circulatory compromise

3. **Initial workup**
   a. Arterial blood gas to evaluate for hypercarbia, respiratory/metabolic acidosis and A–a gradient.
   b. 12-lead ECG to assess for myocardial ischemia and laboratory studies as indicated (hemoglobin, coagulation profile, troponin)
   c. Chest x-ray for focal infiltrates, pneumothorax, and pulmonary edema. Ideally, the radiograph is taken with the patient positioned sitting upright. If pneumothorax is suspected, x-ray taken at end-expiration helps to emphasize the pneumothorax.
   d. Fiberoptic bronchoscopy may be diagnostic and therapeutic for bronchial obstruction and lobar atelectasis because of secretion, blood, or tissue.
4. **Treatment**
   a. Oxygen therapy with or without positive airway pressure is the mainstay of treatment for hypoxemia
      1. Patients with underlying heart and lung disease may require higher concentration of inspired oxygen to maintain adequate delivery of oxygen content
      2. Endotracheal intubation (to ensure delivery of 100% oxygen) may be necessary in severe hypoxemia while establishing the cause.
   b. Further treatment of hypoxemia is directed at the cause.

Suggested Readings

Eugene SF, Downs JB, Schweiger JW, et al. Supplemental oxygen impairs detection of hypoventilation by pulse oximetry. *Chest* 2004;126:1552–1558.

Jakob TM, Minna W, Sophus HJ. Hypoxaemia in the postanaesthesia care unit: an observer study. *Anesthesiology* 1990;73:890–895.

Jones JG, Sapsford DJ, Wheatley RG. Postoperative hypoxaemia: mechanisms and time course. *Anaesthesia* 1990;45:566–573.

Kluger MT, Bullock MF. Recovery room incidents: a review of 419 reports from the Anaesthetics Incident Monitoring Study (AIMS). *Anaesthesia* 2002;57:1060–1066.

Smetana GW, Lawrence VA, Cornell JE. Preoperative pulmonary risk stratification for noncardiothoracic surgery: a systematic review for the American College of Physicians. *Ann Intern Med* 2006;144:581–595.

Squadrone V, Coha M, Cerutti E, et al. Continuous positive airway pressure for treatment of postoperative hypoxemia: a randomized controlled trial. *JAMA* 2005;293:589–595.

Tyler IL, Tantisira B, Winter PM, et al. Continuous monitoring of arterial oxygen saturation with pulse oximetry during transfer to the recovery room. *Anesth Analg* 1985;654:1108–1112.

Warner MA, Warner ME, Weber JG. Clinical significance of pulmonary aspiration during the perioperative period. *Anesthesiology* 1993;78:56–62.

Perioperative Cardiac Complications

Milad Sharifpour and Kenneth Shelton

The likelihood of postoperative cardiac complications is influenced by the type of surgery, the patient's preexisting comorbid state, and perioperative management. Postoperative complications can be general or specific to particular operations and can also be classified according to their time of onset: immediate, early, and late. This chapter will outline a range of common postoperative cardiac complications.

Cardiac complications including nonfatal myocardial infarction (MI), cardiac arrest, and death occur in up to 5% of the patients undergoing noncardiac surgery, and up to 8% in patients undergoing major vascular surgery. Patients who experience an MI after noncardiac surgery have a 15% to 25% in-hospital mortality rate and are at increased risk of cardiovascular death and nonfatal MI during the 6 months following the surgery.

Common cardiac complications in the immediate postoperative period include disorders of blood pressure (hypertension and hypotension), arrhythmias, MI, and cardiac arrest.

I. **HYPERTENSION**

Hypertension is defined as systolic blood pressure >140 mm Hg or diastolic blood pressure >90 mm Hg. Hypertension in the postanesthesia care unit (PACU) places patients at a higher risk of intensive care unit admission compared to hypotension.

A. **Common causes of hypertension in the PACU include:**

1. Preexisting hypertension: The most common cause of hypertension in the PACU, especially if the patient did not take his or her morning dose(s) of antihypertensive agent(s)

2. Pain: usually hypertension in association with tachycardia and/or tachypnea

3. Urinary retention and bladder distention: Intraoperative administration of large volumes of intravenous (IV) fluids, history of benign prostatic hyperplasia, inadequate bladder tone because of neuraxial anesthesia, no intraoperative urinary catheter

4. Hypercapnia

5. Hypoxemia

6. Fluid overload: Administration of large volume of IV fluids, intraoperative blood transfusion, and/or large volume of irritation fluid during urologic procedures (prostate surgery)

7. Drug withdrawal (β-blocker, angiotensin-converting enzyme (ACE) inhibitor, opioids, and benzodiazepines)

8. Alcohol withdrawal: Can occur as early as 24 hours after the last alcoholic beverage

9. Anxiety, agitation, or emergence delirium

B. **Treatment**

1. Administer the patient's outpatient antihypertensive medications to prevent/treat rebound hypertension.

2. Treat postoperative pain adequately with acetaminophen, nonsteroidal anti-inflammatory drugs (if not contraindicated), and opioids as needed.
3. Measure bladder residual volume and insert urinary catheter if needed.
4. Provide supplemental oxygen via nasal prongs, facemasks, high-flow nasal cannula, constant positive airway pressure (CPAP), or reintubate if needed.
5. In case of hypercapnia, assist ventilation by inserting an oral or a nasopharyngeal airway, start noninvasive ventilation, or reintubate if needed.
6. Administer diuretics in case of fluid overload.
7. Administer benzodiazepines or barbiturates if alcohol withdrawal is suspected.
8. Assess and treat reversible causes of anxiety such as pain, bladder distention, or hypoxemia. Administer IV haloperidol and/or IV physostigmine to treat anxiety, emergence delirium, or agitation.

II. HYPOTENSION

Hypotension in the PACU is caused by decreased preload, decreased cardiac contractility, or decreased vascular tone (decreased systemic vascular resistance).

A. Common causes of hypotension in the PACU include:

1. Hypovolemia secondary to intra- or postoperative hemorrhage, and/or inadequate volume replacement. Check chest tubes, surgical drains, and urinary catheter bags for excessive output.
2. Arrhythmias
3. Myocardial infarction (MI)
4. Pulmonary embolus (PE)
5. Tension pneumothorax
6. Septic or anaphylactic shocks
7. Residual anesthetic effect
8. Neuraxial anesthesia (epidural and spinal)
9. Residual effects of long-acting antihypertensive medications (ACE inhibitors and angiotensin receptor blockers [ARBs])

B. Treatment

1. Treat hypovolemia with a 500 mL IV fluid bolus and assess the patient's response and repeat this as needed. Avoid excessive volume administration to patients with left- or right-sided heart failure with decreased ejection fraction.
2. For detailed treatment of arrhythmias, please refer to Section III.
3. For detailed treatment of MI, please refer to Section IV.
4. To treat PE provide supplemental oxygen, administer vasopressors (norepinephrine > phenylephrine) to ensure adequate coronary perfusion, administer inotropes (dobutamine or milrinone) to maintain adequate cardiac output and reduce right ventricular afterload, and notify the vascular medicine and cardiac surgery teams to administer IV/IA thrombolytics (if not otherwise contraindicated), perform mechanical thrombectomy, or evaluate for extracorporeal membrane oxygenation (ECMO) cannulation. Avoid volume loading because it can worsen the right ventricle failure.
5. In case of tension pneumothorax, perform needle thoracostomy to stabilize the patient before a chest tube can be inserted.
6. Treat septic or anaphylactic shock with IV fluids and appropriate vasopressors (norepinephrine and epinephrine drips, respectively).
7. Hypotension due to residual volatile anesthetics and/or neuraxial anesthetics can be treated with IV fluid boluses and low-dose phenylephrine drip, or decreasing the rate of continuous epidural infusion.

8. Residual effects of long-acting antihypertensive medications such as ACE inhibitors and ARBs can be treated with a combination of IV fluid boluses and vasopressors (phenylephrine and/or vasopressin if needed).

III. ARRHYTHMIAS

A. Common causes of arrhythmia in the PACU include electrolyte abnormalities (hypo- or hyperkalemia and hypomagnesemia), hypoxemia, coronary insufficiency, hypercapnia, acid/base abnormalities, irritation of peri- or myocardium (particularly in patients undergoing thoracic surgery), and residual effect of medications.

1. Sinus tachycardia: Common causes of sinus tachycardia in the PACU include inadequate analgesia, hypovolemia, hypoxemia, hypercapnia, and anxiety/agitation.

2. Premature ventricular contractions (PVCs): The most common postoperative arrhythmia.

3. Torsade de Pointes: Polymorphic ventricular tachycardia secondary to medications that prolong QT interval (ondansetron, metoclopramide, haloperidol, droperidol, etc.) in susceptible individuals. Can rapidly deteriorate to ventricular fibrillation and cardiac arrest.

4. Atrial fibrillation: Most common after cardiac or thoracic surgery due to irritation of the pericardium. Majority of the cases of new onset postoperative atrial fibrillation resolve spontaneously within 24 to 48 hours.

5. Ventricular tachycardia/fibrillation: Most common in patients with history of coronary artery disease. Hypoxemia and ongoing ischemia are the most common causes of ventricular tachycardia/fibrillation in the PACU.

6. Bradyarrhythmias: Most commonly secondary to antihypertensive medications (β-blockers and calcium channel blockers), residual effect of cholinesterase inhibitors (neostigmine), or sympathectomy from high epidural/spinal.

7. Cardiac arrest: Most commonly due to hypoxemia, ischemia, and ongoing hemorrhage. Patients experiencing a cardiac arrest after noncardiac surgery have a 65% in-hospital mortality rate.

B. **Treatment**

1. Identify and treat underlying causes of sinus tachycardia (inadequate pain control, hypovolemia, hypoxemia, hypercapnia, emergence delirium, and agitation).

2. PVCs are unlikely to deteriorate to life-threatening arrhythmias and routinely do not require interventions.

3. In case of Torsade de Pointes, correct hypomagnesemia if present. Refer to advanced cardiovascular life support (ACLS) guidelines if the patient becomes hemodynamically unstable (hypotensive, hypoxemic, electrocardiogram evidence of ischemia, altered mental status, chest pain, and shortness of breath).

4. Correct electrolyte abnormalities in patients with atrial fibrillation. In case of rapid ventricular rate, attempt rate control with boluses of IV β-blockers (metoprolol or esmolol) or calcium channel blockers (diltiazem). If unsuccessful, attempt rhythm control with amiodarone bolus and infusion. If the patient is hemodynamically unstable, prepare for direct current cardioversion and refer to ACLS guidelines for management of atrial fibrillation.

5. Ensure adequate oxygenation and coronary perfusion (IV fluid boluses, vasopressors, and venodilators) in patients with ventricular fibrillation. Refer to ACLS guidelines for management of ventricular fibrillation.

6. Majority of the cases of new onset bradyarrhythmias in the PACU are self-limiting and do not require intervention. Treat

hemodynamically unstable patients with anticholinergic agents (IV atropine or glycopyrrolate), inotropes (dopamine or norepinephrine), transcutaneous, or transvenous pacing. Obtain an electrophysiology consult for permanent pacemaker placement if unresponsive to aforementioned measures.

7. Identify and treat underlying causes of cardiac arrest (MI, hemorrhage, etc.) and refer to ACLS guidelines for management of cardiac arrest.

IV. MYOCARDIAL INFARCTION (MI)

A. Perioperative MI after noncardiac surgery has an incidence of 1% to 5%. The pathophysiology of perioperative MI is unclear and likely multifactorial. Small retrospective studies have shown plaque rupture to play a minor role in patients who experienced perioperative death due to MI. Inflammation, hypercoagulability, increased oxygen demand, and decreased oxygen supply place the patients at increased risk of perioperative MI. Oxygen consumption increases up to 50% in the immediate postoperative period. The following risk factors increase oxygen demand and/or decrease oxygen supply and place patient at increased risk for ischemia:

1. Hypertension
2. Anemia
3. Hypovolemia
4. Arrhythmias
5. Inadequate pain control
6. Hypothermia and shivering
7. Surgical stress

B. **Treatment**

Minimizing oxygen demand, maximizing oxygen supply, and reestablishing flow are the cornerstone of managing perioperative MI.

1. Provide supplemental oxygen.
2. Administer acetylsalicylic acid (ASA) orally, rectally, or via naso- or orogastric tubes.
3. Sublingual or IV nitroglycerine if blood pressure tolerates to reduce preload, myocardial wall tension, and induce coronary vasodilation.
4. Use short-acting agents (esmolol, clevidipine, and nitroglycerine) to control heart rate and blood pressure because they may further increase myocardial oxygen demand.
5. Treat tachy- or bradyarrhythmias according to ACLS protocols.
6. Administer IV fluids in case of hypovolemia or packed red blood cells in case of anemia.
7. Provide adequate analgesia because pain-induced hypertension and tachycardia increase myocardial oxygen demand.
8. Provide warm blankets, forced-air warming blankets, and warm IV fluids in case of hypothermia and shivering because shivering increases oxygen consumption.
9. Consult cardiology/MI team for possible percutaneous intervention.

Suggested Readings

Carney A, Dickinson M. Anesthesia for esophagectomy. *Anaesth Clin* 2015;33:143–163.

Chobanian AV, Bakris GL, Black HR, et al. Seventh Report of the Joint National Committee on prevention, detection, evaluation, and treatment of high blood pressure. *Hypertension* 2003;42:1206–1252.

Dawood MM, Gutpa DK, Southern J, et al. Pathology of fatal perioperative myocardial infarction: implications regarding pathophysiology and prevention. *Int J Cardiol* 1996;57:37–44.

Devereaux PJ, Goldman L, Cook DJ, et al. Perioperative cardiac events in patients undergoing noncardiac surgery: a review of the magnitude of the problem, the pathophysiology of the events and methods to estimate and communicate risk. *Can Med Assoc J* 2005;173:627–634.

Glick DB. Overview of complications occurring in the post-anesthesia care unit. Available at: https://www.uptodate.com/contents/overview-of-post-anesthetic-care-for-adult-patients. Accessed February 27, 2015.

Landsberg G, Beattie WS, Mosseri M, et al. Perioperative myocardial infarction. *Circulation* 2009;119:2936–2944.

Lee TH, Marcantoni ER, Mangione CM, et al. Derivation and prospective validation of a simple index for prediction of cardiac risk of major noncardiac surgery. *Circulation* 1999;1000:1043–1049.

Maia PC, Abelha FJ. Predictors of major postoperative cardiac complications in a surgical ICU. *Rev Port Cardiol* 2008;27:321–328.

Mangano D, Layug EL, Wallace A, et al. Effect of atenolol on mortality and cardiovascular morbidity after noncardiac surgery. *N Engl J Med* 1996;335:1713–1720.

Postoperative Central Nervous System Dysfunction

Meredith Miller and Ala Nozari

Changes in mental function after anesthesia and surgery were described more than 50 years ago. Because these phenomena have been elucidated in subsequent years, they have been categorized into the distinct syndromes of delirium and postoperative cognitive dysfunction (POCD). This chapter describes the epidemiology of, risk factors for, clinical significance, and, when applicable, management of these syndromes.

I. EPIDEMIOLOGY

Patient populations at increased risk of emergence delirium include those with preexisting structural brain disease (e.g., patients with a history of stroke or Alzheimer dementia), those with existing psychiatric disorders or intellectual impairment, intoxicated patients, children and young adults, those with high levels of preoperative anxiety regarding their procedures, those given psychoactive medications pre- or intraoperatively, and those with preexisting communication difficulties or communication difficulties related to their procedures (nonnative speakers, hearing impaired patients, or those with jaw immobilization as part of their procedure). Anesthetic and surgical factors that increase the risk of postoperative delirium include surgical blood loss, number of intraoperative blood transfusions, intraoperative hemodynamic derangements such as hypotension, intraoperative physiologic derangements such as hypoxia, high intraoperative narcotic use, and general (as opposed to regional) anesthesia.

II. CLINICAL SIGNIFICANCE

Altered mental status postoperatively places patients at risk of significant medical complications such as accidental trauma, dislodgement of equipment needed for treatment (lines, tubes, dressings), and interference with care. In addition, altered mental status in the postanesthetic care unit (PACU) is disturbing to nursing staff and other patients. Significantly altered mental status postoperatively can delay discharge from PACU and increase the care burdens on PACU staff. Emergence delirium can run the gamut from lethargy and confusion to physical combativeness and extreme agitation. In an Australian study, 8% of recovery room incidents reported related primarily to central nervous system dysfunction.

It is important in classifying a patient with altered mental status postoperatively to distinguish between emergence delirium and POCD. Emergence delirium occurs acutely after surgery and involves altered levels of consciousness and level of attention. POCD may be short or long term, appearing in the days to weeks to months following surgery. POCD involves normal level of consciousness but involves a subtle cognitive decline in attention, memory, and ability to learn from the preoperative state. POCD may be temporary or may be permanent.

III. DIFFERENTIAL DIAGNOSIS

It is important to consider the differential diagnosis of altered sensorium postoperatively in order to assess for an underlying pathology. The differential diagnosis of emergence delirium includes residual medication effect (inhaled anesthetics, narcotics, sedatives including premedications, and anticholinergics), hypoxia, residual neuromuscular blockade mimicking depressed consciousness, hypothermia, hypoglycemia, hyperglycemia with resultant hyperglycemic hyperosmolar coma, hyponatremia, and carbon dioxide narcosis. Rare causes of altered sensorium include local anesthetic toxicity either from overdose or inadvertent subarachnoid injection, nonconvulsive seizures, anoxic brain injury, acute cerebrovascular accident, or, in the correct setting, unrecognized intracranial process such as cerebral hemorrhage, tension pneumocephalus, or other causes of elevated intracranial pressure following neurosurgery. It is also important to evaluate the patient for underlying encephalopathy related to renal or hepatic dysfunction, which may have been exacerbated by surgery.

Postoperative pain or discomfort is an important consideration in the differential diagnosis of postoperative agitation. Less commonly recognized sources of discomfort should be considered such as bladder distention, gastric distention, tight dressings, corneal abrasion, intravenous line infiltration, small objects forgotten underneath the patient, and patient body part malpositioning.

IV. WORKUP

A. Clinical Assessment

1. Vital signs with particular attention to pulse oxygenation, blood pressure, and temperature
2. Quick delirium screening tools such as CAM-ICU or brief confusion assessment method (CAM) have a high specificity but lower sensitivity and can be administered by allied health care providers like PACU nurses
   a. CAM-ICU criteria: acute onset or fluctuating mental status, inattention (letters test), altered consciousness (RASS other than 0), and disorganized thinking (erroneous question answers, unable to follow two-part command)
3. Physical exam including assessment of adequacy of ventilation and oxygenation such as color and quality of respiratory efforts, assessment of strength to check for residual neuromuscular blockade, examination of skin and extremities to evaluate for unusual causes of patient discomfort (foreign object beneath patient, limb malpositioning, intravenous line infiltration)
4. Focused neurologic exam, with a special attention to the size, reactivity, and symmetry of pupils, and lateralizing signs (e.g., gaze deviation when eyelids passively opened, moving one side of the body less than the other). Detailed neurologic exam is often difficult and the goal of exam should be a screening to determine the need for further workup such as brain imaging (e.g., computerized tomography [CT]) or electroencephalogram (EEG) for underlying primary CNS process.
5. ECG findings which could indicate electrolyte disturbance or ischemic changes

B. Laboratory Assessment

1. Arterial or venous blood gas to assess for adequacy of oxygenation and ventilation, serum sodium, serum glucose, and serum lactic acid because acidemia can cause anxiety and may reflect a state of global hypoperfusion.

C. Imaging

V. For high-risk patients for primary intracranial process causing altered mental status, especially in the presence of focal neurologic signs, noncontrast head CT or EEG may be indicated to assess for intracranial bleeding or mass effect, acute cerebrovascular accident, or seizure. Examples of high-risk patients include postcraniotomy, carotid endarterectomy or stenting, cardiac surgery, or thoracic aortic dissection repair, a history of known severe carotid stenosis or atrial fibrillation, and intra-op hemodynamic instability with labile blood pressure and/or prolonged hypoxia.

VI. MANAGEMENT OPTIONS

Treatment will of necessity depend on the most likely etiology of altered mental status postoperatively. Immediate correction of any physiologic derangements such as hypoxia, hypercarbia, or hypotension by ensuring adequate oxygenation, respiratory efforts, and blood pressures. Patients with preexisting hypertension may require augmentation of a "normal" blood pressure to achieve adequate cerebral perfusion. Pain may be treated with opioids and examination for unusual causes of discomfort such as bladder distention. Anxiety may be treated with benzodiazepines. Residual drug effects causing altered mental status may be treated with antagonists of the responsible medication: opioid antagonists (20 to 40 μg doses of naloxone to effect), benzodiazepine antagonists (flumazenil), and physostigmine to treat residual effects of anticholinergic agents such as scopolamine, glucose for hypoglycemia, additional reversal agents for residual neuromuscular agents, and intralipid for suspected local anesthetic toxicity. Unusual causes of altered mental status such as seizure, intracranial hemorrhage or intracranial hypertension, hypothermia, and electrolyte derangements should also be evaluated and treated.

VII. OUTCOMES

Although distressing to the patient and health care provider, emergence delirium is generally self-limited and responsive to treatment of the underlying cause such as pain, anxiety, respiratory distress, hypoglycemia, etc. Emergence delirium is distinct from POCD, which is a lasting CNS insult caused by surgery and anesthesia. However, even self-limited emergence delirium increases risks of long-term POCD and discharge to an institution for patients who were previously living independently. In addition, the presence of early delirium in the recovery room is a strong predictor for the development of POCD.

POCD represents the subtle decline in cognitive function that can occur following surgery, typically in the timeframe of days to weeks, although it is possible for POCD to present in the PACU. Typically subtle declines in cognition occur in the areas of attention, memory, and ability to learn. The definition of POCD varies in the literature, but many studies use a standard of a 20% decline in 20% of neurophysiologic tests comparing the patient postoperatively and preoperatively, with each patient therefore serving as his or her own control.

POCD has been reported since the 1950s when a study by Bedford reported on elderly patients being subjectively "demented" following general anesthesia. It is a well-described phenomenon in the literature following cardiac surgery, occurring in 50% to 70% of patients in the first week and 20% to 40% at the 1 year mark, but it also occurs following noncardiac surgery. Risk factors related to the procedure in cardiac surgery have been attributed to length of time of cardiopulmonary bypass, lower hematocrit, hyperglycemia, hyperthermia on rewarming, absence of arterial line filters, use of bubble oxygenators, and failure to use the epiaortic ultrasound for cannula placement in patients with atheromatous disease. Its etiology has been generally attributed in part to the showering of the brain with microemboli, both solid and gaseous.

POCD has also been described following noncardiac surgery. Risk factors after noncardiac surgery include advancing age, especially greater than age 60, anesthetic duration, postoperative respiratory or infectious complications, preexisting cognitive dysfunction or depression, lower educational levels preoperatively, major versus minor surgery, and general versus regional anesthesia. Explanations for the etiology include central nervous system toxicity of anesthetic agents, activation of the stress response with increased stress hormone production, systemic inflammation, and intraoperative physiologic or metabolic derangements such as hypoxia or brain hypoperfusion related to hypotension or hypoglycemia.

Suggested Readings

Card E, Pandharipande P, Tomes C, et al. Emergence from general anaesthesia and evolution of delirium signs in the post-anaesthesia care unit [published online ahead of print December 23, 2014]. *Br J Anaesth* 2015;115(3):411–417. doi:10.1093/bja/aeu442.

Fowler MA, Spiess BD. Post anesthesia recovery. In: Barash P, ed. *Clinical Anesthesia*. 7th ed. Philadelphia, PA: Lippincott Williams & Wilkins; 2013:1421–1443.

Neufield KJ, Leoutsakos JMS, Sieber FE, et al. Outcomes of early delirium diagnosis after general anesthesia in the elderly. *Anesth Analg* 2013;117:471–478.

Nicholau D. The postanesthesia care unit. In: Miller RD, Eriksson LI, Fleisher LA, et al, eds. *Miller's Anesthesia*. 7th ed. Philadelphia, PA: Churchill Livingstone; 2010:2708–2729.

Rasmussen L, Stygall J, Newman SP. Cognitive dysfunction and other long-term complications of surgery and anesthesia. In: Miller RD, Eriksson LI, Fleisher LA, et al, eds. *Miller's Anesthesia*. 7th ed. Philadelphia, PA: Churchill Livingstone; 2010:2805–2820.

Sharma PT, Sieber FE, Zakriya KJ, et al. Recovery room delirium predicts post-operative delirium after hip fracture repair. *Anesth Analg* 2005;101:1215–1220.

Acute Perioperative Urinary and Renal Dysfunction

Michael Hermann and Sheri Berg

EPIDEMIOLOGY

The exact percentage of patients who suffer from some degree of acute kidney injury (AKI) is difficult to assess, because the number will vary depending upon which definition for AKI is used for determining whether or not AKI is present. The **incidence** varies depending on the type of procedure that was performed; however, about 25% of all hospital-acquired AKI occurs in the surgical setting.

There are known preoperative risk factors that will increase the patient's chance of developing AKI. These include:

1. Age > 55 years
2. Male sex
3. Active congestive heart failure
4. Presence of ascites
5. Diabetes requiring oral therapy or insulin therapy
6. Hypertension
7. Mild or moderate perioperative renal insufficiency
8. Nephrotoxic agents (contrast dyes)

With regard to intraoperative risk factors, procedures that are performed emergently involve cardiopulmonary bypass, and many vascular surgical procedures all carry an increased risk of developing AKI, likely secondary to relative intraoperative hypovolemia and renal ischemia.

Inadequate hydration, perioperative hypotension, and urinary obstruction can instigate possible postoperative AKI.

PATHOPHYSIOLOGY

The etiology of AKI is conventionally separated into prerenal, intrinsic renal, and postrenal considerations (Table 20.1).

Kidney dysfunction in the perioperative period is frequently multifactorial, with acute tubular necrosis (ATN) as the most common cause, given preoperative risks of hypotension and hypovolemia.

Perioperative kidney hypoxia that occurs intraoperatively is a result of anesthetic-induced decreases in kidney perfusion and function; this is usually reversible and without permanent damage.

Prerenal injury to the kidneys can be caused by decreased perfusion, which is a known common complication of hypotension and hypovolemia. In addition, increased intra-abdominal pressure during surgery (laparoscopy) can create a hypotensive state to the kidneys.

Normally renal blood flow (RBF) is 20% of the cardiac output, and 90% of RBF supplies the renal cortex. The kidney is very sensitive to hypoperfusion, because the medulla extracts ~80% of the delivered oxygen. Blood flow to the kidney is autoregulated between a blood pressure of 80 and 160 mm Hg. Medullary blood flow is normally controlled by vasodilators (nitric oxide,

TABLE 20.1	Causes of Acute Kidney Injury	
Prerenal	**Intrinsic Renal**	**Postrenal (Obstructive)**

Intravascular volume depletion
• GI fluid loss (e.g., vomiting, diarrhea, EC fistula)
• Renal fluid loss (e.g., diuretics)
• Burns
• Blood loss
• Redistribution of fluid (e.g., "third spacing," pancreatitis, cirrhosis)
	Acute tubular necrosis
	• Ischemic
	• Toxin induced
	  • Drugs
	  • IV contrast
	  • Rhabdomyolysis
	  • Massive hemolysis
	  • Tumor lysis syndrome
		Upper urinary tract obstruction
		• Nephrolithiasis
		• Hematoma
		• Aortic aneurysm
		• Neoplasm

Decreased renal perfusion pressure • Shock (e.g., sepsis) • Vasodilatory drugs • Preglomerular (afferent) • Postglomerular (efferent) arteriolar vasodilation	Acute interstitial nephritis • Drug induced • Infection related • Systemic diseases (e.g., SLE) • Malignancy	Lower urinary tract obstruction • Urethral stricture • Hematoma • Benign prostatic hypertrophy • Neurogenic bladder • Malpositioned urethral catheter • Neoplasm
Decreased cardiac output • Congestive heart failure • Myocardial ischemia	Acute glomerulonephritis • Postinfectious • Systemic vasculitis • TTP/HUS • Rapidly progressive GN Vascular • Atheroembolic disease • Renal artery or vein thrombosis • Renal artery dissection • Malignant hypertension Hepatorenal syndrome Increased intra-abdominal pressure	

GI, gastrointestinal; EC, enterocutaneous; IV, intravenous; SLE, systemic lupus erythematosus; TTP, thrombotic thrombocytopenic purpura; HUS, hemolytic uremic syndrome; GN, glomerulonephritis.

prostaglandins, adenosine, dopamine), vasoconstrictors (endothelia, angiotensin II, antidiuretic hormone), and tubuloglomerular feedback (reflex mechanism from insufficient sodium reabsorption causing glomerular afferent vasoconstriction, thus reducing filtration). Blood flow and glomerular filtration rate (GFR) are maintained to a mean arterial pressure (MAP) as low as 60. Autoregulation is maintained by decreasing afferent glomerular arteriolar resistance with prostaglandins as well as increasing efferent arteriolar resistance with angiotensin II. Below the autoregulatory range, endogenous vasoconstrictors increase afferent arteriolar resistance, which in turn decreases GFR, causing **prerenal azotemia**.

Hypoxia disrupts several pathways in cellular metabolism coalescing in cytoskeletal disruption. This mechanism can result in the sloughing of cells and can possibly lead to tubular obstruction. Further oxidant injury causes an increased amount of vasoconstriction and propagates the cycle of further damage, ultimately culminating in ATN, see below. Vasoconstrictors can cause significant renal ischemia, because α_1 activation is unopposed given the absent β_2 receptors in the renal vascular bed. Cardiopulmonary bypass produces ischemia repercussion injury secondary to hypovolemia and low cardiac output. Aortic surgery, with cross-clamping, decreases RBF by up to 40%, causing renal vascular resistance to increase by 75%.

Persistent hypovolemia and hypoxemia result in intrarenal injury, namely ATN. ATN is usually triggered by hypoperfusion and ischemia, which disrupt metabolic pathways. Endothelial cells in capillaries are also damaged. Decreased ATP and hypoxia activate proteases and phospholipases with resultant oxidant destruction.

Adhesion molecules and cytokines are expressed in response to the cycle of vasoconstriction and low perfusion, thus attracting leukocyte infiltration causing microcirculatory obstruction. Leukocytes also express their own reactive oxygen species, enzymes, and cytokines, causing further damage.

Other causes include contrast-induced nephropathy, drugs, rhabdomyolysis, hemolysis, glomerulonephritis, and vascular causes, among others.

Postrenal injury is a result of obstruction distal to the tubules and collecting ducts (obstructed urinary tract or kinked foley, benign prostatic hyperplasia, or other factors). Diffusion of urea from renal tubules, not creatinine, into the blood causes an increase of the blood urea nitrogen (BUN) to Cr ratio.

CLINICAL SIGNIFICANCE

AKI serves as an independent predictor of mortality in hospitalized patients at 30 days and long-term mortality. An increase in creatinine by 0.5 mg/dL is associated with a 6.5 times increase in death, 3.5 day increase in hospital stay, and $7,500 increase in hospital costs.

An AKI risk index for patients undergoing general surgery has been developed with 11 risk factors including:

1. Age greater than 56 years, male sex, emergency surgery, intraperitoneal surgery, diabetes requiring oral therapy, diabetes requiring insulin therapy, active CHF, ascites, hypertension, mild preoperative renal insufficiency, and moderate preoperative insufficiency,
2. Six or more risk factors have a 9% postoperative risk of AKI.

WORKUP

A focused history should be obtained to evaluate the predisposing factors or events that might have precipitated renal injury. A focused physical examination can guide the assessment of volume status.

Typical signs of hypovolemia include (but are not limited to): skin tenting/decreased skin turgor, decreased capillary refill, collapsed veins, cool extremities postural hypotension, and tachycardia. Other adjuncts may include central venous pressure (CVP), pulmonary artery wedge pressure (PAWP), transesophogeal echocardiography (TEE), or abdominal ultrasound to examine inferior vena cava (IVC) width.

Placement of a urinary catheter is helpful to accurately measure hourly urine output. A basic metabolic panel with BUN and Cr is essential to diagnose

	Prerenal	Renal
Microscopy	Hyaline casts	Abnormal
Specific gravity	>1,020.0	~1,010.0
Uosmol (mOsmol/kg)	>500.0	<350.0
Urine/plasma urea	>8.0	<3.0
Urine/plasma creatinine	>40.0	<20.0
UNa (mmol/L)	<20.0	>40.0
Fe_{Na} (%)*	<1.0	>2.0
Renal failure index†	<1.0	>2.0

*Fractional sodium excretion Fe_{Na} = [urinary Na × plasma creatinine × 100]/[plasma Na × urinary creatinine].
†Renal failure index = [urinary sodium × plasma creatinine]/urinary creatinine.

decreased GFR as well as the etiology of AKI. However, serum creatinine is not sensitive for acute changes in renal function as an abrupt decrease in GFR causes a slow and delayed rise in serum creatinine (2 to 3 days). Baseline serum creatinine is also affected by age, hydration status, and body habitus (Table 20.2). The gold standard to quantify GFR is a 24-hour creatinine clearance; however, this is rarely used given the time necessary to collect this test. Other necessary studies include urine sodium and creatinine to evaluate the fractional sodium excretion (though unreliable in the setting of diuretic administration), urine microscopy to evaluate for the presence of active glomerular disease, to evaluate for intrinsic renal injury, as well as a renal ultrasound to evaluate for signs of obstruction (including hydronephrosis).

MANAGEMENT OPTIONS

Prevention of AKI is perhaps the best method in averting renal dysfunction. Patients at high risk (above) for renal insult during operative procedures should be afforded "adequate" volume resuscitation, which will routinely vary depending upon the patient's preexisting comorbidities as well as the surgical procedure itself. It should be noted that the optimum MAP for renal perfusion is not known. Excessive volume infusion may place patients at risk for prolonged mechanical ventilation and impaired wound healing. In addition, excessive intra-abdominal pressure, or intra-abdominal hypertension (IAH), secondary to third spacing and volume overload, may actually predispose patients to AKI. A cycle of decreased renal function and fluid overload may continually worsen AKI. Goal-directed therapy and preoperative hemodynamic optimization, to avoid the deleterious effects of volume overload and IAH, is a potential management strategy to reduce postoperative renal impairment. Potential variables to optimize include cardiac index, pulmonary artery occlusion pressure, systemic vascular resistance, and DO_2. Interestingly, choice of hydration fluid does not seem to have an effect on outcome.

Certain medications have been shown to predispose patients to AKI. Contrast dyes are nephrotoxic by a suspected variety of mechanisms (vasospasm, direct nephrotoxicity, and reactive oxygen species). Preprocedure hydration with normal saline (NS; with or without bicarbonate) and *N*-acetylcysteine is the only current method of preventing contrast-induced nephropathy. Antibiotics such as vancomycin, cephalosporins, and aminoglycosides have been speculated to worsen kidney secondary to the development of acute interstitial nephritis. Nonsteroidal anti-inflammatory drugs (NSAIDs) have been shown to decrease RBF by altering prostaglandin synthesis. In addition, they can also cause acute interstitial nephritis. Chronic usage also places patients at risk for progression to end-stage renal disease. However, NSAIDs likely do not cause significant alterations in kidney function in patients with normal renal function. Other drugs that decrease RBF are angiotensin-converting enzyme inhibitors and angiotensin blockers.

TREATMENT

In addition to adequate hydration, treatment of AKI depends on the etiology and the removal of potential insults such as nephrotoxic drugs and relieving any obstruction. AKI is difficult to diagnose in the setting of true hypovolemia, whether due to surgical blood loss or redistributive intravascular volume depletion secondary to altered capillary permeability (sepsis). Fluid repletion options include crystalloids, colloids, or blood products. However, as in prevention, there is no advantage of crystalloids over colloids. Given the expense of colloid resuscitation and the lack of added benefit, crystalloids are recommended. Blood products are recommended when indicated (low hemoglobin/hematocrit, coagulopathy, etc.). Although NS is often chosen over lactated Ringer's (LR) given the concern for LR potentiation of hyperkalemia, current evidence does not support this recommendation. Historically, it was theorized that furosemide may reduce the metabolic demand of the kidneys and convert oliguric renal failure to nonoliguric renal failure, which was thought to improve outcomes. However, diuretics have not been shown to provide any benefit in decreasing the duration of renal failure, the eventual need for dialysis, or improved survival, and, in fact, may actually worsen outcomes. Titratable fluid goals may be similar to those in septic shock and include blood pressure control (MAP > 65–70), HR < 110, CVP around 15, urine output >0.5 cc/kg/hour.

Initiation of renal replacement therapy may be necessary in the setting of severe, persistent hyperkalemia and metabolic acidosis that prove refractory to conventional medical therapy, pulmonary edema/volume overload, uremia (encephalopathy, pericarditis), and toxin removal.

Suggested Readings

Abuelo JK. Normotensive ischemic acute renal failure. *N Engl J Med* 2007;357(8): 797–805.

Bihorac A, Yavas S, Subbiah S, et al. Long-term risk of mortality and acute kidney injury during hospitalization after major surgery. *Ann Surg* 2009;249(5):851–858.

Brienza N, Giglio MT, Marucci M, et al. Does perioperative hemodynamic optimization protect renal function in surgical patients? A meta-analytic study. *Crit Care Med* 2009;37:2079–2090.

Brienza N, Giglio MT, Massimo M. Preventing acute kidney injury after noncardiac surgery. *Curr Opin Crit Care* 2010;16:353–358.

Carmichael P, Carmichael AR. Acute renal failure in the surgical setting. *ANZ J Surg* 2003;73(3):144–153.

Dalfino L, Tullo L, Donadio I, et al. Intra-abdominal hypertension and acute renal failure in critically ill patients. *Intensive Care Med* 2008;34:707–713.

Jones DR, Lee HT. Perioperative renal protection. *Best Pract Res Clin Anaesthesiol* 2007;22(1):193–208.

Kheterpal S, Tremper KK, Heung M, et al. Development and validation of an acute kidney injury risk index for patients undergoing general surgery: results from a national data set. *Anesthesiology* 2009;110(3):505–515.

Mangano CM, Diamondstone LS, Ramsay JG, et al. Renal dysfunction after myocardial revascularization: risk factors, adverse outcomes, and hospital utilization. *Ann Intern Med* 1998;128(3):194–203.

Moran SM, Myers BD. Acute renal failure studied by a model of creatinine kinetics. *Kidney Int* 1985;27:928–937.

Navar LG. Renal autoregulation: perspectives from whole kidney and single nephron studies. *Am J Physiol* 1978;234(5):F357–F370.

Novis BK, Roizen MF, Aronson S, et al. Association of preoperative risk factors with postoperative acute renal failure. *Anesth Analg* 1994;78(1):143–149.

O'Malley CM, Frumento RJ, Hardy MA, et al. A randomized, double-blind comparison of lactated Ringer's solution and 0.9% NaCl during renal transplantation. *Anesth Analg* 2005;100(5):1518–1524.

Sear JW. Kidney dysfunction in the postoperative period. *Br J Anaesth* 2005;95(1):20–32.

Vincent JL, Gerlach H. Fluid resuscitation in severe sepsis and septic shock: an evidence-based review. *Crit Care Med* 2004;32(11):S451–S454.

Wijeysundera DN, Karkouti K, Beattie WS, et al. Improving the identification of patients at risk of postoperative renal failure after cardiac surgery. *Anesthesiology* 2006;104(1):65–72.

Postoperative Hemorrhage

Matthew Tichauer, Martha DiMilla,
and D. Dante Yeh

I. INTRODUCTION

Perioperative bleeding, a risk with any operation, presents a challenge for both the surgeon and anesthesiologist. While mortality associated with most surgical procedures typically ranges between 0.1% and 8%, depending upon the nature of the operation, postoperative bleeding significantly affects mortality risk with estimates as high as 20%. In addition to the associated increase in morbidity and mortality, postoperative bleeding, if not identified and managed expediently, may lead to unintended intensive care unit admission and prolonged hospital stays.

II. RISK FACTORS FOR PERIOPERATIVE BLEEDING

A. Surgical and Patient-Based Risk Factors

Among all sources of perioperative bleeding, failure to establish surgical hemostasis intraoperatively is the most common cause. Although this is never the intention of the surgeon, it underscores the importance of due diligence and careful attention to detail in the planning and execution of all surgical procedures (Table 21.1). While most operations carry the risk of bleeding, certain factors increase the likelihood of severe bleeding.

1. Surgical procedures such as trauma, cardiac/cardiovascular, and cancer surgery
2. Massive blood loss resulting in disorders of coagulation (e.g., dilutional coagulopathy, factor deficiencies, platelet loss, or consumption)
3. Drug-induced coagulation disorders (e.g., warfarin)
4. Liver disease
5. Inherited disorders of coagulation (e.g., hemophilias and von Willebrand disease)

TABLE 21.1	Causes of Intraoperative and Postoperative Hemorrhage	
Intraoperative	Early Postoperative (Days 0–2)	Delayed Postoperative (Days 2–7)
Structural/technical defects	Structural/technical defects	Thrombocytopenia
Disseminated intravascular coagulation	Thrombocytopenia Inherited or acquired platelet disorders	Acquired platelet disorders Vitamin K deficiency
Heparin overdose		Multiorgan failure
Hyperfibrinolysis	Mild to moderate inherited coagulation disorder	
Antibodies to factor V following use of bovine thrombin in fibrin		

Marietta M, Facchini L, Pedrazzi P, et al. Pathophysiology of bleeding in surgery. *Transplant Proc* 2006; 38(3):812–814.

6. Hypothermia
7. Acidemia

III. PATHOPHYSIOLOGY OF HEMOSTASIS AND ASSESSMENT OF COAGULOPATHY

The vessel wall, platelets, and plasma proteins (coagulation factors), acting in conjunction, form the basis for hemostasis.

A. Primary hemostasis, occurring within seconds of vessel wall injury, results in the formation of a platelet plug. There are four steps involved in formation of the platelet plug:

Platelet activation → adhesion → degranulation → aggregation

B. Secondary hemostasis involves coagulation factors of the intrinsic and extrinsic cascade, resulting in the formation of fibrin. Factor VIIa represents the convergence of the intrinsic and extrinsic cascade.

1. **Partial thromboplastin time (PTT) or activated PTT (aPTT):** Measures the functionality of the intrinsic coagulation system. Decreased intrinsic coagulation factors, heparin, and autoimmune/anticoagulants antibodies result in increased PTT values.

2. **Prothrombin time (PT):** Measures the functionality of the extrinsic coagulation system. Its value is derived by the addition of thromboplastin reagent to the sample. Both PT and PTT are affected by factors V and X and are sensitive to low levels of factor VII.

3. **International normalized ratio (INR):** Created as a means to standardize PT values across laboratories in determining response to warfarin. Additionally, the INR is used to determine coagulopathy in liver disease.

4. **Fibrinogen:** It is a protein produced by the liver essential in clot formation. Fibrinogen is depleted in disseminated intravascular coagulation (DIC) and massive hemorrhage. Fibrinogen is also an acute phase reactant, and is often elevated in the postoperative setting and in the presence of inflammation. Fresh frozen plasma, cryoprecipitate or fibrinogen concentrate may be transfused to replace depleted fibrinogen levels.

5. **Activated clotting time (ACT):** The ACT measures the inhibiting effect that heparin has on the body's clotting system. It can be performed at the bedside and is often utilized to manage the administration of heparin in the setting of invasive vascular and cardiac surgeries.

IV. DISORDERS OF HEMOSTASIS AND COAGULATION

A. **Disseminated Intravascular Coagulation (DIC)**

DIC develops as a consequence of systemic activation and consumption of the clotting factors. It does not occur by itself but as a complicating factor from another underlying condition such as sepsis, trauma, head injury, burns, hemorrhage, end-stage liver disease, and snake envenomation. Clinically, it can range from mild to severe, and may lead to massive bleeding, the formation of thrombi, and multiple organ dysfunction/failure. Regardless of the inciting event once initiated, the pathophysiology of DIC is similar in all conditions. Tissue factor (TF), presumably from monocytes and vascular subendothelium, triggers the development of DIC. After exposure to inflammatory proteins, TF is believed to activate the coagulation cascade throughout the vascular system. Extensive clot formation results in both clotting and coagulopathy. PT and PTT are both prolonged and fibrinogen levels are low because of the extensive formation of fibrin.

B. **Hemophilia**

Hemophilias are hereditary diseases characterized by deficiency in isolated coagulation factors, for example, factor VIII (hemophilia A) or factor IX (hemophilia B). Patients with hemophilia typically have a prolonged PTT and normal PT. Platelet function is intact, so there is normal formation of the initial clot; however owing to an inability to stabilize the clot with the coagulation cascade, bleeding recurs.

C. **von Willebrand Disease**

von Willebrand disease is a relatively common genetic bleeding disorder resulting from the lack of von Willebrand factor production, leading to the inability of platelets to anchor to exposed collagen as well as failure of platelets to aggregate. Depending on the subtype of von Willebrand disease, DDAVP, cryoprecipitate, or fresh frozen plasma (FFP) may be administered to treat the disease.

D. **Liver Disease**

Decreased hepatic production of coagulation factors (all except factor VIII and von Willebrand factor, which are produced by the endothelium) results in coagulopathy. Thrombocytopenia commonly manifests in patients with liver disease requiring platelet transfusion in bleeding situations (see Section VI).

V. **POSTOPERATIVE ASSESSMENT**

A. **Physical Examination**

A thorough physical examination in the setting of presumed hemorrhage is of paramount importance. Early recognition of clinical signs of bleeding and identification of the site of hemorrhage may be life-saving.

Clinical signs of bleeding include tachycardia, hypotension, cool extremities, weak peripheral pulses, prolonged capillary refill (defined as >2 seconds), narrowed pulse pressure (<25 mm Hg), and altered mental status.

The clinician must be proactive in assessment of surgical sites. Active bleeding directly at the surgical site (pulsating, oozing, etc.), saturated dressings, and peri-incisional fullness usually warrants urgent re-exploration. Additionally, monitoring output from surgical drains (i.e., chest tubes, Jackson–Pratt drains, mediastinal drains, etc.) must be assessed noting trends in output and character of the output (serosanguinous, sanguinous, etc.).

Ultrasound has become a popular tool for assessment of acute bleeding. Although more sensitive diagnostic tests such as computed tomography (CT) are often included in the standard assessment of a patient with concerns for bleeding (particularly in the abdomen), the ability to obtain a rapid and reliable assessment with ultrasound, particularly in a patient with hemodynamic instability, has become invaluable.

VI. **TREATMENT OF HEMORRHAGE AND TRANSFUSION MEDICINE**

A. Standard management of hemorrhage control typically involves one of the following surgical techniques: packing or tamponade, vessel ligation, or angioembolization of the bleeding vessel.

B. Aprotinin, aminocaproic acid, tranexamic acid (TXA), DDAVP, blood-derived products, and other hemostatic agents are regularly used to improve hemostatic balance in bleeding patients. Recombinant-activated factor VII has been shown to be effective for the treatment of surgical or traumatic massive bleeding unresponsive to conventional therapy in hemophiliac patients. Administration of TXA in the setting of trauma has shown to be improve survival if given within 3 hours of injury.

C. **Whole blood** is rarely used in civilian practice. Whole blood requires identical ABO and Rh pairing versus that of red blood cells (RBCs) requiring only ABO compatibility.

D. **RBCs** are typically transfused as 1 unit of red blood cells (RBCs) with a volume of approximately 250 mL. In the absence of ongoing bleeding, 1 unit of RBCs should increase the recipient's hemoglobin by 1 g/dL. ABO compatibility is critical to avoid hemolysis owing to antibody production against surface antigens. If the blood type of the patient is not known, "emergency release" blood, type O Rh-negative red cells, should be transfused (Note: It is important to begin transfusing type-specific blood as soon as the patient's blood type has been determined to avoid the buildup of anti-A and anti-B antibodies.)

E. **FFP** contains components of coagulation, fibrinolytic, and complement systems, and is the liquid part of blood that is frozen following centrifugation. ABO compatibility is necessary for transfusion of FFP. It is rich in factors II, V, VII, IX, X, and XI; thus, it is indicated in patients who are bleeding or require invasive procedures and are on warfarin. Fibrinogen levels typically increase by 1 mg/mL of plasma administered.

F. **Cryoprecipitate** is formed by thawing FFP at a specific temperature and is rich in factor VIII and fibrinogen (200 to 300 mg). Additionally, it contains von Willebrand factor, factor XIII, and fibronectin, and it is indicated in patients with significant hypofibrinogenemia, von Willebrand disease, and hemophilia A. Cryoprecipitate raises the plasma fibrinogen approximately 50 mg/dL (if administered at a dose of 1 U/10 kg).

G. **Platelets** are transfused in "6 packs". ABO compatibility is not required for platelet transfusion; however, it may have a better result in particular patients (i.e., alloimmunization). Patients who are actively bleeding with thrombocytopenia should be transfused to a platelet count greater than 50,000 and greater than 100,000 in the setting of DIC.

Suggested Readings

Dagi TF. The management of postoperative bleeding. *Surg Clin North Am* 2005;85(6): 1191–1213.

Peitzman AB, Schwab CW, Yealy DM, et al. *The Trauma Manual: Trauma and Acute Care Surgery*. 4th ed. Philadelphia, PA: Lippincott Williams & Wilkins; 2013.

Shakur H, Roberts I, Bautista R, et al; The CRASH-2 Collaborators. Effects of tranexamic acid on death, vascular occlusive events, and blood transfusion in trauma patients with significant haemorrhage (CRASH-2): a randomised, placebo-controlled trial. *Lancet* 2010;376(9734):23–32.

Tanaka KA, Key NS, Levy JH. Blood coagulation: hemostasis and thrombin regulation. *Anesth Analg* 2009;108(5):1433–1446.

Temperature Abnormalities

Craig S. Jabaley and Kathryn L. Butler

I. INTRODUCTION

A. **Temperature abnormalities** are frequently encountered postoperatively because anesthetic, surgical, and environmental factors work in concert to disrupt thermostasis. Although normothermia is not a component of frequently utilized postanesthesia care unit (PACU) scoring systems (see Chapter 36), normothermia is often preferred and commonly required prior to discharge from the PACU, especially with ambulatory surgery patients. Evidence has mounted over the past two decades implicating hypothermia as a contributor to numerous adverse outcomes. Not surprisingly, the establishment and maintenance of normothermia has garnered increased regulatory attention.

B. Measurement of temperature in the PACU is a **practice standard** as outlined by the American Society of Anesthesiologists and must be documented as an element of the postanesthesia evaluation as mandated by the Centers for Medicare & Medicaid Services (CMS).

C. Normal human core temperature is 37°C (98.6°F) and ranges between 36.5°C and 37.5°C. **Hypothermia** is defined as core temperature less than 36°C and **hyperthermia** or **fever** as a temperature greater than 38°C.

II. THE PHYSIOLOGY OF THERMOREGULATION

A. Understanding the **mechanisms of heat transfer** is critical when conceptualizing both the physiology of thermoregulation and the disruption thereof.

1. **Radiation** refers to heat emission and absorption by means of electromagnetic waves, which occurs owing to atomic and molecular movement in all matter above absolute zero. Classic whole-body calorimetry studies have suggested that radiation accounts for about two-thirds of heat loss in a cold environment. Accordingly, it is felt to be the primary contributor to perioperative hypothermia.

2. Heat transfer by **convection** occurs by the movement of fluid or air across a surface and is the second greatest contributor to intraoperative heat loss. The use of surgical drapes is thought to mitigate convective heat loss owing to restricted motion of air over body surfaces.

3. **Conduction** describes heat transfer between adjacent surfaces in thermal contact and can be mitigated by insulation. The use of foam pads intraoperatively diminishes heat loss due to conduction.

4. The **evaporation** of water into gas is one example of a matter state change that leads to latent heat loss. The skin and upper airways both serve as barriers to this process. Appreciable skin incisions, bowel exposure, and the introduction of dry air into the respiratory tract during mechanical ventilation have all been postulated to increase evaporative heat loss.

B. For practical purposes, the body can be divided into two thermal **compartments**: the **core** and the **periphery**. Tissues comprising the core are well perfused, thermally homogeneous, and maintained within a very narrow range of temperatures. In contrast, temperatures across the peripheral compartment are variable. Practically, the core refers to the visceral contents of the head, thorax, and abdomen, whereas the periphery consists of the skin and appendages.

C. **Regulatory pathways** and **responses** have evolved to counteract changes in environmental temperature through complex and incompletely understood mechanisms. Despite this tight regulation, thermostasis is readily disrupted by anesthesia.

1. **Afferent** signals originate from widely distributed peripheral—including cutaneous and visceral—and central thermoreceptors. Although little is known about the nature of visceral thermoreceptors in humans, discrete cold and warm-sensitive cutaneous thermoreceptors have been identified. Electrical conduction is facilitated by means of Aδ and C fibers for cold receptors and warm receptors, respectively. Following some degree of preprocessing and modulation based on the input of spinal thermoreceptors, these signals are transmitted cephalad via the spinothalamic tract.

2. The hypothalamus facilitates **central** integrative processing of afferent inputs. Lesion studies have demonstrated that the anterior hypothalamic nucleus works to oppose hyperthermia, whereas the posterior nucleus coordinates thermogenesis in response to hypothermia.

3. **Efferent** responses are variable in their progression and intensity depending on environmental stimuli. They can be broadly categorized as follows:

   a. **Vasomotor tone** can be altered rapidly and at a low energy cost. As such, it is the first response to a change in environmental temperature. The goal of variable vasomotor tone is to shunt blood either toward or away from the core to facilitate the respective preservation or elimination of heat. Notably, cutaneous blood flow can nearly equal resting cardiac output under maximal vasodilatation.

      1. **Sweating** quickly accompanies vasodilatation and is the primary response to an increase in core temperature.

   b. **Behavioral** modifications are extremely effective at counteracting environmental changes but come at a high energy cost.

   c. **Thermogenesis** occurs when other compensatory mechanisms fail to correct hypothermia.

      1. **Shivering** generates heat by means of oscillatory skeletal muscle activity at the cost of increased oxygen consumption and discomfort.

      2. **Nonshivering** thermogenesis that occurs through increased mitochondrial oxidative metabolism within brown adipose tissue is an important thermostatic mechanism in infants and children, because they cannot shiver effectively.

D. Patients at both **extremes of age** demonstrate impaired thermoregulation.

1. The **elderly** are prone to hypothermia when subjected to mild environmental or physiologic stress owing to decreased muscle mass with concomitant impaired vasoconstrictive and shivering responses. Additionally, these compensatory mechanisms do not occur until a lower temperature threshold is reached in comparison to younger patients.

2. **Infants** are prone to hypothermia secondary to a high ratio of body surface area to core mass (radiation), ineffective shivering (impaired thermogenesis), and a thin skin barrier (evaporation). Therefore, nonshivering thermogenesis plays a significant role in the maintenance of normothermia.

III. TEMPERATURE MONITORING SITES AND MODALITIES

A. Assessment of **core temperature** should be the goal of any measurement modality. Although heat is distributed heterogeneously throughout the body, perturbations in the comparatively stable core compartment provide the best insight into total body thermal status. Core temperature can be measured **directly** at the tympanic membrane, nasopharynx, pulmonary artery, or (distal) esophagus. Although these sites are frequently chosen intraoperatively or in critical care environments, they are too invasive for routine postoperative monitoring of extubated patients in the PACU.

B. A more practical approach to temperature monitoring in the PACU relies on the high degree of **concordance** between less invasive sites and core temperature.

1. **Bladder** temperature, as measured by a Foley catheter, has long been excluded from the list of core temperature sites because it can lag behind rapid changes in total body heat, such as during cardiopulmonary bypass and deliberate hypothermia. However, under most every other condition, bladder temperature very closely approximates core temperature. For patients who require a Foley catheter, placement of one with an integrated thermistor or thermocouple is a practical approach to facilitate accurate and **continuous** postoperative temperature assessment. For these reasons, bladder temperature is often chosen as the investigational standard against which other modalities are compared for postoperative patients.

2. **Oral** temperature measurement, although not practical for intubated patients, is a low-cost and reliable modality in the PACU. Postoperatively, it has demonstrated a high degree of accuracy compared to bladder temperature measurement. Avoiding contemporaneous per os intake, keeping the mouth closed during measurement, and placement of the thermometer deep in the rear sublingual pocket yield the most accurate readings.

   a. **Axillary** measurement should be considered only when oral measurement is not feasible. Accuracy can be increased by positioning the thermometer near the axillary artery and keeping the arm adducted.

3. **Skin temperature** measurement, although convenient, should be considered an option of last resort given the heterogeneous nature of heat distribution in the periphery. Of all sites, the forehead with its thin skin and relatively high vascularity is the most commonly utilized.

4. **Rectal temperature**, more so than bladder temperature, lags behind core temperature during periods of rapid flux. Furthermore, its measurement in the PACU is often impractical.

C. As no single thermometry modality or monitoring site is without its caveats, using a single method of temperature monitoring in the perioperative period can allow for more accurate comparison of readings. Clinicians should always be suspicious of extreme temperature values, and in such instances a second modality can be useful.

IV. HYPOTHERMIA

A. Hypothermia is defined as a core body temperature **less than 36°C** (96.8°F) and is the **most common** perioperative temperature derangement. In the recent past, it was common practice to permit a modest degree of intraoperative hypothermia. Although hypothermia does confer benefits in a few discrete instances, its strong association with numerous adverse outcomes has drawn clinical and regulatory attention to the avoidance and treatment of hypothermia.

1. The **incidence** of unintended postoperative hypothermia was estimated at over 60% in the era before forced air warming, and more recently ranges between 5% and 20% of patients. Variable patient populations, anesthetic techniques, surgical procedures, temperature measurement modalities, and attentiveness to intraoperative normothermia cloud the true incidence.

2. **Benefits** to **mild** hypothermia include a reduction in the cerebral metabolic rate of oxygen (~7%/°C), improved neurologic outcomes following cardiac arrest, and a potential, although controversial, protective role in patients with traumatic brain injury.

3. The **risks** of hypothermia mount with even a 1°C drop in core temperature.
   a. **Cardiac morbidity** has been associated with hypothermia. In one study, normothermia conferred a 55% risk reduction in the pooled incidence of ischemia, infarction, and arrest.
   b. **Coagulopathy** is an inevitable complication of hypothermia that begins with platelet dysfunction and progresses to overt dysfunction of the coagulation cascade. Increased blood loss and transfusion requirements, especially in orthopedic surgery, have been consistently associated with hypothermia.
   c. **Drug metabolism** is impaired because hypothermia reduces both hepatic and renal blood flow. The effects of multiple drug classes are prolonged, including neuromuscular blockers, intravenous anesthetics, and volatile agents.
   d. **Discomfort** is an obvious but underappreciated effect of hypothermia that leads to both increased circulating catecholamines and poor patient satisfaction.
   e. **Length of stay** in the PACU is prolonged, which contributes to increased healthcare costs and compromised operating room workflow. Furthermore, hypothermia is an important contributor to **delayed emergence**.
   f. **Surgical site infection** is one of the most costly and potentially devastating consequences of hypothermia. The risk appears to be highest in patients undergoing abdominal surgery.

4. As healthcare delivery becomes increasingly focused on **quality of care**, the avoidance of hypothermia has become one of the first metrics that directly affects anesthesiologists. The first such impetus came from the CMS Surgical Care Improvement Project (SICP), which tracked compliance with either the achievement of postoperative normothermia or use of forced air warming. Although this metric is no longer tracked as of 2015 owing to high compliance rates, normothermia remains an element of the CMS Physician Quality Reporting Initiative.

B. Unintended or **inadvertent perioperative hypothermia** (IPH) is, by far, the most common cause of hypothermia on admission to the PACU. Given its deleterious effects and relatively high incidence as outlined earlier, all PACU practitioners must be familiar with the treatment of hypothermia.

1. The **etiology** of IPH is multifactorial and stems from increased heat loss. General anesthesia affects all efferent compensatory mechanisms in the setting of hypothermia. As such, patients will invariably develop IPH when subjected to a sufficiently lengthy anesthetic in the absence of any active warming efforts. Intraoperative core temperature trends have been described as **triphasic** with steep initial decline because heat is **redistributed** from the core compartment to the periphery. Heat loss continues over the next 2 to 4 hours, in the

second phase, owing to blunted compensatory mechanisms and environmental exposure until a final steady state is reached around 33°C to 35°C, which is often sufficient to prompt an increase in vasomotor tone despite anesthetics.

a. **Neuraxial** and **regional** techniques disrupt thermoregulation in a similar fashion and also block peripheral thermoreceptor input, which can further contribute to hypothermia even in awake or lightly sedated patients.

2. Several **treatment** modalities can be employed in the PACU to correct IPH. Notably, the cessation of general anesthesia gradually restores many of the body's compensatory mechanisms. Vasoconstriction, although normally helpful, slows the rewarming of postoperative patients due to shunting of blood away from the periphery, which is the site of surface warming modalities. As such, the **prevention** of IPH intraoperatively is easier than postoperative rewarming.

a. **Prewarming** of patients prior to general anesthesia not only improves patient comfort but avoids peripheral vasoconstriction and can thus blunt the magnitude of heat redistribution that accompanies induction. Attention to temperature preoperatively and the prompt implementation of warming strategies even before induction can aid in this effort. Disposable gowns with integrated forced air warming channels can facilitate warming before, during, and after procedures.

b. **Surface warming** is the cornerstone of temperature management. As a general principle, efforts should be made to warm as much of the patient's surface area as can be practically accomplished. Even thin stretcher mattresses are sufficient to insulate against dorsal heat loss; therefore, efforts to warm the dorsum should be pursued only when ventral warming efforts prove inadequate.

1. **Forced air warming** is the most common, effective, and comfortable way to warm patients. The disposable plastic covers not only act as a conduit for convective warming but also help to reduce radiant heat loss. The covers are safe and most effective when used in direct contact with skin. However, the heated air output of the combined heater/blower unit should **never** be directed onto patients or used with paired patient covers from another manufacturer. Both of these practices have resulted in thermal injury.

a. **Resistive heating** with electric blankets has largely been replaced by forced air warming over concerns for sterility. Although resistive heating is highly effective, older devices require heightened vigilance to avoid thermal injury. A new offering combines resistive polymer in several topical and wraparound configurations with a control unit that monitors a temperature feedback loop to reduce the likelihood of thermal injury.

2. **Circulating water** devices come in many variations including mattresses, blankets, and pads with or without gel coatings. Postoperatively, the application of these devices **on top** of patients is preferable because they are more safe, effective, and comfortable in this configuration. (The placement of these devices under patients intraoperatively represents a trade-off between easy facilitation of surgical exposure and efficacy.) Wraparound circulating water garments and pads have recently become available, but remain expensive. Regardless of application, water temperature should never exceed 40°C.

3. Use of **passive insulation,** such as blankets, helps to minimize heat loss, but will **not effectively treat** hypothermia in the absence of active warming. The use of modest insulation **on top** of warming devices can help to increase their efficacy.

4. **Ambient temperature** can be increased to aid in the maintenance of normothermia, but is typically impractical in a large PACU. Furthermore, ambient temperatures high enough to actively rewarm patients will be uncomfortable for staff with associated reduced performance and vigilance.

c. **Fluid warming** alone is insufficient to actively warm patients, but plays an important role in the avoidance of hypothermia. Patients undergoing aggressive fluid resuscitation or transfusion of cold blood products should receive warmed fluids. Furthermore, fluid warming should be implemented in conjunction with other warming strategies in the face of persistent hypothermia.

d. The **heating and humidification** of inhaled gases can help to minimize the small degree of heat lost from associated mucosal surfaces. Intubated patients or those with tracheostomies are most likely to benefit, because in these circumstances inhaled gases bypass the mucosa-lined upper airways.

3. **Rewarming vasodilatation** is typically well tolerated. However, patients with marked intraoperative hypothermia may have achieved a reasonable degree of vasoconstriction despite anesthetic effects, which can not only mask hypovolemia but present as hypertension upon arrival to the PACU. Tachycardia and hypotension during rewarming should prompt clinical evaluation and consideration of volume resuscitation.

C. **Other etiologies** of hypothermia should be considered in patients with a low likelihood of IPH. Such scenarios include previously normothermic patients, patients with specific disease states, or when conventional warming strategies fail to effectively increase core temperature.

1. The **systemic inflammatory response syndrome** (SIRS) or **sepsis** can present with a multitude of symptoms, including hypothermia. Although fulminant sepsis is uncommon in the immediate postoperative period, surgical stress leading to SIRS is frequently encountered. Hypothermia carries a poor prognosis in sepsis, and these patients should be rewarmed in addition to immediate treatment with appropriate antibiotics and attention to source control. (Please see further discussion of sepsis and SIRS later.)

2. Several **endocrine** disturbances can contribute toward hypothermia, including adrenal insufficiency, hypopituitarism, and hypothyroidism. However, these entities are unlikely to present as acute isolated hypothermia. Please refer to Chapter 25 for further discussion.

3. **Nutritional** aberrations, such as malnutrition, place patients at a greater risk for hypothermia owing to decreased heat production. Patients with profound **hypoglycemia** are often hypothermic, but are more likely to present with altered mental status.

4. **Neurologic** insults frequently contribute toward hypothermia. Patients with neurologic trauma including those with spinal cord injuries and blunt head trauma are at the greatest risk. Wernicke's encephalopathy, cerebrovascular accident, and hypothalamic damage have also been associated with hypothermia.

5. Patients with **neuromuscular disease** often demonstrate impaired heat production and thus are predisposed to hypothermia.

D. **Shivering** is a common problem in the PACU, with an estimated incidence of about 50% following general anesthesia and over 30% for neuraxial anesthesia. Although shivering is a normal physiologic response to hypothermia, both general and neuraxial anesthesia produce physiologic sequelae that contribute to the development of similar tremors. Accordingly, **postanesthetic tremor** may be the more technically correct name.

1. Shivering has numerous **deleterious** effects. It nearly doubles oxygen consumption, but is only weakly associated with myocardial ischemia. Hypothermia itself may better explain the relationship between shivering and adverse cardiac outcomes. Shivering is not only uncomfortable but increases intraocular pressure, intracranial pressure, and incisional pain.

2. **Treatment** should be directed toward surface warming, correction of hypothermia, and consideration of pharmacologic modalities when conservative treatment fails. **Meperidine** has been a mainstay of treatment for many years and is more effective than other opioids even at equipotent doses. However, it has come under increasing scrutiny from regulatory agencies and is no longer available at some institutions. Please refer to Table 22.1 for a review of treatment options.

V. **Hyperthermia** and **fever**, although often used interchangeably in reference to an elevated core temperature, describe two different physiologic processes.

A. **Fever** represents an increase in the hypothalamic set point mediated by pyrogens and is often initiated in response to inflammation or infection. Fundamentally, true fever should result in cold discomfort, vasoconstriction, and shivering.

TABLE 22.1 Pharmacologic Treatment of Postanesthetic Shivering

Drug	Class	Dose (IV Route)	Availability in USA	Strength of Evidence
Butorphanol	Opioid	1 mg IV	+	+
Clonidine	α agonist	75–150 μg IV	+	+++
Dexmedetomidine	α agonist	1 μg/kg IV	+	++
Doxapram	CNS stimulant	100 mg IV	+	+++
Ketamine	NMDA antagonist	0.5 mg/kg IV	+	+
Ketanserin	5-HT$_{2A}$ antagonist	10 mg IV	−	++
Magnesium sulfate	Inorganic salt	30 mg/kg IV	+	++
Meperidine	Opioid	25 mg IV	+	+++
Nalbuphine	Opioid	0.08 mg/kg	+	+
Nefopam	Nonopioid analgesic	0.15 mg/kg IV	−	++
Ondansetron	5-HT$_3$ antagonist	4–8 mg IV	+	+
Physostigmine	AChE inhibitor	0.04 mg/kg IV	+	++
Tramadol	Opioid	1 mg/kg IV	− (IV)	+

IV, intravenous; CNS, central nervous system; AChE, acetylcholinesterase; NMDA, *N*-Methyl-D-aspartate.

1. Briefly, the **febrile response** is marked by cytokine-mediated effects that include not only fever (in response to altered hypothalamic regulation) but also the release of acute-phase reactants. Accordingly, fever is just one of the many physiologic perturbations that accompany the **acute-phase response**. Pyrogenic cytokines are classified as either endogenous (IL-1, IL-6, TNF, etc.) or exogenous.

2. A traditional approach to the **differential diagnosis** of postoperative fever is to consider five common etiologies: pulmonary (wind), genitourinary (water), deep venous (walking), surgical site (wound), and medications (wonder drugs). However, these so-called "5 Ws" are of limited utility when evaluating febrile patients in the PACU because fever within the first few hours postoperatively has a relatively narrow differential.

   a. A benign **cytokine-mediated** febrile response is commonly encountered postoperatively. In response to the duration of surgery and magnitude of operative or antecedent trauma, IL-6 and other cytokines are released and trigger an increase in the hypothalamic temperature set point. The average postoperative core temperature in one study was 38°C ± 0.7°C, with less than one quarter of patients demonstrating a maximum temperature greater than 39°C. Accordingly, many clinicians rarely investigate postoperative fever less than 38.5°C on the basis that some degree of febrile response should be expected. Furthermore, testing for other causes may be both unwarranted and wasteful when coupled with low clinical suspicion.

      1. **SIRS** is a pathologic cytokine response leading to fever, tachycardia, tachypnea, and white blood count abnormalities. These patients warrant increased vigilance and monitoring because SIRS can progress to shock and organ system dysfunction.

   b. **Infection** should always be considered when faced with fever in postoperative patients. However, the likelihood of fever representing a true surgically related infection in the **immediate** postoperative period is low, especially in the case of a single fever of modest intensity. Concern for infection at least warrants prompt **clinical** evaluation including physical examination and a review of the patient's history and operative course.

      1. **Preoperative infection** should be considered both in ambulatory and previously hospitalized patients. Numerous studies have demonstrated that true postoperative infection is unlikely prior to postoperative day 3. Accordingly, patients with clinical signs of infection should be evaluated for both operative and nonoperative sources.

      2. **Transient bacteremia** has been described following burn surgery, soft tissue debridement, oral surgery, and genitourinary procedures. Bacteremia is more likely following any procedure involving a contaminated or dirty surgical site. These patients will typically be covered with a perioperative antimicrobial regimen, and fever does not necessarily require further workup or antimicrobial coverage extension.

      3. **Necrotizing soft tissue infection** (NSTI) is unlikely to present immediately postoperatively, but warrants consideration because it is potentially life threatening. If left untreated, NSTI can progress to **toxic shock syndrome** because bacterial toxins prompt a marked cytokine response and multiple organ system dysfunction. High fever in the early postoperative period mandates examination of any operative incisions in consultation with the surgical team.

4. **Sepsis** in the PACU typically marks the progression of either a preexisting infection or the progression of perioperative bacteremia as discussed previously. The timely administration of appropriate antibiotics is of the utmost importance followed by attention toward source control and possible transfer to an intensive care unit (ICU).

   c. **Allergic reactions** are often associated with fever, as discussed in Chapter 27.

   d. **Epidural** anesthesia and analgesia are frequently associated with mild fever both in pregnant and nonpregnant patients. Although the mechanism is unclear, epidural analgesia may not blunt the febrile response effectively compared to alternative analgesic regimens.

   e. Fever may represent a reaction to **blood products**, including those transfused in the OR. Refer to Chapter 28 for further discussion.

   f. **Atelectasis** is often cited as a common cause of early postoperative fever; however, investigational evidence does not support this assertion. Presumed atelectasis with concomitant shunt physiology should be managed even in the absence of fever.

   g. **Deep venous thrombosis** and **pulmonary embolus** may both present as an indolent fever. However, both are unlikely in the immediate postoperative period.

B. **Hyperthermia** refers to either exogenous heat gain or endogenous production that exceeds thermoregulatory compensation. Unlike fever, hyperthermia should be accompanied by heat discomfort, vasodilatation, and sweating.

1. **Malignant hyperthermia** (MH) is a pharmacogenetic syndrome marked by extreme skeletal muscle metabolism that can quickly lead to circulatory collapse and death. MH is a medical emergency that mandates immediate intervention. However, **postoperative MH** is exceedingly **rare**, and other causes of elevated temperature in the PACU must be considered in the absence of symptoms suspicious for MH. The Malignant Hyperthermia Association of the United States (**MHAUS**) should be contacted for all suspected cases of MH, as they maintain a 24-hour telephone hotline for emergent clinical guidance.

   a. Briefly, the **pathophysiology** of MH relates to heritable mutations in genes encoding for proteins that facilitate intracellular calcium transport in skeletal muscle. Abnormal excitation–contraction coupling in response to environmental and pharmacologic triggers, with unchecked sarcoplasmic calcium release, leads to a marked catabolic state accompanied by hyperthermia, muscular rigidity, and metabolic disarray. **Volatile anesthetics** and **depolarizing neuromuscular blockers** are well-established anesthetic agents that can trigger MH.

   b. The **diagnosis** of MH relies on prompt recognition of its associated symptoms followed by laboratory evidence of metabolic abnormalities as summarized in Table 22.2. Clinical grading scales are available to aid clinicians in the diagnosis of suspected MH (see Suggested Readings).

   c. General principles for the **management** of MH in a PACU setting are outlined in Table 22.3. Every PACU should have a MH treatment protocol and access to a MH cart stocked with **dantrolene** as recommended by MHAUS. Clinicians in the PACU may be faced with four conceivable MH-related scenarios as outlined below:

      1. Patients with **fulminant acute** MH that develops intraoperatively should be transferred directly to an ICU following stabilization.

TABLE 22.2	Signs and Symptoms of Malignant Hyperthermia in the PACU
Clinical Findings	**Laboratory Findings**
Tachycardia	Mixed metabolic and respiratory
Tachypnea	acidosis
Respiratory failure	Hyperkalemia
• Hypoxemia	Rhabdomyolysis
• Hypercapnia	• Myoglobinuria
• Hypoxia and cyanosis	• Myoglobinemia
Generalized rigidity	• Elevated CK
Hyperthermia	• Elevated LDH
• Diaphoresis	DIC
Gross myoglobinuria	Markers of shock
Cardiac arrhythmia	Elevated serum lactate
Hypotension	Arterial base deficit
Cardiac arrest	Low SvO_2

CK, creatine kinase; LDH, lactate dehydrogenase; DIC, disseminated intravascular coagulation; SvO_2, mixed venous oxygen saturation.

Admission to the PACU in these cases should only be considered as a bridge to a more definitive treatment environment.

2. In cases of **suspected** intraoperative MH, current MHAUS guidelines recommend at least 24 hours of postoperative monitoring in either a PACU or ICU. Given the level of resources and personnel required to care for these patients, admission to an ICU is appropriate in most instances.

   a. **Masseter spasm** can be an early sign of MH. However, its clinical diagnosis is confounded by the often-observed benign increase in jaw muscle tone following succinylcholine administration. Even if the spasm abates intraoperatively, MHAUS recommends serial serum creatinine kinase and urine myoglobin measurement every 6 hours for 36 hours and close observation in a PACU or ICU for 12 hours.

3. Current MHAUS recommendations state that patients with **known** or **suspected susceptibility** to MH who underwent an **uneventful nontriggering anesthetic** are candidates for routine postoperative monitoring. They suggest monitoring vital signs no less frequently than every 15 minutes for at least 1 hour followed by an additional hour in a Phase 2 or step-down setting. Point-of-care urine testing to document the absence of myoglobin may provide additional confirmation that an MH episode has been avoided.

4. **Postoperative MH** is very uncommon, and in one review it represented less than 2% of all suspected MH cases. A delay between exposure to triggering anesthetics and the symptoms of MH may be because of the ability of hypothermia, hypnotic agents, and nondepolarizing neuromuscular blocking drugs to blunt or prevent the symptoms of MH intraoperatively. In these rare instances, the typical **latency period** appears to be **less than 40 minutes** from the end of general anesthesia to the onset of symptomatology. However, there are scattered case reports of delayed MH that develops many hours after trigger exposure.

TABLE 22.3	Management Principles of Malignant Hyperthermia in the PACU

Immediate Steps

Get Help	Airway Support	Administer Dantrolene
Anesthesia team Notify surgeon Summon personnel MHAUS hotline	Administer 100% oxygen Emergent endotracheal intubation Mechanical hyperventilation	Dantrolene 2.5 mg/kg IV bolus Repeat in 1 mg/kg increments May require 10–30 mg/kg total Large-bore peripheral IV access

Supportive Measures

Metabolic Acidosis	Hyperthermia	Hyperkalemia	Monitoring
Sodium bicarbonate 1–4 mEq/kg empiric OR per ABG results	Cool when >39°C Aggressive surface cooling Cold infusions Cavity lavage	Hyperventilation Glucose and insulin Bicarbonate Calcium if severe	Foley catheter 12-lead EKG Consider arterial and central venous catheterization

Laboratory Studies

Chemistry panel, arterial blood gas, creatine kinase, coagulation studies, urine myoglobin

Ongoing Management

Observation	Dantrolene	Rhabdomyolysis	Counseling
Transfer to ICU Monitor for at least 24 h	Dantrolene 1 mg/kg q4–6 h for 24 h OR 0.25 mg/kg/h infusion	Target urine output >2 mL/kg/h with diuretics and fluid Consider urine alkalinization	Advise patient and family Referral to MHAUS File report with MH registry

PACU, postanesthesia care unit; MHAUS, Malignant Hyperthermia Association of the United States; IV, intravenous; ABG, arterial blood gas; EKG, electrocardiogram; ICU, intensive care unit; MH, malignant hyperthermia.

Tachycardia, tachypnea, rigidity, and respiratory failure are the most common early symptoms of postoperative MH. As with acute intraoperative MH, **hyperthermia** may be a late sign.

2. **Non-Malignant Hyperthermia** describes all causes of hyperthermia unrelated to MH. Nonexertional hyperthermia and classic heat stroke are synonymous descriptions. The term "benign hyperthermia" is a misnomer because hypothermia is generally better tolerated. For example, core temperatures exceeding 41°C are accompanied by progressive organ dysfunction, but even profound hypothermia is often survivable.

a. **Passive hyperthermia** is often encountered following aggressive rewarming. Close attention to core temperature trends postoperatively can help avoid this iatrogenic complication.

b. Several **drug-related** conditions can lead to hyperthermia:

1. **Ethanol withdrawal** and **drugs of abuse** can both present with hyperthermia among other sequelae and should be considered in trauma patients or following emergency surgery. Refer to Chapter 34 for further discussion.

2. **Neuroleptic malignant syndrome** (NMS) is a neurologic emergency marked by altered mental status, hyperthermia, rigidity, and dysautonomia following the administration of antipsychotics. Although the symptoms can mimic those of MH, the onset of NMS is typically more indolent. Notably, dopamine antagonists commonly used as antiemetics can also precipitate NMS. Offending agents should be discontinued immediately if NMS is suspected, and additional personnel should be recruited for aggressive resuscitation prior to transfer to an ICU. Dantrolene has been successfully used to abate hyperthermia associated with NMS.

   a. NMS can be mistaken for serotonin syndrome as both can present with relatively analogous symptoms. Whereas both can cause hyperthermia, mental status changes, and increased muscle tone, patients with NMS typically demonstrate a rigid akinesis, and are more commonly taciturn. The onset of NMS is more protracted as compared to SS, and tends to develop over days rather than hours.

   b. Withdrawal from antiparkinsonian medications and intrathecal baclofen can mimic NMS.

3. **Serotonin syndrome** results from unchecked serotonergic CNS stimulation and manifests with altered mental status, autonomic hyperactivity, and neuromuscular symptoms. Although numerous drugs have been associated with serotonin syndrome, patients taking monoamine oxidase inhibitors (MAOIs) are at an especially increased risk for drug interactions that can precipitate the syndrome. **Methylene blue** and **linezolid** both act as reversible MAOIs and have precipitated serotonin syndrome when administered to patients on psychiatric medications, namely selective serotonin reuptake inhibitors. Removal of the offending agent is essential to minimize further exacerbation of this condition. Specific treatment is usually guided by the severity of presentation, and often supportive measures, such as fluid resuscitation, medications to decrease tachycardia and hypertension, and employing cooling methods, are sufficient. Severe cases may warrant admission to an ICU.

c. **Endocrine** disease can manifest as hyperthermia in combination with other symptoms. Thyroid disease, pheochromocytoma, and acute or chronic adrenal insufficiency are three examples as discussed in Chapter 25.

d. Given the role of the CNS in thermoregulation, it is unsurprising that **intracranial pathology** can contribute to the development of hyperthermia.

1. **Cerebral hemorrhage** has been associated with hyperthermia, especially when blood invades the fourth ventricle following pontine hemorrhage.

2. **Status epilepticus** leads to hyperthermia owing to muscle activity. Transient febrile reactions have been reported following

electroconvulsive therapy despite the administration of neuro-muscular blockade.

3. **Hypothalamic injury** commonly causes fever. Additionally, operations involving suprasellar pituitary tumors may lead to postoperative hypothalamic edema and associated fever.

C. **Treatment strategies** when faced with fever or hyperthermia should first be directed toward resolution of the **underlying cause**.

1. Generally speaking, **fever** can be treated most effectively with antipyretics, which interrupt the influence of interleukins on the hypothalamus. However, there are a few important **caveats** as outlined below.

   a. The use of **antipyretics** in fever secondary to infection is controversial based on experimental evidence in critically ill patients. Fever in response to infection is a normal physiologic response that confers some degree of benefit with regard to both microbial inhibition and immune system function. The balance of evidence suggests that antipyretic therapy in septic critically ill adults either confers no benefit or may be deleterious. The extent to which this assertion applies to stable postoperative patients with concern for fever of infectious etiology is unclear.

   b. Additionally, the role of **active cooling** to control fever in response to infection is not well-defined based on current evidence. Active cooling in patients with intact thermoregulatory mechanisms is often tedious and of limited efficacy.

2. Conversely, **hyperthermia** can be treated by measures that either interrupt heat production or aid in its dissipation. Treatment of the underling etiology leading to hyperthermia will help to abate heat production, and **active cooling** facilitates heat dissipation.

   a. When faced with modest degrees of passive hyperthermia following overwarming, **exposure** of the patient is often sufficient to gradually restore normothermia.

   b. Many **forced air** devices can be set to deliver ambient temperature room air to their paired covers. However, **circulating water** options are often able to achieve a greater magnitude of core temperature reduction.

   c. The induction of **deliberate hypothermia** postoperatively is often pursued in patients with neurologic or myocardial injury. The degree of core temperature reduction required often necessitates advanced cooling devices, such as intravascular heat exchange catheters or temperature-targeted circulating water garments. These patients require a high level of nursing care and aggressive management of side effects. Accordingly, arrangements should be made for transfer to an ICU.

Suggested Readings

De Witte J, Sessler DI. Perioperative shivering: physiology and pharmacology. *Anesthesiology* 2002;96:467–484.

Frank SM, Fleisher LA, Breslow MJ, et al. Perioperative maintenance of normothermia reduces the incidence of morbid cardiac events. A randomized clinical trial. *JAMA* 1997;277:1127–1134.

Frank SM, Kluger MJ, Kunkel SL. Elevated thermostatic setpoint in postoperative patients. *Anesthesiology* 2000;93:1426–1431.

Hardy JD, Milhorat AT, Du Bois EF, et al. Basal metabolism and heat loss of young women at temperatures from 22°C. to 35°C. Clinical calorimetry No. 54. *J Nutr* 1941;21:383–404.

Horn EP, Sessler DI, Standl T, et al. Non-thermoregulatory shivering in patients recovering from isoflurane or desflurane anesthesia. *Anesthesiology* 1998;89:878–886.

Hynson JM, Sessler DI, Moayeri A, et al. The effects of preinduction warming on temperature and blood pressure during propofol/nitrous oxide anesthesia. *Anesthesiology* 1993;79:219–228; discussion 21A–22A.

Kimberger O, Cohen D, Illievich U, et al. Temporal artery versus bladder thermometry during perioperative and intensive care unit monitoring. *Anesth Analg* 2007;105:1042–1047; table of contents.

Kimberger O, Thell R, Schuh M, et al. Accuracy and precision of a novel non-invasive core thermometer. *Br J Anaesth* 2009;103:226–231.

Kranke P, Eberhart LH, Roewer N, et al. Pharmacological treatment of postoperative shivering: a quantitative systematic review of randomized controlled trials. *Anesth Analg* 2002;94:453–460; table of contents.

Kurz A, Sessler DI, Lenhardt R. Perioperative normothermia to reduce the incidence of surgical-wound infection and shorten hospitalization. Study of Wound Infection and Temperature Group. *N Engl J Med* 1996;334:1209–1215.

Larach MG, Localio AR, Allen GC, et al. A clinical grading scale to predict malignant hyperthermia susceptibility. *Anesthesiology* 1994;80:771–779.

Lee BH, Inui D, Suh GY, et al. Association of body temperature and antipyretic treatments with mortality of critically ill patients with and without sepsis: multi-centered prospective observational study. *Crit Care* 2012;16:R33.

Lenhardt R, Marker E, Goll V, et al. Mild intraoperative hypothermia prolongs postanesthetic recovery. *Anesthesiology* 1997;87:1318–1323.

Litman RS, Flood CD, Kaplan RF, et al. Postoperative malignant hyperthermia: an analysis of cases from the North American Malignant Hyperthermia Registry. *Anesthesiology* 2008;109:825–829.

Melling AC, Ali B, Scott EM, et al. Effects of preoperative warming on the incidence of wound infection after clean surgery: a randomised controlled trial. *Lancet* 2001;358:876–880.

Sessler DI. Perioperative heat balance. *Anesthesiology* 2000;92:578–596.

Sun Z, Honar H, Sessler DI, et al. Intraoperative core temperature patterns, transfusion requirement, and hospital duration in patients warmed with forced air. *Anesthesiology* 2015;122:276–285.

Fluid and Electrolyte Disorders

Kevin Blackney and Jonathan Charnin

I. INTRODUCTION

A. Multiple systems are used to regulate fluids and electrolytes during "normal" states of health. In the perioperative period, homeostatic regulation may become unbalanced by periods of fasting, blood loss, medication effects, and blood pressure changes. Perioperatively, clinicians must use all the available data to assist their patients in achieving and maintaining fluid and electrolyte balance. Failure to do so may result in delayed discharge from the postanesthesia care unit (PACU), unanticipated transfer from the PACU to the intensive care unit (ICU), and increased morbidity or mortality. Factors to be considered when replacing fluids or electrolytes include:

1. The type of surgical procedure performed and estimated blood loss
2. The volume and type of fluid administered intraoperatively
3. Baseline medical conditions (i.e., cardiac, pulmonary, and renal disease)

B. Many strategies for fluid management have been proposed. Recently, two strategies have risen to prominence, sometimes referred to as "liberal" and "restrictive."

1. Liberal fluid administration can cause the following complications:
   a. Interstitial and pulmonary edema
   b. Poor wound healing
   c. Delayed gastric emptying/prolonged resumption of bowel function
   d. Cardiovascular overload
2. Restrictive fluid administration can potentially lead to:
   a. Hypotension and shock
   b. Increased postoperative nausea/vomiting
3. The best approach to perioperative fluid management is still under debate.

C. Water in the human body resides in two fluid compartments: intracellular fluid (ICF) and extracellular fluid (ECF). The ICF constitutes approximately 67% of total body water (TBW), whereas the ECF consists of the remaining 33% TBW. The ECF is further broken down into the interstitial compartment (75% of the ECF) that surrounds cells and the plasma compartment, which comprises the remaining 25%. Excess fluid in the interstitial compartment leads to edema formation. The electrolyte composition in the ICF and ECF will differ, but the osmolarity will be the same.

1. The "third space" refers to fluids, known as transcellular fluids, that are normally low in volume and high in turnover. Examples include pleural, peritoneal, and cerebrospinal fluid.

D. Movement of water between the compartments is governed by osmotic forces.

1. The cell membrane between the *intracellular* (ICF) and *interstitial* (ECF) compartments is a charged lipid bilayer that prevents free

movement of cations such as sodium and potassium. Movement of these ions is strictly through charged protein channels. This creates a transmembrane voltage potential for cell function. The lipid bilayer does allow water to freely pass from hyperosmolar to hypo-osmolar areas, thus creating an osmotic pressure gradient.

2. In contrast, the capillary endothelium allows for free passage of both water and ions between the *interstitial* (ECF) and *plasma* (ECF) compartments. Therefore, the driving force for water movement here is the concentration of plasma proteins, especially albumin, which creates osmotic (i.e., oncotic) pressure, shifting water between these two compartments.

   a. Starling's law is used to describe fluid movement in this manner.

   $$J_v = K_{fc}[(P_c - P_i) - \delta(\pi_c - \pi_i)]$$

   J_v is the transcapillary fluid flux, K_{fc} is the filtration coefficient across the capillary wall, P_c and P_i are the capillary and interstitial hydrostatic pressures, respectively, δ is the reflection coefficient, and π_c and π_i are the capillary and interstitial oncotic pressures. δ is the permeability of a substance through a capillary membrane.

   b. In inflammatory states, δ is increased, allowing more proteins to leave the plasma compartment and enter the interstitial compartment. *This creates an oncotic driving force toward interstitial accumulation and edema formation.*

E. The electrolyte differences between the fluid compartments create membrane potentials important for cellular function.

1. The predominant ECF electrolyte creating an osmotic gradient is sodium. Chloride, calcium, and bicarbonate are also in higher concentration in ECF.

2. The predominant ICF cation is potassium. Proteins provide neutrality.

3. Gastrointestinal (GI) tract fluids contain elevated concentrations of potassium, chloride, and hydrogen ions. Thus, postoperative nausea and vomiting or gastric suctioning results in a hypokalemic, hypochloremic metabolic alkalosis.

II. ASSESSMENT OF FLUID STATUS

A. There is no single physiologic or biochemical marker that can act as a perfect indicator of fluid status and resuscitation. Clinicians therefore utilize assessment of vital signs, physical exam findings, and additional physiologic and biochemical testing.

B. *Vital signs* are likely the first indication of suboptimal fluid resuscitation in the postoperative patient.

1. Assuming the patient is not on a nodal blocking agent and other causes of tachycardia are ruled out, an increase in heart rate (HR) is often the first vital abnormality indicating hypovolemia (Table 23.1).

TABLE 23.1	Stages of Hypovolemic Shock			
	Stage I	**Stage II**	**Stage III**	**Stage IV**
% Blood volume lost	<15%	15%–30%	30%–40%	>40%
Heart rate	<100	>100	>120	>140
Blood pressure	Normal	Normal	Decreased	Decreased
Capillary refill	Normal	Delayed	Delayed	Delayed

This is a normal physiologic response to hypovolemia, and treatment should be aimed at repleting fluid losses.

2. As in evaluation of HR, assessing the blood pressure must be done after ruling out other causes of hypotension when assessing volume status in the PACU. Other causes include blood pressure–lowering medications, neuraxial anesthesia, and effects of residual anesthetic agents, to name a few.

3. Delta down (DD) and delta pulse pressure (DPP) are both effective *dynamic* indicators of hypovolemia *in mechanically ventilated* patients with *arterial line* monitoring. These correlate best when the patient is resting on a mechanical ventilator with 8 mL/kg tidal volumes, and positive end-expiratory pressure (PEEP) between 0 and 5 cm H_2O. DD is defined as the difference in the systolic blood pressure (sBP) after a 5-second respiratory pause from the minimum sBP during a positive pressure breath. A *difference of 5 mm Hg* or more is considered a positive finding of hypovolemia. DPP is the difference of the maximal and minimal pulse pressure (PP_{max} and PP_{min}) during mechanically assisted breathing divided by the mean. A *value of 13%* or greater is considered a positive test for hypovolemia (Fig. 23.1).

   In the proper patient (i.e., no significant restrictive or valvular cardiac disease, no arrhythmias, no acute respiratory distress syndrome, normal abdominal compartment pressures, adequate sedation, closed chest), both of these methods correlate well in identifying patients with hypovolemia. The sensitivity and specificity of DPP for predicting hypovolemia has been shown to be as high as 94% and 96%, respectively, and DD has been shown to correlate well with DPP.

4. Urine output (UOP) can be difficult to analyze with reference to volume status in the PACU. Medications, physiologic changes from PPV, as well as the stress response induced by surgery that alters

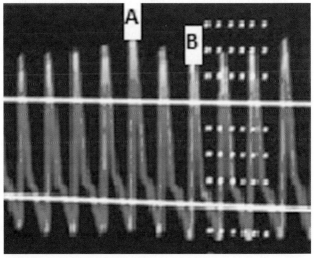

FIGURE 23.1 Measurement on an arterial tracing through a respiratory cycle of PP_{max} and PP_{min} with calculation of DPP (DPP = 100 × (PP_{max} − PP_{min})/[(PP_{max} + PP_{min})/2]). "A" represents PP_{max} and "B" represents PP_{min}. A DPP of 13% indicates hypovolemia.

release of antidiuretic hormone (ADH) and the renin–angiotensin system (RAS), can all affect normal UOP. In the first 48 hours postoperatively, the patient may continue to be oliguric, defined as a UOP < 0.5 mL/kg/hour. Furthermore, the serum concentration of ADH increases 50- to 100-fold during surgery and remains elevated for 3 to 5 days postoperatively. UOP should not be used as the lone indicator of fluid status.

5. Orthostasis is defined as an increase in HR of at least 10 beats per minute, or a decrease in SBP of at least 20 mm Hg when standing for 3 minutes after lying flat and supine. Performing orthostatic vital signs in the PACU is often not possible, and the accuracy of orthostatic vital signs in determining hypovolemia is poor.

C. The *physical exam*, when evaluating volume status, can include lung and heart auscultation, evaluation for jugular venous distension (JVD), hepatojugular reflex (HJR), and the skin. All of these can be difficult in the PACU. With the exception of pulmonary auscultation in fluid overload, none of these should be used as isolated findings.

1. Lung auscultation in fluid overload and pulmonary edema present as crackles. Crackles are nonmusical sounds heard in mid- to late inspiration and are gravity dependent. Studies about the accuracy of identifying pulmonary edema through auscultation of crackles vary, some showing a sensitivity and specificity of only 50% each. Identifying pulmonary edema early is important. A large retrospective study of 8,195 patients found that 7.6% of those undergoing major surgery developed pulmonary edema. Of that cohort, 11.9% died because of excessive fluid administration, especially in the first 36 hours postoperatively.

2. Heart auscultation may yield an S3 heart sound in overload states, but is otherwise of little yield in evaluating volume status.

3. JVD can be used as a surrogate for central venous pressure (CVP) measurement. JVD observed 5 cm or greater above the sternal angle, with the patient reclined at 45 degrees, may be indicative of fluid overload. The basis for this finding is that the right atrium lies, on average, 5 cm below the sternal angle. Therefore, using the ratio of 1 cm height = 1 cm H_2O, if JVD, or a peak jugular venous pulse, is 5 cm above the sternal angle, then the CVP is estimated to be at least 10 cm H_2O. Conversely, if no JVD is observed, evaluate the patient in the horizontal position and if still absent, then hypovolemia may be suspected. The specificity of the HJR (jugular distension with palpation of the liver) in volume overload has been reported as high as 94%.

4. Skin findings indicating hypovolemia include cold temperature, mottling, and poor turgor. Multiple factors postoperatively confound these observations, making its utility in isolation poor.

D. Other tools used to assess volume status after surgery include use of transthoracic echocardiography (TTE), passive leg raise (PLR), CVP, pulmonary artery occlusion pressure (PaOP), and laboratory evaluation.

1. Many studies have shown the benefit of TTE in the assessment of volume status. Changes in the distensibility of the inferior vena cava with respiration are highly accurate in both mechanically ventilated and spontaneously breathing patients. This is done via a subcostal image in M-mode (Fig. 23.2). The amount of variability to be considered indicative of hypovolemia is 18%, which has a 90% sensitivity and specificity.

2. PLR is both an effective assessment and intervention for hypovolemia and fluid responsiveness. To perform a PLR, the patient is placed in a horizontal and supine position and then the legs are raised at a

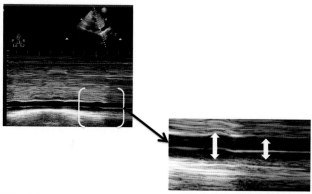

FIGURE 23.2 Image of a subcostal view of the inferior vena cava in M-mode showing differences in height with respiration. A respiratory variation of 18% indicates hypovolemia.

45-degree angle at the hips. This has been shown to have the same hemodynamic changes as a 500 mL fluid bolus. Improvement in cardiac parameters such as SV with a PLR has as much as an 86% and 90% sensitivity and specificity, respectively. PLR is effective in both mechanically ventilated and spontaneously breathing patients.

3. Use of CVP and PaOP monitoring to dictate fluid management has fallen out of favor after mounting evidence has shown poor correlation with fluid responsiveness.

4. Volume status can alter laboratory values as well.

   a. Hemoconcentration is seen in hypovolemic states.

   b. Brain natriuretic peptide (BNP) is elevated in volume overload, but is not very specific. A normal BNP, indicating no cardiac stress/stretch, is, however, reassuring that the patient is not volume overloaded.

   c. A hypovolemic patient could have elevations in both lactate and a base deficit.

   d. Central venous oxygen saturation (CvO_2) can also be used as a marker of perfusion and oxygen delivery. A value less than 70% may indicate hypovolemia; however, the base deficit has been shown to be a more accurate marker.

III. FLUID REPLACEMENT STRATEGIES

A. As noted earlier, the two most commonly used fluid replacement strategies are liberal and restrictive. There is a lack of definition of what constitutes each approach, which has made high-quality studies difficult. Although each has benefits in a variety of situations, overall, there is no difference in mortality between liberal and restrictive fluid administration.

B. When prescribing a fluid regimen, it is beneficial to consider one basic question: Does the patient need fluids? If the answer is "yes," then answering the following questions is imperative:

   1. Is it to replace a fluid deficit?

   2. Is it to replace ongoing losses?

   3. Is it to maintain a daily balance? The average adult requires 25 to 35 mL/kg/day of water, 0.9 to 1.5 mmol/kg/day of sodium, 1 mmol/kg/day of potassium, and 100 g of dextrose per day to avoid starvation ketosis.

C. At a minimum, the strategy utilized should correct fluid deficits and replace potential ongoing losses.

1. Large-volume resuscitation is based on the concept that expanding the intravascular space will improve organ perfusion. This includes large fluid volumes without hemodynamic parameters and goal-directed therapy, which is fluid titration based on specific hemodynamic endpoints. Both strategies result in higher volumes of fluid administration compared to restrictive approaches.

2. Restrictive fluid management also has several definitions. This approach is preferred in multiple types of surgeries where edema formation would lead to adverse outcomes, typically plastic, thoracic, and bowel surgery. This method is used in outpatient "fast-track" surgery, like the Enhanced Recovery Partnership in Europe, where low volumes help expedite patient discharge.

3. Fluid challenge is an additional method that is employed either independently or to accentuate the above. A fluid challenge is defined as an increase in CO following administration a fixed amount of intravenous (IV) fluid. It is used to determine if the patient is on the steep portion of the Frank–Starling curve and thus "preload dependent." Three parameters must be met to assess if a fluid challenge is successful; the patient must have low PEEP, normal right ventricular function, and assumed to be hypovolemic. Four steps have been suggested for proper use and interpretation of a fluid challenge:

   a. Select a fluid to bolus, typically crystalloid because of cost
   b. Select a rate and volume, usually 300 to 500 mL over 20 to 30 minutes
   c. Select an objective, what response is considered positive?
   d. Consider safety parameters. Is the patient at risk for pulmonary edema?

   Using a fluid challenge to guide therapy has been shown to reduce mortality 37% in the perioperative setting and reduce hospital length of stay.

IV. CRYSTALLOIDS VERSUS COLLOIDS

A. The ideal resuscitation fluid, one that is predictable in its intravascular expansion and metabolism, is cost-effective, is chemically equal to the extracellular compartment, and does not produce any metabolic derivations, does not exist. Studies favoring use of crystalloids point to the lower cost of these solutions as well as higher rates of coagulopathy and anaphylaxis with colloids. Proponents of colloids note the higher rates of tissue edema with use of crystalloids. For instance, use of salt-containing crystalloids in septic patients can result in retention of up to 12 L of excess water, which takes up to 3 weeks to excrete. No studies, either in the postoperative or critical care setting, have conclusively shown one type of fluid to be superior to the other in terms of mortality.

B. Crystalloids can be classified based on their tonicity relative to blood as well as if they are buffered, such as lactated ringers (LR), or nonbuffered like normal saline (NS). Though dextrose-containing solutions are not commonly used for resuscitation, it should be noted that isotonic dextrose (i.e., 5% or 50 g glucose per liter) is used for maintenance or free water replacement, whereas hypertonic dextrose solutions (i.e., 25% or 50% in water) are used to acutely treat hypoglycemic patients. Dextrose solutions have also been shown to promote diuresis faster than other crystalloids.

1. NS is made by adding 0.9 g of NaCl to 1 L of water. The major complication with large-volume replacement with saline is the

development of hyperchloremic metabolic acidosis. This phenomenon is best explained using the strong ion difference (SID). The SID,
also known as the Stewart Approach, simply equates fully dissoci-
ated major cations minus anions in plasma. A normal value is between 38 and 46 mmol/L.

$$SID = (Na + K + Ca + Mg) - (Cl + lactate) = 38–46 \text{ mmol/L}$$

When the gap increases, a metabolic alkalosis is present, and when
the gap narrows, it is due to a metabolic acidosis. Thus NS, which has
an SID of zero (sodium = chloride) leads to metabolic acidosis. Large
volumes of NS and the resultant derangements lead to:
  a. Reduced UOP, because of hyperchloremia causing renal vasocon-
     striction
  b. Sodium retention that lasts several days because of suppression
     of RAS
  c. Reduced cardiac contractility
  d. Coagulopathy
2. LR is considered a balanced solution because the chemical composition more closely approximates the ECF. LR is hypotonic because of
   lower concentration of sodium. LR is now the preferred crystalloid
   for resuscitation; however, among crystalloids, NS has a more prolonged intravascular volume expansion. This effect is due to NS suppressing RAS and because LR is slightly hypotonic, which reduces
   the release of ADH. Additionally, LR contains calcium, which limits
   use with citrated blood because of the formation of calcium citrate.
   PlasmaLyte, a calcium-free balanced solution with a pH of 7.4, has
   been shown to have lower rates of acute kidney injury compared
   to NS.
C. Colloids consist of human albumin and semisynthetic colloids. Most
   are made by dissolving the osmotically active material in NS.
   1. Albumin, first used clinically in the treatment of burn victims fol-
      lowing the attack on Pearl Harbor in 1941, is derived from fraction-
      ation of blood, which is then heat-treated to prevent transmission of
      disease. Studies evaluating whether replacement of serum albumin
      improves postoperative outcomes compared with crystalloids have
      not shown benefit.
   2. Semisynthetic colloids include gelatins, dextrans, and hetastarch.
      Hetastarch solutions have become more popular, especially in
      Europe. In the United States, concerns about bleeding and kidney
      failure have called the use of hetastarch into question. All semisyn-
      thetic colloids can increase bleeding either by reduced or impaired
      coagulation factors and platelets. They also have a significant risk
      of anaphylaxis.

V. ELECTROLYTES
A. Often associated with fluid abnormalities, electrolyte disturbances are
   frequently more acutely fatal than fluid perturbations.
B. *Sodium* balance is likely a reflection of free water imbalance than of
   sodium stores.
   1. Hyponatremia can have significant morbidity and/or mortality
      if not correctly managed. A significantly increased risk of death
      30 days postoperatively has been shown with a preoperative so-
      dium <135 mEq/L. Surgical procedures where hyponatremia is
      more commonly seen include urologic procedures, especially trans-
      urethral resection of the prostate (TURP) known as TURP syndrome.
      Symptoms of hyponatremia include nausea/vomiting, but can pro-
      gresses to headache, lethargy, seizure, and coma with lower sodium

levels. Significant hyponatremia warrants admission to an ICU. Correction of sodium levels less than <120 mEq/L should not occur faster than 8 to 12 mEq/L/day to avoid risk of central pontine myelinolysis (CPM). Acute onset (<48 hours) can be more rapidly corrected with smaller risk of CPM. In chronic hyponatremia, treatment generally starts with fluid restriction and consideration for ICU admission. Evaluation begins with assessing the volume status. Following this, a measurement of urine sodium levels is conducted to aid in diagnosis.

   a. Hypovolemia
      1. U_{Na} < 30 mEq/L (extrarenal: loss through skin or GI, pancreatitis)
      2. U_{Na} > 30 mEq/L (renal: cerebral salt wasting, diuretics, Addison's)
   b. Euvolemia
      1. U_{Na} > 30 mEq/L (Syndrome of inappropriate antidiuretic hormone secretion [SIADH], water overload, hypothyroid, hypopituitarism)
   c. Hypervolemia
      1. U_{Na} < 30 mEq/L (congestive heart failure, nephrotic syndrome, cirrhosis)
      2. U_{Na} > 30 mEq/L (chronic renal failure)

2. Symptoms of hypernatremia present when sodium levels reach 158 mEq/L, beginning with restlessness, nausea, and vomiting and progressing to lethargy, stupor, and coma. Due to shrinkage of the brain, subarachnoid hemorrhage can occur. Correction should occur no faster than 1 mEq/L/hour, slower in chronic hypernatremia, and begins with calculating the free water deficit:

$$\text{Free water deficit} = \text{dosing factor} \times \text{weight (kg)} \times ((\text{serum Na}/140)-1)$$

$$\text{Dosing factor: 0.6 for males, 0.5 for females}$$

Like hyponatremia, diagnosing the cause of hypernatremia includes evaluating the fluid status.

   a. Hypovolemia (skin/GI/renal, diuretics, hyperosmolar nonketotic coma)
   b. Euvolemia (diabetes insipidus, fever, hyperventilation)
   c. Hypervolemia (hyperaldosteronism, hypertonic saline, tube feeds)

C. *Potassium* is primarily an intracellular cation where levels are maintained by a sodium–potassium pump. A decrease of ECF potassium increases the electrical gradient (aka the membrane potential), whereas an increase in ECF potassium decreases the membrane potential of the cell. This effect is most profoundly seen in cardiac myocytes where a decrease in the membrane potential decreases excitability at the sinoatrial node and decreases the threshold to ventricular fibrillation. Hyperkalemia can be abruptly lethal.

1. Hyperkalemia is present in 1% to 10% of all hospitalized patients. Cases where this may be seen include vascular surgery, liver transplantation, prolonged surgery that can result in rhabdomyolysis, or malignant hyperthermia. Symptoms include fatigue, distal paresthesias, respiratory depression, and cardiac arrhythmias. On electrocardiogram (ECG), hyperkalemia presents with peaked T-waves that progress to widening of the QRS complex, decreased amplitude of the P-waves, merging of the QRS and T-waves, and ultimately ventricular fibrillation. Treatment with a *combination therapy with insulin/glucose and an inhaled β-agonist* is an effective medical

TABLE 23.2	Treatment of Hyperkalemia
10% calcium chloride	Give when ECG changes are first observed. Administer 10 mL (1 g)
Insulin/glucose	Improvement in 15 min. Administer 10 U regular insulin w/an amp D50
β-agonist	Improvement in 30 min, 20 mg total dose over 2 h is best
Hemodialysis	Instituted if medical therapy fails, high flows best
Bicarbonate infusion	Insufficient evidence that this is effective even in combination
Resins	Typical dose 30 g with repeat. Not effective acutely, requires 24 h
Other	Not enough data to support diuretic therapy or aminophylline

therapy to acutely lower serum potassium levels. Administration of calcium chloride helped prevent cardiac arrhythmias. Treatment options are discussed in Table 23.2.

2. Hypokalemia can be a reflection of depleted total body stores or an alkalosis. Potassium levels <3.0 mEq/L lead to development of a U-wave (additional positive deflection after the T-wave) on the ECG and can progress to arrhythmias such as ventricular tachycardia. It is believed that the total body deficit has a linear relationship with serum potassium levels, with each 100 mEq total body potassium decrease equating to a 0.27 mEq/L decrease in serum levels on lab testing. This holds true up to a 500 mEq total body deficit. A replacement dose of 0.5 mEq/kg should be expected to correct the serum potassium by 0.6 mEq/L, with a rate of 40 mEq/hour infusion via central access being considered safe.

D. *Calcium* abnormalities predominantly affect cardiac, smooth muscle, and coagulation. Calcium is integral to the heart for both generating the action potential and increasing the interaction between actin and myosin for cardiac contraction. In the vasculature, calcium is necessary for smooth muscle contraction. Additionally, platelets and coagulation factors require calcium for normal functioning. Fifty percent of the total serum calcium is in the free, ionized state. This form is also sensitive to changes in pH with acidosis, leading to increased levels of ionized calcium because of dissociation from plasma proteins, predominantly albumin.

1. Hypercalcemia is seen most commonly in patients with hyperparathyroidism and malignancy, though numerous other causes (end-stage renal disease, adrenal insufficiency, immobilization) are possible. Symptoms include GI (nausea, vomiting, acute pancreatitis), renal (polyuria), neurologic (lethargy, stupor, agitation), and cardiac (shortening of the QT interval, hypertension, arrhythmia). Treatment includes hydration with calcium free solutions, diuretic therapy, and monitoring of cardiac function and electrolytes.

2. Hypocalcemia can be seen postoperatively following parathyroidectomy, thyroidectomy, after cardiopulmonary bypass, and following large infusions of citrated blood. Findings include Chvostek's and Trousseau's sign, muscle cramps, QT prolongation/arrhythmia, and

laryngo-/bronchospasm. Treatment includes replacement with 100 to 200 mg elemental calcium over 10 minutes followed by a continuous infusion of 1 to 2 mg/kg/hour; 10 mL of 10% calcium gluconate contains 9.3 mg of elemental calcium, whereas 10% calcium carbonate in the same volume contains 27.2 mg of calcium.

E. *Magnesium* plays an important role in protein synthesis, neuromuscular function, generation of adenosine triphosphate (ATP), and regulation of many other electrolytes. Centrally, magnesium antagonizes *N*-methyl-D-aspartate (NMDA) receptors, glutamate receptors, and catecholamine release. Magnesium has been suggested to help lower anesthetic and pain levels because of these effects on NMDA receptors.
   1. Hypermagnesemia is relatively rare and usually associated with iatrogenic administration. Treatment is usually hydration and administration of calcium.
   2. Hypomagnesemia occurs in up to 11% of hospitalized and 65% of critically ill patients. Symptoms include nausea, vomiting, lethargy, convulsions, prolonged PR/QT intervals, and arrhythmias. It is more common following thyroidectomies and major abdominal surgery. Treatment is usually IV replacement in doses of 2 g over 30 minutes.

F. *Phosphorous* is a major intracellular electrolyte that is integral in maintaining the integrity of the cell membrane, storages energy as ATP, controls oxygen delivery to tissues by regulating hemoglobin affinity for oxygen, and is a key cofactor for many enzymes and second-messenger systems. Hypophosphatemia is more common in the postoperative period. This is seen in malnourished patients when high-carbohydrate enteral feeding is reinstituted abruptly, known as refeeding syndrome, or with chronic abnormalities of bone metabolism. Symptoms include myopathy, decreased cardiac contractility, respiratory failure, and encephalopathy. Acute hyperphosphatemia is likely due to overcorrection and can cause hypocalcemia because of calcium deposition in soft tissues.
   1. Refeeding syndrome occurs when a malnourished patient resumes taking either enteral or parenteral nutrition after several days of fasting. In all hospitalized patients, there is a 0.43% incidence of severe hypophosphatemia, but in patients receiving total parenteral nutrition, even with phosphorous supplementation, there is an 18% incidence. Under starvation, the body changes from using carbohydrates to using fat and protein for energy. As starvation continues, the body depletes stores of many important electrolytes, though the plasma levels remain unchanged. Once refeeding begins, the body once again uses carbohydrates for energy, which leads to an insulin surge and depletion of phosphorous levels because of phosphorous being a cofactor for glucose utilization.

Suggested Readings

Aguilera IM, Vaughan RS. Calcium and the anesthetist. *Anaesthesia* 2000;55:779–790.
Annane D, Siami S, Jaber S, et al. Effects of fluid resuscitation with colloids vs crystalloids on mortality in critically ill patients presenting with hypovolemic shock: the CRISTAL randomized trial. *JAMA* 2013;310(17):1809–1817.
Canneson M, Aboy M, Hofer CK, et al. Pulse pressure variation, where are we today? *J Clin Monit Comput* 2010;25(1):45–56.
Corcoran T, Rhodes JEJ, Clarke S, et al. Perioperative fluid management strategies in major surgery: a stratified meta-analysis. *Anesth Analg* 2012;114(3):640–651.
Deflandre E, Bonhomme V, Hans P. Delta down compared to delta pulse pressure as an indicator of volemia during intracranial surgery. *Br J Anaesth* 2008;100(2):245–250.
Grocott MPW, Mythen MG, Gan TJ. Perioperative fluid management and clinical outcomes in adults. *Anesth Analg* 2005;100:1093–1106.

Herroeder S, Schonherr ME, De Hert SG, et al. Magnesium—essentials for anesthesiologists. *Anesthesiology* 2011;114(4):971–993.

Kobayashi L, Constantini TW, Coimbria R. Hypovolemic shock resuscitation. *Surg Clin North Am* 2012;92:1403–1423.

Lobo DN, Lewington AJP, Allison SP. *Basic Concepts of Fluid and Electrolyte Therapy*. Melsungen, Germany: Bibliomed; 2013.

Lobo DN, MaCafee DAL, Allison SP. How perioperative fluid balance influences postoperative outcomes. *Best Pract Res Clin Anaesthesiol* 2006;20(3):439–455.

Mahoney BA, Smith WAD, Lo D, et al. Emergency interventions for hyperkalemia. The Cochrane Collaboration. *The Cochrane Library* 2009.

Mehanna HM, Moledina J, Travis J. Refeeding syndrome: what it is and how to prevent and treat it. *BMJ* 2008;336:1495–1498.

Michard F. Changes in arterial pressure during mechanical ventilation. *Anesthesiology* 2005;103:419–428.

Myburgh JA, Mythen MG. Resuscitation fluids. *N Engl J Med* 2013;369:1243–1251.

Peacock WF, Soto KM. Current technique of fluid status assessment. *Congest Heart Fail* 2010;16(4):S45–S51.

Pearse RM, Ackland GL. Perioperative fluid therapy. *BMJ* 2012;344:e2865.

Rassam SS, Counsell DJ. Perioperative electrolyte and fluid balance. *Anaesth Crit Care Pain* 2005;5(5):157–160.

Reynolds RM, Padfield PL, Seckl JR. Disorders of sodium balance. *BMJ* 2006;332:702–705.

Taylor AE. Capillary fluid filtration. *Circ Res* 1981;49(3):557–575.

Tetzlaff JE, O'Hara JF, Walsh MT. Potassium and anesthesia. *Can J Anaesth* 1993;40(3):227–246.

Acid–Base Disorders

Kevin H. Zhao and Kathryn L. Butler

Acid–base disorders arise in a wide variety of postoperative scenarios and have severe consequences on organ function and perfusion. An abnormal pH can alter enzyme function, electron transport, membrane stability, and endanger patients to arrhythmias, hemodynamic instability, and organ ischemia.

Clinicians caring for postoperative patients with acid–base disorders must diagnose the underlying cause to provide effective treatment. Classification schemes to aid understanding of acid–base disorders include:

1. acidosis versus alkalosis
2. metabolic versus respiratory
3. anion-gap versus nonanion-gap acidosis
4. acute versus chronic
5. iatrogenic versus secondary to a disease process

Understanding the appropriate categorization of acid–base disorders guides not only the therapeutic options, but also the urgency of treatment (Fig. 24.1).

I. PATHOPHYSIOLOGY

A. Various *acid–base paradigms* help to quantify acid–base relationships. *Traditional acid–base* teaching focuses on the generation of protons (H^+) and their neutralization through bicarbonate (HCO_3^-) buffers.

$$H^+ + HCO_3^- \leftrightarrow H_2CO_3 \leftrightarrow H_2O + CO_2$$

The body regulates this equilibrium through the enzyme carbonic anhydrase. With regard to by-products, the kidneys eliminate bicarbonate, whereas lung ventilation removes carbon dioxide. The *Henderson–Hasselbalch* equation quantifies this equilibrium through the interaction of weak acids and their conjugate bases:

$$pH = pK_a + \log_{10}([A^-]/[HA])$$

Making the appropriate substitutions from the bicarbonate–carbon dioxide equilibrium yields:

$$pH = pK_{a\,H_2CO_3} + \log\{[HCO_3^-]/[H_2CO_3]\}$$

Substituting and converting numerical variables yields:

$$pH = 6.1 + \log\{[HCO_3^-]/(PaCO_2{}^*0.03)\}$$

Understanding the role of bicarbonate as a buffer and the Henderson–Hasselbalch equation provides clinically useful values such as base excess and base deficit. A base excess reflects an alkalotic condition, whereas a base deficit indicates an acidotic condition. Base excess and base deficit are the amount of strong acid or strong base, respectively, that must be added to each liter of blood to return the pH to 7.40 at

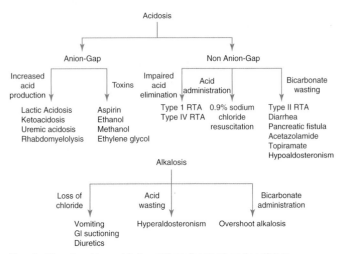

Flow chart for categorizing metabolic acid-base disorders based on etiology
and mechanism.

FIGURE 24.1 Algorithm for categorizing metabolic acid–base disorders based on etiology
and mechanism.

37°C. These values can be used to trend the severity and resolution of
acid–base disorders.

B. Acidosis and alkalosis have unique and varied clinical effects
(Table 24.1). The severity of these effects depends on the magnitude
of the acid–base disturbance and each patient's preexisting medical

TABLE 24.1	Clinical Effects of Acidemia and Alkalemia	
	Acidemia	**Alkalemia**
Cardiovascular	Decreased cardiac contractility	Reduced coronary blood flow
	Blunted catecholamine response	Increased cardiac contractility
	Hypotension	Increased arrhythmias
	Increased arrhythmias	
Pulmonary	Increased pulmonary vascular resistance	Hypoventilation
	Hyperventilation	
Cerebral	Cerebral vasodilation	Cerebral vasoconstriction
	Increased cerebral blood flow	Decreased cerebral blood flow
	Increased intracranial pressure	Decreased intracranial pressure
Metabolic	Hyperkalemia	Hypokalemia
	Increased protein catabolism	Hypomagnesemia
		Hypophosphatemia

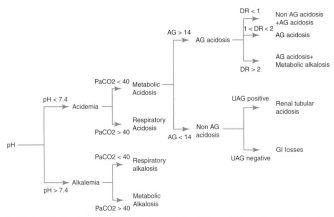

FIGURE 24.2 Algorithm for differentiating and classifying acid–base disorders based on laboratory results. AG, anion-gap; UAG, urine anion-gap; DR, δ ratio.

conditions. Acid–base abnormalities can be iatrogenic or due to underlying disease. Although an alkalosis caused by aggressive diuresis or an acidosis caused by permissive hypercapnia will self-resolve with discontinuation of therapy, acid–base disturbances due to lactic acidosis or hypoventilation may be life-threatening and warrant immediate intervention. Understanding the laboratory values associated with acid–base disorders provides useful diagnostic information (Fig. 24.2). Under typical circumstances, the body will attempt to compensate for the underlying disorder and minimize clinical consequences. In rare cases, the effects of an altered pH may be therapeutic and desired. For example, mild hyperventilation-induced cerebral vasoconstriction offers short-term intracranial pressure relief until a more definitive treatment can occur. Management of acid–base disorders mandates consideration of each patient's unique clinical context.

II. METABOLIC DISORDERS

A. **Metabolic acidosis** can be caused by increased acid production, increased bicarbonate elimination, or exogenous acid administration. These categories can then be sorted into anion-gap and nonanion-gap disorders (Table 24.2).

1. The *anion-gap* represents unmeasured anions in the plasma, which is primarily composed of negatively charged proteins.

$$\text{Anion-gap} = [Na^+] - [Cl^-] - [HCO_3^-]$$

In pathologic states, an increase in unmeasured anions (e.g., lactate) will cause an increased anion-gap. Because albumin is a negatively charged protein, hypoalbuminemia will result in a falsely low anion-gap and will need to be accounted for in the final calculation. The anion-gap will decrease by approximately 2.5 mEq/L for every 1 g/dL less of albumin below 4 mEq/L. A normal anion-gap is between 7 and 14 mEq/L, although it will be 11 to 18 mEq/L if the anion-gap equation includes $[K^+]$.

2. The *etiology* of the anion-gap acidosis influences time until resolution. In lactic acidosis, appropriate resuscitation causes lactate conversion to bicarbonate and resolution within hours. In the case

TABLE 24.2	Metabolic Acidosis Causes
Anion-gap acidosis	Increased acid production • Lactic acidosis • Ketoacidosis • Uremia • Rhabdomyolysis Intoxication • Aspirin • Ethanol • Methanol • Ethylene glycol • Paraldehyde
Nonanion-gap acidosis	Increased base loss • Diarrhea • Renal tubular acidosis • Ureterosigmoidostomy • Pancreatic fistula • Acetazolamide use • Topiramate use Exogenous acid administration • Normal saline

of excessive bicarbonate loss, such as diarrhea or renal tubular acidosis, resolution will require endogenous bicarbonate production that may take days.

3. *Alkali therapy* is a temporizing measure to correct a metabolic acidosis. Commonly given in the form of intravenous bicarbonate, alkali therapy can raise the pH and limit the consequences of severe acidemia (Table 24.1). The evidence supporting alkali therapy is limited, and the underlying cause must still be corrected to prevent further acid production. Sodium bicarbonate therapy is also not without risks. Bicarbonate is converted to carbon dioxide and elevates $PaCO_2$, which may increase a patient's respiratory acidosis if ventilation is impaired. In shock states, correction of acidosis can worsen oxygen delivery to peripheral tissues. A sodium bicarbonate preparation can also worsen hypernatremia. Tromethamine (THAM) is an alternative to sodium bicarbonate that does not increase $PaCO_2$, but it has serious electrolyte side effects, and evidence does not show improvement in clinical outcomes.

B. **Metabolic alkalosis** can be caused by chloride losses, increased bicarbonate absorption, or bicarbonate administration. A metabolic alkalosis can be sorted into chloride-responsive or chloride-unresponsive disorders. Most chloride-responsive disorders are caused by chloride loss through the gastrointestinal tract or kidneys. Chloride-unresponsive alkalosis is less common and caused by increased mineralocorticoid activity.

C. *Compensation*, or the secondary response, refers to the body using the metabolic or respiratory system to shift the pH toward 7.40 during an acid–base disorder. Although metabolic changes to an underlying respiratory disorder may take days to adequately compensate, a respiratory response to a metabolic disorder can occur within hours. The degree of expected compensation is often predictable and can be calculated (see Table 24.3). It is important to remember that some

TABLE 24.3	Predicted pH, PaCO₂, and HCO₃– Interaction and Compensation	
Respiratory acidosis	Change in pH ($PaCO_2 \to pH$)	Acute: $PaCO_2$ increases 1 mm Hg → pH decreases 0.008 Chronic: $PaCO_2$ increases 1 mm Hg → pH decreases 0.003
	Metabolic compensation	Acute: $PaCO_2$ increases 10 mm Hg → HCO_3^- increases 1 mEq/L Chronic: $PaCO_2$ increases 10 mm Hg → HCO_3^- increases 5 mEq/L
Respiratory alkalosis	$PaCO_2 \to pH$	Acute: $PaCO_2$ decreases 1 mm Hg → pH increases 0.008 Chronic: $PaCO_2$ decreases 1 mm Hg → pH increase 0.003
	Metabolic compensation	Acute: $PaCO_2$ decreases 10 mm Hg → HCO_3^- decreases 2 mEq/L Chronic: $PaCO_2$ decreases 10 mm Hg → HCO_3^- increases 5 mEq/L
Metabolic acidosis	$HCO_3^- \to pH$	HCO_3^- decreases 1 mEq/L → pH 0.015 decrease
	Respiratory compensation	$PaCO_2$ (mm Hg) = 1.5 * HCO_3^- (mEq/L) + 8
Metabolic alkalosis	$HCO_3^- \to pH$	HCO_3^- increases 1 mEq/L → pH 0.015 increase
	Respiratory compensation	$PaCO_2$ (mm Hg) = 0.7 * HCO_3^- (mEq/L) + 20

patients may mask or exacerbate an acute acid–base disorder by living in a chronic acidemic or alkalemic state because of their preexisting medical conditions.

III. ANION-GAP METABOLIC ACIDOSIS

A. Increased Acid Production

1. *Lactic acidosis* is one of the most common and ominous acid–base disorders seen postoperatively. Suggestive of impaired tissue oxygenation, lactic acidosis is a marker of circulatory failure. The etiology can be a hypovolemic, septic, cardiogenic, or obstructive perfusion abnormality. Depending on the cause, circulatory support may need to be directed toward volume resuscitation, improved oxygenation, afterload reduction, and inotropic support. Other resuscitative measures may include the need for antibiotics and operative intervention. It is important to note that a mild to moderate lactic acidosis (3 to 5 mmol/L) may not be sufficient to trigger an anion-gap outside of the normal reference range, and ordering a lactate value will be necessary to detect the disorder. Timing of lactate resolution correlates well with survival.

2. *Ketoacidosis* can be caused by insulin deficiency in type I diabetics as well as nutritionally deficient states such as severe alcohol use and starvation. In type I diabetics, insufficient insulin results in the impairment of normal glucose metabolism and subsequent ketone formation. Diabetic ketoacidosis (DKA) requires treatment with volume resuscitation, insulin, electrolyte repletion, and normalization of the anion-gap. DKA in a type II diabetic is rare, but has been reported. In the postoperative period, DKA can occur either due to insulin being inappropriately withheld perioperatively or increased insulin requirements from the stress of surgery. Starvation ketosis and alcoholic ketoacidosis are less common causes of ketoacidosis. Unlike DKA, starvation ketosis and alcohol ketoacidosis rarely present with elevated serum glucose levels. In these nutritionally deficient states, treatment with intravenous fluids and dextrose will stimulate insulin secretion and resolution of the ketoacidosis.

3. *Uremic acidosis* occurs in severe and end-stage renal disease. Due to the inability of the kidney to excrete anions, there is an anion-gap metabolic acidosis. In most cases, the acidosis is not severe because of buffering by other organ systems. In cases of mild or early uremic acidosis, patients may first present with a nonanion-gap acidosis.

4. *Rhabdomyolysis*, which can occur after trauma or operative positioning, can cause a metabolic acidosis through the release of anions directly from muscle cell lysis.

B. **Toxins**

1. *Aspirin* overdose requires substantial ingestion, often greater than 300 mg/kg. The increase in plasma salicylate levels inhibits the Krebs cycle and mitochondrial oxidative phosphorylation, resulting in lactic acid and ketoacid production. Salicylate is a direct respiratory stimulant, causing a mixed respiratory alkalosis and metabolic acidosis. Treatment involves resuscitation, alkalinization of urine, gastric decontamination, and potentially hemodialysis.

2. *Ethanol* ingestion at toxic levels results in the production of lactic acidosis, ketoacidosis, and acetic acidosis. Patients may also present with a hypochloremic metabolic alkalosis from protracted vomiting, creating a mixed acid–base disorder. Treatment should be targeted toward volume resuscitation, thiamine, and electrolyte repletion.

3. *Methanol* ingestion can occur accidently or as an ethanol substitute. The liver metabolizes methanol into formaldehyde and then formic acid. The toxic metabolites can produce a profound anion-gap and are implicated in blindness. Patients initially present with an osmolar gap that evolves into a gap acidosis as methanol is metabolized. Treatment involves resuscitation, inhibition of alcohol dehydrogenase through ethanol or fomepizole, and potentially hemodialysis.

4. *Ethylene glycol*, commonly used in antifreeze, can cause a metabolic acidosis through the production of glycolic and oxalic acid at the liver. Treatment is the same as methanol toxicity.

IV. **NONANION-GAP METABOLIC ACIDOSIS**

A. Increased base loss through the gastrointestinal tract or kidneys is the primary mechanism for a nonanion-gap metabolic acidosis. In cases where it is challenging to determine the source, a *urine anion-gap (UAG)* may be helpful.

$$UAG = Na_{urine} + K_{urine} - Cl_{urine}$$

UAG is positive if the cause is renal in origin and negative if gastrointestinal in origin. In normal patients, the UAG is approximately zero. In a metabolic acidosis of gastrointestinal origin, ammonium (NH_4^+) is

TABLE 24.4	Renal Tubular Acidosis Classification			
RTA Type	Location of Defect	Mechanism	Urine pH	Potassium
Type I	Distal tubules	Insufficient H^+ secretion	>5.3	Hypokalemia
Type II	Proximal tubules	Insufficient HCO_3^- reabsorption	<5.3	Hypokalemia
Type IV	Adrenal glands	Aldosterone deficiency or resistance	<5.3	Hyperkalemia

excreted with chloride in the kidneys, causing an elevation in the Cl_{urine} and a negative UAG. If the etiology is renal, ammonium excretion at the kidneys is impaired and Cl_{urine} will not be elevated.

1. *Renal tubular acidosis (RTA)* denotes a group of disorders where the kidneys fail to appropriately excrete acids into the urine. Kidney function, including glomerular filtration rate, is otherwise unaffected. There are three common types of RTA based on the location and etiology of the disorder (Table 24.4). Type I RTA presents with an inability to acidify urine at the distal tubule, a mechanism that utilizes the H^+/K^+ pump. As a result, protons are retained in circulation, whereas potassium is excessively eliminated. A Type II RTA is caused by failure of the proximal tubule to reabsorb bicarbonate. Because the distal tubule is intact, the urine can still be acidified to a pH < 5.3. A Type IV RTA is due to hypoaldosteronism and a reduction in ammonium excretion. Although Type I and IV RTAs represent decreased acid elimination, a Type II RTA causes a nonanion-gap acidosis by increasing bicarbonate elimination.

2. Chronic *diarrhea* can cause bicarbonate loss through the gastrointestinal tract, causing a nonanion-gap acidosis.

3. *Ureterosigmoidostomy* is a treatment for bladder cancer where urine is diverted to the sigmoid colon following a cystectomy. The urine chloride that reaches the colon is exchanged for bicarbonate, causing base elimination through the gastrointestinal tract.

4. A *pancreatic fistula* can result in the loss of pancreatic fluid high in bicarbonate.

5. *Acetazolamide* is a diuretic with multiple medical uses. Due to its activity as a carbonic anhydrase inhibitor, acetazolamide increases bicarbonate excretion at the kidney.

6. *Topiramate*, a drug used for seizures and migraines, can cause a nonanion-gap metabolic acidosis through inhibition of both bicarbonate absorption and proton excretion at the kidneys, mimicking a combined Type I and Type II RTA.

B. Exogenous Acid Administration

1. *Normal saline (0.9%)* has a pH of 5.5 and a chloride concentration of 154 mEq/L. Because the chloride levels exceed those in plasma, patients can develop an iatrogenic hyperchloremic metabolic acidosis following significant volume resuscitation. As a result, this condition is commonly seen in ORs, PACUs, and ICUs that choose normal saline as their primary resuscitation fluid; 5% albumin is formulated in normal saline, so significant 5% albumin resuscitation can cause

a hyperchloremic metabolic acidosis as well. Although the acidosis is generally mild and cleared rapidly in otherwise healthy individuals, it can be hazardous in the critically ill when conditions such as hyperkalemia or hyperventilation to compensate for the acidosis are not well tolerated.

V. METABOLIC ALKALOSIS

A. Metabolic alkalosis can be caused by loss of chloride, increased bicarbonate absorption, or inhibited proton absorption. Attention should be paid to not only the alkalosis, but also the electrolyte imbalances and clinical consequences that occur in the setting of an elevated pH (Table 24.1).

1. *Gastrointestinal losses* can cause a metabolic alkalosis through the loss of chloride from the stomach. Whether through protracted vomiting or iatrogenic suctioning (e.g., continuous nasogastric suctioning), patients can develop a hypochloremic metabolic alkalosis.

2. *Diuretics* can cause a contraction alkalosis through chloride loss. Although the exact mechanism for the alkalosis is not clear, suggested mechanisms include the loss of chloride without a proportional loss of bicarbonate and a compensatory increase in aldosterone levels that causes an increase in bicarbonate absorption.

3. *Hyperaldosteronism*, such as Conn syndrome, can cause an alkalosis through increased activity of a Na^+/H^+ transporter with sodium retention and hydrogen elimination at the kidneys.

4. *Overshoot alkalosis*, or excessive bicarbonate administration, to correct a metabolic acidosis can also cause a metabolic alkalosis.

B. Treatment should be targeted at the underlying cause. If vomiting is the etiology, antiemetics and promotility agents may be beneficial. If loop diuretics are the culprit and diuresis is still necessary, acetazolamide and free water repletion may improve the contraction alkalosis. Hypochloremic alkalosis can be treated using normal saline for chloride repletion. In rare cases, an acid infusion or dialysis can be used when other options have failed.

VI. RESPIRATORY ACIDOSIS

A. Respiratory acidosis is caused by insufficient ventilation to adequately clear carbon dioxide. $PaCO_2$ is determined by both ventilation and carbon dioxide production.

$$PaCO_2 = CO_2 \text{ production/alveolar ventilation}$$

Although a respiratory acidosis from residual anesthetics will resolve with time, a respiratory acidosis in the setting of respiratory distress may also be a sign of impending respiratory collapse.

1. *Increased CO_2 production* can be caused by several factors in the perioperative period. An increased metabolic rate from inflammation or infection can create a hyperdynamic state that produces increased carbon dioxide. In cases of laparoscopic surgery, carbon dioxide for insufflation can cause a profound respiratory acidosis, especially if the patient is difficult to ventilate because of poor respiratory mechanics.

2. *Acute alveolar hypoventilation* can be caused by medications or preexisting patient conditions. There are a variety of pulmonary, central nervous system, and neuromuscular disorders that limit ventilation (Table 24.5). Anesthetics can also play a significant role in alveolar hypoventilation. Hypnotic agents, such as volatile anesthetics and propofol, are potent respiratory depressants. Even though modern

Category	Causes
Anesthetic/surgical	Residual inhalational or intravenous anesthetic
	Opioids
	Benzodiazepines
	Residual neuromuscular blockade
	Pain/splinting
	Airway obstruction
Respiratory disease	COPD exacerbation
	Asthma exacerbation
	Obstructive sleep apnea
	Obesity hypoventilation syndrome
	Restrictive lung disease
	Aspiration
	Pneumonia
	Pulmonary embolism
Gastrointestinal	Abdominal compartment syndrome
Neurological and neuromuscular disease	Myasthenia gravis
	Amyotrophic lateral sclerosis
	Muscular dystrophy
	Guillain–Barré
	Spinal cord injuries
	Stroke

anesthetic agents have quick clearance, patients still retain anesthetics in the PACU that can cause hypoventilation. Opioids and other respiratory depressants depress ventilation by raising the $PaCO_2$ threshold for breathing. In the perioperative period, patients at high risk of respiratory depression should have judicious use of opioids, benzodiazepines, and long-acting anesthetics.

3. Chronic alveolar hypoventilation may be present in patients with chronic obstructive pulmonary disease. In such cases, patients develop a chronic respiratory acidosis with a compensatory metabolic alkalosis. Chronic alveolar hypoventilation should be suspected in patients with elevated serum bicarbonate levels. A higher $PaCO_2$ should be expected and tolerated as long as mental status is preserved.

B. Treatment of respiratory acidosis is directed at the underlying cause. The patient should be assessed for signs of respiratory distress. If an airway obstruction is suspected, diagnosing whether the obstruction is in the upper or lower airway is essential to guide therapy. Aspiration should be considered postoperatively, especially in patients at risk for an ileus or too sedated to protect their airway. Prolonged PACU monitoring may be warranted to prevent hypoxic events in patients with obstructive sleep apnea. Because $PaCO_2$ displaces oxygen, supplemental oxygen is a critical part of therapy to maintain a PaO_2 compatible with organ perfusion.

$$P_aO_2 = FiO_2*(P_b-H_2O) - P_aCO_2/\text{respiratory quotient}$$

Interventions to ease the work of breathing include bronchodilators, head of bed elevation, and chest physical therapy. In cases of severe limitation, bronchoscopy to clear secretions or mechanical ventilation may be necessary.

C. *Permissive hypercapnia* is a unique scenario where intentional hypoventilation is part of the treatment for acute respiratory distress syndrome (ARDS). Due to the barotrauma caused by high tidal volume ventilation, adequate minute ventilation to normalize $PaCO_2$ may not be possible. As a result, hypercapnia and its associated respiratory acidosis are tolerated until the underlying lung disease resolves. Low tidal volume lung-protective ventilation may be used in cases of ARDS postoperatively or in cases where ARDS is anticipated.

VII. RESPIRATORY ALKALOSIS

A. Respiratory alkalosis is due to hyperventilation. It is normal in several conditions, such as high-altitude adaptation and pregnancy. In the perioperative period, it can be due to anxiety and be relieved with reassurance or sedation. A high respiratory rate may also be a sign of postoperative pain and should be treated with analgesics. However, a clinical assessment of the patient is essential because a respiratory alkalosis can also be a sign of hypoxemia. In hypoxemia, peripheral chemoreceptors at the aortic and carotid bodies stimulate ventilation in response to low PaO_2 levels. Hypoxemia-induced respiratory alkalosis could also be a sign of a pulmonary embolism or pneumonia.

VIII. MIXED ACID–BASE DISORDERS

A. *Mixed acid–base disorders* can occur in the critically ill and should be suspected when appropriate metabolic or respiratory compensation does not occur. Under normal circumstances, the body will attempt to shift the pH toward 7.40 through buffering, renal elimination, and respiratory adjustments. It is important to know the interactions between pH, $PaCO_2$, and HCO_3^- in order to properly diagnosis whether appropriate compensatory adjustments are being made (Table 24.3).

B. *δratio*, also referred to as a *δ–δ* or *δ*gap, is used to determine if there is a mixed acid–base disorder. If a patient has a suspected anion-gap and nonanion-gap acidosis simultaneously, a *δ*gap can be used to determine if both types of acidosis are present.

$$\delta\text{ratio} = (\text{measured anion-gap} - \text{normal anion-gap})/(\text{normal serum bicarbonate} - \text{measured serum bicarbonate})$$

A *δ*gap less than one signifies the bicarbonate drop is more pronounced than expected by the anion-gap acidosis. As a result, a nonanion-gap acidosis must also be contributing to the decrease in bicarbonate. A *δ* ratio of 1 to 2 is likely a pure anion-gap acidosis. The range is present because bicarbonate clears at 0.6 mmol/L per 1.0 mmol/L of lactate, whereas the ratio is closer to 1:1 for ketoacidosis. A *δ*ratio greater than 2 suggests that the change in bicarbonate is not significant relative to the change in anion-gap. As a result, the increased buffering must be due to a metabolic alkalosis in addition to the anion-gap acidosis.

C. There are numerous clinical scenarios for mixed metabolic and respiratory disorders where the expected compensation does not occur. The mixed picture can be attributed either to a single disease or multiple simultaneous disease processes. The list of potential interactions is extensive (Table 24.6).

TABLE 24.6	Examples of Mixed Acid–Base Disorders
Disorder	**Example(s)**
Anion-gap and nonanion-gap acidosis	Lactic acidosis and RTA
	Ketoacidosis and severe diarrhea
Anion-gap acidosis and metabolic alkalosis	Lactic acidosis and chronic diuretic use
	Ketoacidosis and continuous vomiting
Nonanion-gap acidosis and metabolic alkalosis	Gastrointestinal illness with vomiting and diarrhea
Anion-gap metabolic acidosis and respiratory acidosis	Lactic acidosis in a COPD patient
	Cardiopulmonary arrest
Anion-gap metabolic acidosis and respiratory alkalosis	Aspirin intoxication

Suggested Readings

Adrogue JH, Madias NE. Management of life-threatening acid-base disorders. First of two parts. *N Engl J Med* 1998;338:26–34.

Adrogue JH, Madias NE. Management of life-threatening acid-base disorders. Second of two parts. *N Engl J Med* 1998;338:107–111.

Berend K, de Vries AP, Gans RO. Physiological approach to assessment of acid–base disturbances. *New Eng J Med* 2015;371:1434–1445.

Corey HE. Stewart and beyond: new models of acid-base balance. *Kidney Int* 2003;64:777–787.

Fencl V, Jabor A, Kazda A, et al. Diagnosis of metabolic acid–base disturbances in critically ill patients. *Am J Respir Crit Care Med* 2000;162:2246–2251.

Fidkowski C, Helstrom J. Diagnosing metabolic acidosis in the critically ill: bridging the anion-gap, Stewart, and base excess models. *Can J Anaesth* 2009;56:247–256.

Guaran C, Steele D. Fluid, electrolytes, and acid–base management. In: Bigatello LM, Alam H, Allain RM, et al, eds. *Critical Care Handbook of the Massachusetts General Hospital*. 5th ed. Philadelphia, PA: Lippincott Williams & Wilkins; 2010:141–149.

Kaplan LJ, Frangos S. Clinical review: Acid–base abnormalities in the intensive care unit. *Crit Care* 2005;9:198–203.

Kellum JA. Clinical review: reunification of acid–base physiology. *Crit Care* 2005;9:500–507.

Neligan P, Deutschman CS. Perioperative acid–base balance. In: Miller RD, Eriksson LI, Fleisher LA, et al, eds. *Miller's Anesthesia*. 7th ed. Philadelphia, PA: Churchill-Livingstone; 2010:1557–1572.

Noritomi DT, Soriano FG, Kellum JA, et al. Metabolic acidosis in patients with severe sepsis and septic shock. a longitudinal quantitative study. *Crit Care Med* 2009;37:2733–2739.

Ring T, Frische S, Nielsen S. Clinical review: renal tubular acidosis—a physicochemical approach. *Crit Care* 2005;9:573–580.

Tiruvoipati R, Botha JA, Pilcher D, et al. Carbon dioxide clearance in critical care. *Anaesth Intensive Care* 2013;41:157–162.

25 Endocrine Abnormalities: Glucose Control, Adrenal Insufficiency, and Thyroid Storm

Alana B. Birner and Kathryn L. Butler

I. INTRODUCTION

A. Recognition of endocrine disorders requires a high index of suspicion among clinicians in the postoperative period. The effects of anesthesia often mask initial symptoms of endocrine abnormalities in the postoperative anesthesia care unit (PACU), necessitating vigilance upon the part of caregivers to initiate early treatment and prevent complications. Ideally, a comprehensive preoperative evaluation of patients alerts clinicians to preexisting endocrine disease and lowers the risk of postoperative adverse events.

II. GLUCOSE CONTROL

A. **Effects of Surgery on Blood Glucose Levels**

1. General anesthesia and surgery trigger a neuroendocrine stress response, with release of epinephrine, glucagon, cortisol, growth hormone, and inflammatory cytokines into the systemic circulation. These hormones function to increase insulin resistance, decrease peripheral glucose utilization, decrease insulin secretion, and increase lipolysis and protein catabolism, ultimately creating a hyperglycemic state. The degree of this hyperglycemia varies between patients and depends upon the type of anesthesia, preoperative comorbidities, and the extent and type of surgery. General anesthesia, for example, disrupts metabolism to a greater extent than epidural anesthesia. Disruption of caloric intake prior to and during surgery also alters the normal hyperglycemic response. Such factors impede prediction of final glycemic balance in the postoperative period.

2. **Hyperglycemia**

   a. Definition: >200 mg/dL in the postoperative area.

   1. associated with increased risk of stroke, congestive heart failure, and morbidity/mortality

   2. associated with increased surgical site infections

   3. associated with cardiac cell death and reduced coronary collateral blood flow by triggering an exaggerated ischemia–reperfusion cellular injury

   4. triggers platelet hyperactivity, increasing thrombosis. This results in increased levels of interleukin-6, interleukin-8, and tumor necrosis factor-α, creating a pro-inflammatory response.

   5. leads to endothelial cell dysfunction, inactivation of nitric oxide, decreased synthesis of prostacyclin, and increased synthesis of endothelin 1, which all decrease local blood flow.

   6. decreases renal tubular absorption capabilities, resulting in hypovolemia secondary to an osmotic diuresis

b. Maintain glycemic target <180 mg/dL for all surgical patients
　　1. More stringent protocols increase the risk of hypoglycemic events, resulting in increased mortality.
　　　　a. Intensive insulin therapy with target blood glucose of 80 to 110 mg/dL increases incidences of severe hypoglycemia and increases mortality when compared to the more permissive blood glucose ranges of 140 to 180 mg/dL (7.8 to 10 mmol/L) and 180 to 200 mg/dL (10 to 11.1 mmol/L).
　　2. General hospitalized population: Aim for fasting glucose of <140 mg/dL (7.8 mmol) and random glucose levels <180 mg/dL (10 mmol/L)
c. Maintain nutrition and electrolyte balance

B. Hypoglycemia

1. Definition: random glucose <40 mg/dL (2.2 mmol/L).
2. "Cut off value" is often debated, but PACU medical staff should be concerned with a level <70 mg/mL.
3. Causes: Most commonly long-acting insulin in patients with difficult to control diabetes
4. Potentially life-threatening: Underdiagnosed in the PACU setting due to sedation and anesthesia. If left untreated, can result in lethal cardiac arrhythmias and death.
　　a. Preoperative identification of patients prone to hypoglycemia significantly lowers risk.
　　　　1. High-risk patients: Past medical history of difficult to control diabetes requiring strict glucose monitoring, a history of uncontrolled glucose levels, or documented frequent hypoglycemic episodes
　　b. Preoperative titration of home diabetes regimen helps to avoid episodes of hypoglycemia in the postoperative setting
　　c. Regular measurement of glucose levels (point of care [POC]) postoperatively ensures prompt treatment of abnormalities
5. Postoperative clinical manifestations
　　a. Early recovery (Phase 1): Symptoms are usually nonspecific, and difficult to recognize. Frequently first detected by monitoring blood glucose levels upon arrive to PACU (in patients with known diabetes)
　　b. Late recovery (Phase 2): Recognition of the following symptoms:
　　　　1. tremor, palpitations, increased arousal, anxiety, sweating, and hunger
　　c. If left untreated, hypoglycemia can result in:
　　　　1. changes in level of consciousness, seizures, coma, and death
6. Treatment
　　a. Early recovery (Phase 1): sedated, anesthetized patient with blood glucose of <70 mg/dL
　　　　1. administer intravenous (IV) dextrose 25 g and repeat blood glucose test in 5 to 10 minutes
　　b. Late recovery (Phase 2): In an awake patient with an intact swallow and gag reflex
　　　　1. 15 g of carbohydrates (glucose tablet, sweetened fruit juice), recheck in 10 minutes or if symptoms resolve
　　c. Late recovery (Phase 2): patients unable to ingest by mouth
　　　　1. 25 g of 50% dextrose IV, recheck blood glucose in 5 to 10 minutes

III. DISORDERS OF GLUCOSE HOMEOSTASIS

A. Hyperglycemia

1. Causes
　　a. Stress hyperglycemia (Hyperglycemic Stress Syndrome)

1. transient elevations in blood glucose due to a catecholamine-induced stress response that occurs during acute illness, in patients with and without a history of diabetes mellitus (DM)
  b. Medication-induced hyperglycemia
    1. caused or aggravated by glucocorticoids, octreotide, vasopressors, and immunosuppressants, in patients with and without a history of DM
  c. Dextrose-containing IV fluids administered in the perioperative phase
  d. Excess counterregulatory hormones, as detailed above
  e. Pancreatic disease with insufficient circulating insulin
  f. Preoperative diabetes
2. Postoperative clinical manifestations
  a. Early recovery (Phase 1): Unexplained diuresis, tachycardia, hypotension, anion gap metabolic acidosis, hyponatremia, and hyperkalemia.
  b. Late recovery (Phase 2): Clinical signs and symptoms are vague, especially following administration of anesthetic agents. At baseline, one-third of patients with DM are asymptomatic. Most common symptoms include polyphagia, polydipsia, polyuria, confusion, and coma.
3. Treatment
  a. Corrective insulin
    1. Sliding scale for stable population
    2. IV insulin infusion for critically ill population (Table 25.1)

B. Diabetic Ketoacidosis (DKA)

1. Precipitated from stress of surgery, or from the peri-operative use of mediations that alter metabolism. DKA is a medical emergency, requiring immediate recognition and intervention.
  a. Triad of hyperglycemia, anion gap metabolic acidosis, and ketonemia. Serum glucose >800 mg/dL (44 mmol/L), predominately 350 to 500 mg/dL (19.4 to 27.8 mmol/L). Can exceed 900 mg/dL (50 mmol/L) in the presence of coma. Commonly evolves rapidly, over a 24-hour period.
  b. Medications that can precipitate DKA include:
    1. glucocorticoids, high-dose thiazide diuretics, sympathomimetic agents, and second-generation "atypical" antipsychotic agents
2. Postoperative clinical manifestations
  a. Neurologic deterioration is seen at a plasma osmolality above 320 to 330 mOsmol/kg. Often are masked by effects of recent anesthesia.

Glucose Values (mg/dL/mmol/L)	Insulin Sensitive		Usual		Insulin Resistant	
	AC	HS	AC	HS	AC	HS
<150/8.3	0	0	0	0	0	0
151–200/8.4–11.1	0	0	2	0	4	2
201–250/11.2–13.9	2	0	4	0	8	4
251–300/13.9–16.6	3	1	6	2	12	6
301–350/16.7–19.4	4	2	8	4	16	8
351–400/19.5–22.2	5	3	10	6	20	10

TABLE 25.1 Sample Subcutaneous Sliding Scale Using Short-Acting Insulin

AC, before meals; HS, bedtime.

b. Physical exam will show decreased skin turgor, dry axillae and oral mucosa, low jugular venous pressure, and tachycardia. If severe, hypotension due to volume depletion. Kussmaul respirations and fruity odor on breath due to compensatory hyperventilation and exhaled acetone. Abdominal pain is common, and requires reevaluation if it does not resolve with treatment of the acidosis.

c. Nitroprusside testing is done to determine if serum ketone levels are responsible for anion gap acidosis. A 4+ reaction with serum diluted 1:1 is highly suggestive of ketoacidosis. A 4+ reaction in more diluted serum provides evidence of even higher concentrations of acetoacetic acid.

d. Laboratory changes: Hyperglycemia, hyperosmolality, a high anion gap metabolic acidosis, mild hyponatremia, and potassium deficit around 300 to 600 mEq.

3. Treatment
   a. Correction of the fluid and electrolyte abnormalities and the administration of insulin
      1. Fluid repletion with isotonic saline to expand extracellular volume and stabilize cardiovascular status
         a. without presence of shock: rate of 15 to 20 mL/kg lean body weight per hour, for the first few hours, with a maximum of <50 mL/kg in the first 4 hours
         b. Potassium replacement
      2. Initiate immediately if the serum potassium is <5.3 mEq/L.
      3. IV KCl at 20 to 40 mEq/hour
         a. Hyperglycemia correction
      4. Low-dose IV insulin should be given to all patients in DKA with a serum potassium ≥3.3 mEq/L. The only indication for delaying insulin therapy is serum potassium below 3.3 mEq/L, because insulin will worsen the hypokalemia.
      5. IV bolus of regular insulin (0.1 U/kg body weight) followed within 5 minutes by continuous infusion of regular insulin of 0.1 U/kg/hour
   b. Metabolic acidosis
      1. if arterial pH <6.90, treat with 100 mEq of sodium bicarbonate in 400 mL sterile water with 20 mEq of potassium chloride (if the serum potassium is less than 5.3 mEq/L) administered over 2 hours.
      2. Anion gap should correct with volume repletion and correction of hyperglycemia.
      3. Close monitoring of phosphorus levels should be initiated

C. **Diabetes Insipidus (DI)**
   1. Central DI is most commonly seen in PACU setting
      a. Decreased release of antidiuretic hormone (ADH) from hypothalamus, causing excretion of a relatively dilute urine.
   2. Nephrogenic DI
      a. Inadequate response of the kidney to ADH.
   3. Causes
      a. History of traumatic brain injury, stroke, or lithium dependence. Administration of sodium bicarbonate solutions. Renal water loss due to renal disease or the use of diuretics. Gastrointestinal fluid losses through nasogastric suction. Water losses through fever, drainages, and open wounds.
   4. Postoperative manifestations
      a. Changes in mental status, restlessness, irritability, lethargy, confusion, and somnolence. Patients complain of intense thirst.

5. Management
   a. Desmopressin: two-amino acid substitute of ADH with potent antidiuretic activity, but no vasopressor activity. Can be administered intranasally, in an oral tablet form or in a parenteral formulation at a dose of 5 μg. This can be titrated in 5 μg increments depending upon the response. The daily maintenance dose is about 5 to 20 μg once or twice a day.

D. **Specific Postoperative Patient Populations and Considerations**
   1. DM
      a. Patients with a history of DM (types 1 and 2) are more frequently hospitalized and are more likely to undergo surgical procedures with extended hospital length of stay than patients without DM.
         1. Schedule surgery as early in the day as possible, to minimize disruption of management routine while being nil per os.
         2. If the patient is tolerating a normal diet postoperatively, it is usually acceptable to return to standard home medication management
         3. Meformin should NOT be reinitiated in patients with a history of renal insufficiency, hepatic impairment, or congestive heart failure, until documentation of return to baseline function
         4. Sulfonylureas increase risk the risk for hypoglycemia, and should only be given after eating is tolerated
         5. Thiazolidinediones should be held if concerns for congestive heart failure, fluid retention, or liver function abnormalities arise.
         6. Glucagon-like peptide-1 (GLP-1) analogs may alter gastrointestinal motility, increasing the risk of postoperative nausea and vomiting
         7. Patients with DM are more susceptible to postoperative infections.
   2. DM type 1/insulin-dependent type 2
      a. Increases risk of ketoacidosis and hyperglycemic events
      b. Management for short procedures (less than 2 hours):
         1. continue subcutaneous insulin regimen postoperatively
         2. resume home dose of short- or rapid-acting insulin postoperatively, prior to eating
      c. Patients who require an intraoperative insulin (regular) infusion:
         1. Continue infusion postoperatively in patients who do not resume eating
         2. POC testing should be done every hour, or more frequently if unstable
         3. When solid food is tolerated, patients can be switched to subcutaneous insulin and the infusion discontinued
         4. The first dose of subcutaneous insulin should be given prior to discontinuing an IV infusion
      d. Patients who require insulin (subcutaneous or IV) in the early postoperative phase:
         1. should be given IV dextrose (5 to 10 g of glucose/hour in water or in one half isotonic saline solution) to prevent hypoglycemia
   3. Non–insulin-dependent diabetes
      a. Patients with DM II who are managed with diet alone:
         1. Usually do not require insulin therapy postoperatively
         2. Laboratory or POC glucose levels should be obtained immediately in the PACU
         3. If glucose levels rise over target range, supplemental short- (regular) or rapid-acting insulin (lispro and glulisine) may be considered to correct abnormality

    b. Patients with DM II managed with oral hypoglycemic agents or non-insulin injectables:

      1. Patients with glycated hemoglobin A1C <7.0% do not require insulin therapy for procedures under 2 hours

      2. If hyperglycemia does develop, treat with supplemental short- or rapid-acting insult, subcutaneously every 6 hours.

      3. Supplemental insulin should be administered until patient is tolerating a diet and can resume home oral agents

    c. Non-diabetic patients:

      1. unanticipated rises in postoperative glucose levels may signal undiagnosed DM or pre-diabetes, and should be evaluated post-discharge

  4. Recent history of glucocorticoid use

    a. Exogenous glucocorticoids worsen known DM and can induce hyperglycemia in patients with or without a history of DM

  5. Emergency surgery

    a. Increases the risk of type 1 diabetics developing DKA

    b. Increases the risk of type 2 diabetics developing nonketotic hyperosmolar syndrome

    c. In emergency situations, patients often miss their home insulin dose. In addition, decreased normal consumption of calories and excessive pathologic stress can disrupt the normal counter-regulatory hormone balance. Diabetic patients cannot mount an appropriate insulin increase in response to these changes, with resultant hyperglycemia

IV. POSTOPERATIVE ADRENAL INSUFFICIENCY (AI)

A. Effects of Surgery on Adrenal Hormones

1. Adrenal insufficiency occurs in response to a major emotional or physiologic stressor. In the PACU setting, this includes extreme psychologic stress, trauma, withdrawal from alcohol or opioids, infection, general anesthesia, or surgery. Patients are then unable to secrete adequate amounts of cortisol to maintain hemodynamic stability. During critical periods, increase in circulating cortisol with a decrease in adrenocorticotropic hormone (ACTH) is caused by a decrease in clearance and potentially stimulation of cytokines. Early recognition and treatment are vital, because cortisol deficiency is associated with increased morbidity and mortality during critical illness. Currently, there is no way to consistently identify patients at risk for developing AI during a surgical procedure

2. Secondary AI is the most common form of AI seen in the PACU. Prior to surgical stressors, patients are asymptomatic.

3. Primary AI should be considered in the setting of severe injury (trauma), sepsis, or hemorrhage (Fig. 25.1).

B. Causes

1. Primary AI

    a. Autoimmune (Addisonuffi trauma, infection, fibrosis, bilateral adrenal infarction or hemorrhage, metastatic disease, drugs, and hereditary)

2. Secondary AI

    a. Adrenal atrophy due to acute or chronic glucocorticoid therapies (patient receiving physiologic or pharmacologic doses of glucocorticoid), pituitary/hypothalamic diseases, ACTH deficiency, and surgical interventions

C. Manifestations Following Surgical Stressor

1. Sudden hemodynamic instability (shock)

    a. Potential loss of 20% of circulating volume resulting in decreased tissue perfusion and lactic acidosis

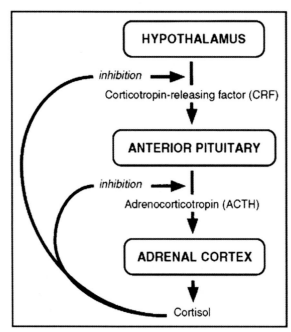

FIGURE 25.1 Primary adrenal insufficiency.

2. Hypotension that is severe and refractory to interventions
   a. High-output circulatory failure with elevated cardiac output and index, normal pulmonary artery occlusion pressure, and decreased systemic vascular resistance
   b. Hypotension refractory to treatment with volume and vasopressors
3. Progressive hyponatremia, hyperkalemia, and hypoglycemia.
4. Nonspecific symptoms (masked following anesthesia): anorexia, vomiting, weakness, fatigue, fever, and confusion
5. Diagnosis should be considered when patient has one or more known risk factors

D. Treatment/Management
1. Rapid infusion of normal saline to correct dehydration and hypovolemia
2. Concurrent therapy focuses on increasing circulating cortisol levels
   a. Laboratory: Obtain baseline plasma cortisol levels (ACTH renin, aldosterone) prior to treatment, as well as serum electrolytes, complete blood count, glucose, blood urea nitrogen, and creatinine to assess electrolyte abnormalities
3. Vigilant correction of any electrolyte abnormalities on an individualized basis. Hyponatremia, hypokalemia, and acidosis are common.
4. Response to medical intervention is usually seen within several hours
5. Identify and treat precipitating cause

E. Specific Patient Populations:
1. Known AI undergoing major procedures
   a. Ensure hydrocortisone 100 mg given preoperatively, followed by IV doses of 50 to 100 mg every 6 to 8 hours, to be tapered until condition improves

F. Suspected AI Without Prior Diagnosis

1. Dexamethasone 4 to 10 mg can be given as an IV bolus immediately
   a. does not cause false reading of serum cortisol levels
   b. Fludrocortisone, a mineralocorticoid, may also be needed for complete correction, because dexamethasone has no aldosterone effect.

V. POSTOPERATIVE THYROID STORM

A. Effect of Surgery on Thyroid Hormones

1. Surgical stressors can cause life-threatening complications when hyperthyroidism is untreated. Unrecognized hyperthyroidism commonly presents postoperatively with severe and sudden thyrotoxicosis. High-risk populations include patients with uncontrolled hyperthyroidism presenting for nonelective or emergency surgery. It is vital that a thorough history and physical be performed, when possible, prior to intervention to evaluate the risk of thyroid abnormalities.

B. Causes

1. Undiagnosed hyperthyroidism (Grave disease, toxic multinodular goiter) or inadequate hyperthyroidism treatment in patients with a surgical stressor

C. Manifestations

1. Physical exam alone is often inadequate to diagnose hyperthyroidism. Nonspecific symptoms of hyperthyroidism include:
   a. mental status changes, sweating, heat intolerance, fatigue, muscle weakness, dry eyes, leg swelling, tachycardia and tachyarrhythmias, warm moist skin, muscle tremor, systolic hypertension, and widened pulse pressure
2. Specific physical indicators include:
   a. thyroid bruits (in the setting of toxic goiter), pretibial edema, and atrial fibrillation
3. Laboratory abnormalities
   a. hypercalcemia, hypokalemia, hyperglycemia, hypocholesterolemia, microcytic anemia, lymphocytosis, granulocytopenia, hyperbilirubinemia, and elevated alkaline phosphatase.
4. Diagnosis
   a. Clinical confirmation with the following serum thyroid studies:

Test	Hyperthyroid
TSH	low
Total T4	high
Total T3	high
Reverse T3	high
Free T4	high

b. Other studies include:
   1. complete blood cell count, electrolyte levels, urinalysis, chest radiograph, and electrocardiogram
   2. Additional studies ruling out infectious processes should be performed prior to confirmation
5. Treatment
   a. Do not wait for laboratory results to begin treatment if there is sufficient clinical suspicion.
   b. General supportive care
      1. IV fluids to restore intravascular volume
      2. Acetaminophen for hyperthermia
      3. Cooling blankets
      4. Magnesium salts to reduce risk of cardiac arrhythmias

    c. Thyroid hormone synthesis inhibition
       1. Proplthiouracil: Up to 1,000 mg loading dose followed by 200 to
          300 mg orally or via nasogastric tube every 4 to 6 hours.
          a. Up to 6 to 8 weeks until return to a euthyroid state
       2. Methimazole: 20 to 30 mg orally or via nasogastric tube every 4 to
          6 hours. Achieves a euthyroid state more quickly than PTU and
          has a lower incidence of agranulocytosis, hepatitis, and vasculitis.
    d. Iodide therapy
       1. Iodide inhibits thyroid hormone synthesis (Wolff-Chaikoff effect).
          Delay iodide therapy at least 4 hours after beginning PTU therapy.

Suggested Readings

American Diabetes Association. Standards of medical care in diabetes—2014. *Diabetes Care* 2014;37(suppl 1):S14–S80.

Canadian Diabetes Association Clinical Practice Guidelines. 2013. Available at: http://guidelines.diabetes.ca/App_Themes/CDACPG/resources/cpg_2013_full_en.pdf. Accessed April 24, 2013.

Clement S, Braithwaite SS, Magee MF, et al. Management of diabetes and hyperglycemia in hospitals. *Diabetes Care* 2004;27(2):553–591.

Connery LE, Coursin DB. Assessment and therapy of selected endocrine disorders. *Anesthesiol Clin North Am* 2004;22:93–123.

Cronin CC, Callaghan N, Kearney PJ, et al. Addison disease in patients treated with glucocorticoid therapy. *Arch Intern Med* 1997;157:456–458.

Cryer PE, Axelrod L, Grossman AB, et al. Evaluation and management of adult hypoglycemic disorders: an Endocrine Society Clinical Practice Guideline. *J Clin Endocrinol Metab* 2009;94:709–728.

Dungan KM, Braithwaite SS, Preiser JC. Stress hyperglycaemia. *Lancet* 2009;373 (9677):1798–1807.

Frisch A, Chandra P, Smiley D, et al. Prevalence and clinical outcome of hyperglycemia in the perioperative period in noncardiac surgery. *Diabetes Care* 2010;33:1783–1788.

Jacobs TP, Whitlock RT, Edsall J, et al. Addisonian crisis while taking high-dose glucocorticoids. An unusual presentation of primary adrenal failure in two patients with underlying inflammatory diseases. *JAMA* 1988;260:2082–2084.

Joshi GP, Chung F, Vann MA, et al. Society for Ambulatory Anesthesia consensus statement on perioperative blood glucose management in diabetic patients undergoing ambulatory surgery. *Anesth Analg* 2010;111:1378–1387.

King JT Jr, Goulet JL, Perkal MF, et al. Glycemic control and infections in patients with diabetes undergoing noncardiac surgery. *Ann Surg* 2011;253:158–165.

Kitabchi AE, Umpierrez GE, Miles JM, et al. Hyperglycemic crises in adult patients with diabetes. *Diabetes Care* 2009;32:1335–1343.

Lattermann R, Carli F, Wykes L, et al. Perioperative glucose infusion and the catabolic response to surgery: the effect of epidural block. *Anesth Analg* 2003;96:555–562.

Mah PM, Jenkins RC, Rostami-Hodjegan A. Weight-related dosing, timing and monitoring hydrocortisone replacement therapy in patients with adrenal insufficiency. *Clin Endocrinol* 2004;61:367–375.

Makaryus AN, McFarlane SI. Diabetes insipidus: diagnosis and treatment of a complex disease. *Cleve Clin J Med* 2006;73(1):65–71.

Moghissi ES, Korytkowski MT, DiNardo M, et al. American Association of Clinical Endocrinologists and American Diabetes Association consensus statement on inpatient glycemic control. *Diabetes Care* 2009;32(6):1119–1131.

Schricker T, Gougeon R, Eberhart L, et al. Type 2 diabetes mellitus and the catabolic response to surgery. *Anesthesiology* 2005;102:320–326.

Seaquist ER, Anderson J, Childs B, et al. Hypoglycemia and diabetes: a report of a workgroup of the American Diabetes Association and the Endocrine Society. *J Clin Endocrinol Metab* 2013;98(5):1845–1859.

The NICE-SUGAR Study Investigators. Hypoglycemia and risk of death in critically ill patients. *N Engl J Med* 2012;367(12):1108–1118.

Umpierrez GE, Hellman R, Korytkowski MT, et al. Management of hyperglycemia in hospitalized patients in non-critical care setting: an Endocrine Society Clinical Practice Guideline. *J Clin Endocrinol Metab* 2012;97(1):16–38.

Gastrointestinal Complications

Christina Anne Jelly and D. Dante Yeh

I. INTRODUCTION

A. Postoperative gastrointestinal (GI) complications occur most commonly following abdominal and pelvic operations. However, GI complications may occur after any type of operation and may be associated with significant morbidity and mortality. Complications range from benign and self-limiting, such as postoperative nausea and vomiting, to severe and life threatening, such as GI bleeding and abdominal compartment syndrome. In this chapter, we will review the causes, risk factors, diagnostic workup, and treatment options for patients with postoperative GI complications that may be encountered in the postanesthetic care unit. Postoperative nausea and vomiting is discussed separately in Chapter 15. We will not discuss postoperative GI complications that occur more remotely postoperatively, such as bowel obstruction due to adhesions, incisional hernias, and enterocutaneous fistulas.

II. GI BLEEDING

A. Significant postoperative GI bleeding is an uncommon but potentially serious complication of surgery. Causes of postoperative GI bleeding may be divided into three broad categories:
   1. Bleeding secondary to the operation or complications of the operation
   2. Bleeding resulting from surgical stress or complications of the operation exacerbating the bleeding risk of a preexisting source
   3. Bleeding unrelated to the operation and occurring incidentally in the postoperative period.

B. In the immediate postoperative period, the most common etiology of bleeding is as a direct result of the operation or complications of the operation.

C. Most episodes of postoperative GI bleeding are self-limited. Minor postoperative bleeding occurs frequently and often without clinical recognition. However, significant GI bleeding, defined as overt bleeding associated with hemodynamic disturbances, demands immediate attention. The initial evaluation of a patient with GI bleeding should focus on hemodynamic stability and resuscitation in parallel with diagnostic evaluation for the cause of bleeding. The initial goals should be to determine the severity of bleeding, triage patients to the appropriate setting, initiate resuscitation, and determine the source of bleeding.

D. The initial assessment includes history, physical exam, surgical and postoperative course review, laboratory data, and vital signs for hemodynamic stability, keeping in mind that tachycardia and hypotension may not manifest until a significant amount of the patient's blood volume has been lost. The amount of blood lost and the rate of ongoing blood loss should be estimated to establish the degree of resuscitative measures. At least two large-bore peripheral intravenous (IVs) should be placed. Management of hemorrhage is detailed in Chapter 21 and may be referred to for further details.

E. GI bleeding is often divided into upper and lower GI bleeding. Upper GI bleeding (UGIB), defined as occurring proximal to the ligament of Treitz, may present with hematemesis or melena. Intubation may be required to protect the airway in cases of high-volume UGIB. Esophagogastroduodenoscopy (EGD) to identify the source of bleeding may be required depending on the preceding operation. Better outcomes are associated with patients who are well resuscitated prior to endoscopic evaluation. If the antecedent surgery involved the upper GI tract, return to the operating room for evaluation may be required, depending on the rate of ongoing bleeding.

F. Acute lower GI bleeding occurs distal to the ligament of Treitz and may present with hematochezia or melena. Urgent colonoscopy is the examination of choice after an UGIB source has been excluded. Treatment depends on the source of bleeding, and often patients with exsanguinating lower GI bleeding will require immediate re-operation.

G. The most common sources of bleeding in postoperative patients include bleeding from intestinal anastomosis, ischemic colitis, and preexisting lesions such as ulcers and diverticuli.

III. STRESS-RELATED MUCOSAL DISEASE

A. Most episodes of GI bleeding in critically ill patients are caused by gastric ulcerations from stress-related mucosal injury. Risk factors for stress-related mucosal ulcerations include prolonged mechanical ventilation, coagulopathy, perioperative hypotension, sepsis, spinal cord injuries, severe burns, shock, hepatic failure, renal failure, polytrauma, organ transplantation, and history of GI bleed or ulcers.

B. Prophylaxis against stress ulceration should be initiated in critically ill patients who are at high risk for GI bleeding. According to guideline recommendations from the American Society of Health Systems Pharmacists, stress ulcer prophylaxis should be administered to patients with any of the following characteristics: coagulopathy (platelet levels below 50,000, INR $>$1.5, prothrombin time (PTT) over 2 times the upper limit of normal), mechanical ventilation $>$48 hours, history of GI bleeding, traumatic brain or spinal cord injury, or burns. Additionally, stress ulcer prophylaxis should also be administered to critically ill patients with two or more of the following minor criteria: sepsis, intensive care unit (ICU) stay over 1 week, occult GI bleeding over 6 days, and steroids (equivalent of 250 mg of IV hydrocortisone or greater).

C. Critically ill patients who are at high risk of GI bleeding should not receive stress ulcer prophylaxis if they are receiving enteral nutrition. Observational data have demonstrated that those on enteral nutrition are unlikely to benefit from pharmacologic stress ulcer prophylaxis and that it may even be harmful.

IV. POSTOPERATIVE ILEUS

A. Postoperative ileus refers to the lack of coordinated propulsive motor activity of the GI tract resulting in intolerance of oral intake and obstipation without any definitive mechanical obstruction that occurs following surgery.

B. Some degree of postoperative ileus is a normal response to abdominal surgery, and is termed *physiologic ileus*. It is usually benign and self-limiting. Pathologic postoperative ileus, however, usually prolongs hospital stay and places a significant burden on the health care system.

C. Risk factors for postoperative ileus include extensive operative manipulation (handling of the bowel and tissue trauma), small bowel injury, perioperative opioid use, open (versus laparoscopic) abdominal surgery, delayed enteral nutrition or nasogastric tube (NGT) placement, intra-abdominal inflammation, intra- and postoperative bleeding, prolonged operative time, and hypoalbuminemia.

D. Postoperative ileus typically presents with abdominal distension, bloating, and diffuse abdominal discomfort. Patients may also have nausea, vomiting, and inability to tolerate an oral diet. Physical exam is usually remarkable for abdominal distension and tympany with variable reduction of bowel sounds and diffuse abdominal tenderness.

E. Ileus is usually diagnosed clinically. Abdominal imaging may be useful if small or large bowel mechanical obstruction is suspected. Upright abdominal radiographic films may demonstrate dilated loops of small bowel with air in the colon and rectum. Abdominal x-rays may differentiate ileus from a small bowel obstruction, which is more likely to demonstrate loops of small bowel with air–fluid levels and an absence of colonic or rectal air.

F. Treatment of ileus is largely supportive. Inciting factors such as opioid use should be removed if possible. Fluid and electrolyte abnormalities should be corrected. Bowel rest and bowel decompression are the usual cornerstones of management of ileus. Depending on the severity and duration of the ileus, the patient may require nutritional support in the form of total parenteral nutrition (TPN). Alvimopan, a novel peripheral μ-opioid antagonist, has also been employed in select circumstances to accelerate GI recovery time and shorten the duration of ileus.

G. Ileus is best prevented by minimizing narcotic use and the inciting surgical risk factors that lead to its development. Thoracic epidural analgesia prior to abdominal surgery has shown promise as a means to prevent postoperative ileus.

V. MESENTERIC ISCHEMIA

A. Mesenteric ischemia is a rare complication; however, when it occurs, diagnosis is often delayed, and thus mortality remains high. Mesenteric ischemia occurs when the intestinal oxygen demand exceeds supply. This sets off a cascade leading to ischemia, inflammation, translocation of gut flora, and eventually septic shock. It can occur in the small intestines, colon, or both, and it may be acute or chronic.

B. Mesenteric ischemia may result from reduction in circulating blood volume, vasoconstriction due to vasoactive medications, or obstruction of blood flow. Thus, it is often divided into nonocclusive and occlusive disease as follows:

1. Nonocclusive disease is caused by inadequate blood flow to the region of ischemia with no definitive obstruction. Examples include hypovolemia, shock, heart failure, or pharmacologically induced constriction caused by vasoactive drugs, all of which result in relative mucosal hypoxia or anoxia.

2. Occlusive disease is caused by a definitive mechanical obstruction that may be in the form of arterial emboli or thrombus, venous thrombus, trauma, or strangulation.

C. Risk factors of acute mesenteric ischemia include surgical devascularization, hypercoagulable states, hypovolemia, and operations associated with a high degree of emboli such as aortic surgery. For example, patients undergoing endovascular aortic aneurysm procedures are at risk not only because of occlusion of mesenteric vessels due to graft placement but also because of dislodgement of atheromatous debris during manipulation of wires or grafts during repair. Patients with underlying risk factors of chronic mesenteric ischemia are even more susceptible to acute mesenteric ischemia. Risk factors for chronic mesenteric ischemia include atherosclerosis, fibromuscular dysplasia, inflammatory disease, and radiation-induced vasculitis.

D. The pathogenesis and natural history of mesenteric ischemia are often divided into three stages: hyperactive, paralytic, and shock. Of note, prior to overt ischemia, small intestinal blood flow may be cut in half, and the bowel can usually compensate by increasing oxygen extraction.

1. The *hyperactive stage* is the first stage and is characterized by abdominal pain and bloody stools. In acute occlusive mesenteric ischemia, this begins shortly after occlusion of the vessel. This is the beginning phase when the patient exhibits the classic "abdominal pain out of proportion to clinical exam." The initial ischemic insult leads initially to hyperperistalsis of the bowel and eventually a spastic reflex ileus.

2. The *paralytic phase* follows and is marked by progression to a hypotonic ileus with dilated loops of small bowel visible on x-ray imaging. Abdominal pain becomes more continuous and diffuse, and as bowel motility decreases, abdominal distension worsens.

3. The *shock phase* develops as fluids begin to leak through the mucosal and serosal linings of the gut and results in intravascular hypovolemia and shock. If ischemia is total or near total for over 8 to 16 hours, transmural infarction results.

E. Diagnosis is often delayed as signs and symptoms of mesenteric ischemia may not develop until late in the disease course. Thus, for those at high risk of mesenteric ischemia, one must have a high degree of suspicion once early nonspecific abdominal symptoms develop.

1. Laboratory studies may demonstrate lactic acidemia or leukocytosis. However, absence of lactatemia or leukocytosis does not rule out mesenteric ischemia.

2. Abdominal radiographic imaging may demonstrate gas in the bowel wall, although this is a late finding. Most commonly, abdominal x-rays are unremarkable.

3. Duplex ultrasonography may be helpful initially; however, as hypotonic ileus and subsequent shock develops, air within the bowel interferes with the exam.

4. Computed tomographic (CT) abdominal studies may be normal, again, depending on the stage. Late CT findings of mesenteric ischemia include bowel dilatation, mesenteric edema, bowel wall thickening, intramural gas, and mesenteric stranding.

5. Angiography is useful to differentiate occlusive from nonocclusive mesenteric ischemia. It is also often therapeutic, because vasodilators may be infused locally to mitigate the effects of nonocclusive mesenteric ischemia.

F. Initial management of patients with suspected acute mesenteric ischemia is to optimize intestinal blood flow and oxygen delivery to ischemic tissues. Patients with mesenteric ischemia should be kept nil per os (NPO), receive nasogastric decompression, and receive fluid therapy to maintain adequate intravascular volume and visceral perfusion. Vasopressors should be avoided, if possible, as they may exacerbate ongoing ischemia. Supplemental oxygen is also recommended to increase oxygen delivery to ischemic tissues. Further treatment options depend on the etiology of the mesenteric ischemia, as well as the hemodynamic stability of the patient.

1. Unless absolutely contraindicated, antithrombotic therapy is initiated to limit thrombus propagation, usually with an unfractioned heparin infusion. Antiplatelets may be added as an adjunct.

Systemic anticoagulation should be initiated only after discussion with the surgical team in the postoperative patient.

2. Thrombolysis via intra-arterial infusion of agents such as streptokinase, urokinase, or recombinant tissue plasminogen activator may be instilled locally to the thrombus or embolus in acute occlusive mesenteric ischemia.

3. Patients with nonocclusive mesenteric ischemia may be treated with intra-arterial instillation of papaverine, a vasodilator and antispasmodic.

4. Patients with peritoneal signs and evidence of bowel ischemia or bowel infarction should undergo exploratory laparotomy and bowel that is infarcted must be resected.

5. Patients often require a "second look" operation in 24 to 48 hours following the index exploratory laparotomy to look for further nonviable bowel.

Suggested Readings

ASHP Therapeutic Guidelines on Stress Ulcer Prophylaxis. ASHP Commission on Therapeutics and approved by the ASHP Board of Directors on November 14, 1998. *Am Health Syst Pharm* 1999;56(4):347–379.

Bohm B, Milsom JW, Fazio VW. Postoperative intestinal motility following conventional and laparoscopic intestinal surgery. *Arch Surg* 1995;130(4):415–419.

Bosch TJA, Teijin JA, Willigendael EM, et al. Endovascular aneurysm repair is superior to open surgery for ruptured abdominal aortic aneurysms in EVAR-suitable patients. *J Vasc Surg* 2010;52(1):13–18.

Cook DJ, Fuller HD, Guyatt GH, et al. Risk factors for gastrointestinal bleeding in critically ill patients. *N Engl J Med* 1994;330(6):377–381.

Holte K, Kehlet H. Postoperative ileus: a preventable event. *Br J Surg* 2000;87(11):1480–1493.

Kingham TP, Pachter HL. Colonic anastomotic leak: risk factors, diagnosis, and treatment. *J Am Coll Surg* 2009;208(2):269–278.

Lewis SJ, Egger M, Sylvester PA, et al. Early enteral feeding versus "nil by mouth" after gastrointestinal surgery: systemic review and meta-analysis of controlled trials. *BMJ* 2001;323(7316):773.

Marik PE, Vasu T, Hirani A, et al. Stress ulcer prophylaxis in the new millennium: a systematic review and meta-analysis. *Crit Care Med* 2010;38(11):2222–2228.

Raff T, Germann G, Hartmann B. The value of early enteral nutrition in the prophylaxis of stress ulceration in the severely burned patient. *Burns* 1997;23(4):313–318.

Wolff BG, Michelassi F, Gerkin TM, et al. Alvimopan, a novel, peripherally acting mu opioid antagonist: results of a multicenter, randomized, double-blind, placebo-controlled, phase II trial of major abdominal surgery and post-operative ileus. *Ann Surg* 2004;240:728–734.

Allergy and Anaphylaxis During the Postoperative Period

Matthew Sigakis

I. INTRODUCTION

Immediate hypersensitivity reactions to anesthetic and associated agents used during the perioperative period have been reported with increasing frequency. The signs and symptoms of allergic reaction range from slight rash or pruritus to significant hypotension, bronchospasm, and cardiovascular collapse. These may be related to exposures prior to arriving in the postanesthesia care unit (PACU), presenting as a delayed phenomenon, or may result from an initial exposure within the PACU. Although certain sources of exposure are more common perioperatively (Table 27.1), it is important to emphasize that any agent may be the cause.

The diagnosis of allergic reaction or anaphylaxis may be delayed because the presenting signs are often nonspecific. Moreover, recent surgical intervention, anesthetic medications, and underlying comorbidities may complicate the clinical picture. Review of procedural, anesthesia, and PACU medical records is usually helpful in determining a potential allergen exposure.

Identification of allergic reaction or anaphylaxis requires a high index of suspicion and constant vigilance in the PACU, enabling the clinician to intervene promptly, stabilize the patient, address the underlying etiology, and enact a safe plan for continued care and follow-up.

II. DEFINITIONS

The World Allergy Organization (WAO) defines *hypersensitivity* as "objectively reproducible symptoms or signs initiated by exposure to a defined stimulus at a dose tolerated by normal persons." The term *allergy*, more specifically, represents an immune-mediated process. *Nonallergic* hypersensitivity reactions (also called pseudoallergic reactions) occur with similar symptoms and signs, but without any known immune system involvement.

TABLE 27.1	Perioperative Exposures Most Commonly Associated with Allergic Reaction	
Medications	**Other Exposures**	
NMBAs	Latex	
Antibiotics	Blood products	
Barbiturates	Aniline dyes	
Opioids	Contrast	
Heparin	Chlorhexidine	
Protamine	Betadine	
NSAIDs	Adhesives/tape	
Oxytocin		

NMBAs, neuromuscular blocking agents; NSAIDs, nonsteroidal anti-inflammatory drugs.

Immune-mediated allergic reactions are either immediate or delayed. There are four classifications:

A. Type I—immediate onset. Due to immunoglobulin E (IgE)-mediated activation of mast cells and basophils.

B. Type II—delayed onset. Due to antibody-mediated cell destruction, immunoglobulin G (IgG) most common.

C. Type III—delayed onset. Due to immune complex (IgG:drug) deposition and complement activation.

D. Type IV—delayed onset. T cell-mediated reaction.

Anaphylaxis traditionally has reflected IgE-mediated reactions, whereas *anaphylactoid* represented IgE independent reactions. However, because the clinical presentation of these conditions is indistinguishable and the terminology is often confused, the WAO recently discarded these definitions in favor of *immunologic anaphylaxis* and *nonimmunologic anaphylaxis* as follows:

A. Immunologic anaphylaxis is immune-mediated; allergic hypersensitivity reaction; mast cell or basophil degranulation involving antibodies or immune complexes.

B. Nonimmunologic anaphylaxis is nonimmune-mediated; nonallergic hypersensitivity reaction; mast cell or basophil degranulation independent of antibodies or immune complexes.

In general, the term *anaphylaxis* represents an acute process with potentially life-threatening symptoms resulting from the release of mediators from mast cells and basophils.

III. **EPIDEMIOLOGY**

While the incidence of immunologic and nonimmunologic anaphylaxis has not been specifically studied in the PACU, prior data indicate that approximately 1:10,000 anesthetics will result in an anaphylactic reaction. However, the nonspecific signs of anaphylaxis likely make it underrecognized and underreported. A recent study determined the overall incidence of intraoperative hypersensitivity reactions to be approximately 1:700 patients, and severe hypersensitivity reactions to be approximately 1:4,500 patients.

Perioperative hypersensitivity reactions have been reported to be higher in females, patients with lower body mass index, preexisting medication allergies, and multiple exposures to the same or related antibiotics. There are also genetic associations between human leukocyte antigen alleles and susceptibility to drug hypersensitivity.

IV. **PATHOPHYSIOLOGY**

A. Immunologic anaphylaxis: Following an initial sensitization, reexposure generates an immune-mediated reaction that results in the release of inflammatory mediators from mast cells and basophils; IgE antibody-mediated reactions being the most rapid in onset. Common perioperative medications/exposures causing immunologic anaphylaxis include neuromuscular blocking drugs, latex, and antibiotics.

B. Nonimmunologic anaphylaxis: Activation of mast cells and basophils occurs without evidence of immunologic involvement and, as a result, may occur on first exposure rather than require a prerequisite exposure for sensitization. Common examples include vancomycin, morphine, and cold temperature exposure. Of note, any agent that can generate a nonimmunologic reaction also has the potential to generate an immune-mediated reaction.

V. **CLINICAL SIGNIFICANCE**

A. **Anaphylaxis**

The National Institute of Allergy and Infectious Disease and the Food Allergy and Anaphylaxis Network have established historic and clinical

TABLE 27.2	Clinical Criteria for Establishing Diagnosis of Anaphylaxis
Any One Below	**Subcriteria**
Acute onset of illness (minutes to hours) with involvement in skin, mucosal tissue, or both (e.g., generalized hives, pruritus or flushing, swollen lips–tongue–uvula)	At least one: a. Respiratory compromise (e.g., dyspnea, wheeze–bronchospasm, stridor, reduced peak expiratory flow, hypoxemia) b. Reduced blood pressure (BP) or associated symptoms of end-organ dysfunction (e.g., hypotonia [collapse], syncope, incontinence)
Two or more of the following that occur rapidly after exposure to a likely allergen for that patient (minutes to several hours)	At least two: a. Involvement of the skin-mucosal tissue (e.g., generalized hives, itch-flush, swollen lips–tongue–uvula) b. Respiratory compromise (e.g., dyspnea, wheeze–bronchospasm, stridor, reduced peak expiratory flow, hypoxemia) c. Reduced BP or associated symptoms (e.g., hypotonia [collapse], syncope, incontinence) d. Persistent gastrointestinal symptoms (e.g., cramps, abdominal pain, vomiting)
Reduced BP after exposure to known allergen for that patient (minutes to several hours)	a. Infants and children: low systolic BP (age specific) or greater than 30% decrease in systolic BP (see symposium report for definitions). b. Adults: systolic BP of less than 90 mm Hg or greater than 30% decrease from that person's baseline

Adapted from the Second Symposium on the Definition and Management of Anaphylaxis: Summary Report—Second National Institute of Allergy and Infectious Disease/Food Allergy and Anaphylaxis Network Symposium, 2006.

criteria to help identify cases of anaphylaxis (Table 27.2). These criteria emphasize the rapid onset (minutes to hours) of cutaneous, respiratory, gastrointestinal, or hemodynamic symptoms that may occur after exposure. Additional signs and symptoms reported in the literature include fever, tachycardia, bradycardia, and pulmonary hypertension. Although cutaneous manifestations are often associated with anaphylaxis, they may not be significant and initially go undetected.

Comorbidities such as asthma, chronic obstructive pulmonary disease, upper respiratory tract infection, and patients taking β-blocker medications may experience exacerbated bronchoconstriction and angioedema during anaphylaxis. Patients with coronary artery disease, cardiomyopathy, or those taking long-acting antihypertensive medications such as angiotensin converting enzyme (ACE) inhibitors/angiotensin receptor blockers may decompensate more rapidly.

B. Transfusion Reactions

Although anaphylaxis during blood product transfusion is rare, it is more common in patients with IgA deficiency. Washed red blood cells should be transfused in patients with a history of transfusion anaphylaxis to remove allergenic plasma proteins. *Acute hemolytic transfusion reaction* is a rare immune-mediated rapid destruction of donor erythrocytes by preformed recipient antibodies - a reaction usually due to ABO blood group incompatibility, most commonly a result of clerical error. This may lead to symptoms of agitation, chest pain, flank pain, headache, dyspnea, and chills along with signs of fever, hypotension, unexplained bleeding, and hemoglobinuria. The most common transfusion reaction is a *febrile, nonhemolytic transfusion reaction.* This is also an immune-mediated reaction where antibodies act against donor white cells or plasma proteins. Signs include fever, flushing, urticaria, tachycardia, and mild hypotension in conjunction with anxiety, pruritus, and dyspnea, and usually respond to treatment with acetaminophen, antihistamines, and glucocorticoids. Leukocyte-poor red cells may be used to avoid reaction (for a more detailed discussion on transfusion reactions, see Chapter 28).

C. Local Anesthetics

Local anesthetics have been reported to cause both immune-mediated and nonimmune-mediated hypersensitivity reactions. Immune-mediated reactions are a result of activated T cells and signs include contact dermatitis and delayed swelling at the site of administration. IgE-mediated urticarial and anaphylactic reactions have been described, but are rare. In many cases, immediate onset hypersensitivity reactions are because of the local anesthetic preservatives methyl- or propyl-parabens (i.e., para-aminobenzoic acid) and metabisulphites. Whereas allergic reactions may appear to be related solely to the local anesthetic, other materials involved with the administration of the local anesthetic, such as latex gloves or antiseptics, may be responsible. Nonimmune-mediated reactions causing psychomotor, anxiety, vasovagal syncope, and sympathetic stimulation may occur, but are difficult to distinguish from dose-dependent systemic toxic effects.

Neuraxial and peripheral nerve blocks using local anesthetic bolus or continuous infusion are common perioperative anesthetic techniques and are often managed in the PACU. Consequently, the aforementioned concerns regarding allergic reactions to local anesthetics should be observed.

D. Neuraxial Opioids and Pruritus

Opioids are often administered in spinal and epidural anesthetics, and pruritus is a commonly associated symptom in the PACU. Whereas systemic opioid administration side effects may be associated with histamine release, facial flushing and pruritus associated with neuraxial administration of opioids is related to an opioid receptor-mediated dysesthesia. Symptoms are frequently located in the nose and upper face because of the μ-opioid and 5-hydroxytryptamine subtype 3 (5-HT3) receptor-rich receptors in the trigeminal nerve. These receptors also play a role in itching through mechanisms in the spinothalamic tract of the dorsal horn in the spinal cord. Thus, these symptoms are not usually improved with antihistamines. Instead, opioid receptor antagonist (naloxone), mixed agonist–antagonist opioids (nalbuphine), and 5-HT3 receptor antagonists (ondansetron and mirtazapine) have the greatest evidence supporting their efficacy.

E. Propofol

Patients may receive propofol in the operating room as part of the general anesthetic and may also arrive in the PACU on a propofol infusion. Data is limited to small studies and case reports of propofol-induced allergic reaction in patients with history of egg, soy, peanut, or milk allergy. Propofol contains egg lethecin and purified soybean oil, which are not thought to be allergenic. Rather, patients with egg, soy, peanut, or milk allergies have sensitivity to egg, soy, peanut, or milk proteins, which are not present in propofol's emulsified solution. The highest quality evidence to date suggests that propofol is safe in patients with mild egg, milk, peanut, and soy allergies. However, conservative practice suggests avoiding propofol in patients with history of severe anaphylaxis to egg, soy, peanut, or milk, or that have multiple IgE-mediated food allergies.

F. Red Man Syndrome
Vancomycin-induced "red man syndrome" occurs in approximately 15% of patients. The mechanism is secondary to direct activation of mast cells and basophils leading to histamine release. Symptoms usually involve the upper body, face, and neck. Cutaneous flushing, erythema, pruritus, muscle pains and, in more severe cases, hypotension has been documented. Risk factors identified include prior use of antihistamines, dose >10 mg/kg, rate of infusion >1 g/100 minutes, concentration >5 mg/cc, age >2 years, Caucasian race, and prior history of "red man syndrome." Other medications associated with nonimmune-mediated histamine release include ciprofloxacin, amphotericin B, rifampin, teicoplanin, opioids (typically morphine, meperidine, and codeine), muscle relaxants, and contrast dye. The combination of any of these medications can exacerbate mast cell or basophil degranulation, and it is prudent to avoid concomitant administration.

G. Dyes
Reactions to dyes such as triarylmethane, patent blue V, isosulfan blue, and methylene blue have been reported and are likely related to sensitization from cosmetics and other household products. Similar to latex, reactions to dyes are often delayed 30 minutes or longer and may present in the PACU.

H. Obstetric Patients
Anaphylaxis occurs in approximately 3:100,000 pregnancies. β-Lactam antibiotics and latex are the most common agents leading to anaphylaxis in parturients. During resuscitation, left lateral uterine tilt >30 degrees is essential to avoid aortocaval compression from the gravid uterus.

I. Dermatologic Reactions
Various immune- and nonimmune-mediated dermatologic reactions may be observed in the PACU. Contact exposure from adhesives, surgical draping, telemetry stickers, or bed sheets, for example, often has a well-demarcated location of reaction. Although typically associated with drug exposures, systemic dermatologic symptoms and signs may also occur from contact exposures. Localized or systemic dermatologic reactions such as drug rash eosinophilia with systemic symptoms (DRESS syndrome) Stevens–Johnson syndrome, and acute febrile neutrophilic dermatosis (Sweet's syndrome) frequently require consultation with specialists in allergy, infectious disease, or dermatology.

VI. DIFFERENTIAL DIAGNOSIS
Many other conditions exhibit the same signs and symptoms as those presenting in hypersensitivity reactions. A comprehensive evaluation of patient history, comorbidities, recent surgical intervention, medication administration, and other exposures must be performed to ensure that the appropriate diagnosis is established. Immediate diagnostic information includes vital signs, electrocardiogram, chest x-ray, laboratory studies, and focused bedside trans-thoracic echocardiography and ultrasound.

VII. **TREATMENT**

Regardless of the trigger, the overarching treatment is the same: identify and discontinue the triggering agent and provide supportive care (circulation, airway and breathing). Although the intensity of treatment is dictated by patient symptoms, it is important to err on the side of caution and mobilize resources early. For anaphylaxis, epinephrine is the drug of choice and should be administered without delay owing to its properties of vasoconstriction (α_1-agonist), inotropy (β_1-agonist), and bronchodilitation (β_2-agonist). Additional vasopressors and bronchodilators may be useful or necessary in the acute treatment of anaphylaxis. Antihistamines and steroids are also useful, but because of their slower onset, they are not considered part of the acute treatment for anaphylaxis.

A. Call for help.

B. Hemodynamic support: Intravenous (IV) fluid bolus, epinephrine, other vasopressors as needed (phenylephrine and norepinephrine), or advanced cardiac life support (ACLS).

C. Respiratory support: 100% inspired oxygen, bronchodilators (β-agonist), positive pressure ventilation, or intubation. Magnesium can also be used as a bronchodilator.

D. Establish large bore IV access, peripheral or central.

E. Establish appropriate monitoring: an arterial line may be helpful for titrating vasopressors and blood gas monitoring.

F. Histamine blockers (diphenhydramine and ranitidine) and corticosteroids should also be administered although these agents are slower in onset and are considered secondary support.

G. Consider transferring the patient to the intensive care unit.

H. Allergy consultation.

VIII. **WORK UP**

A. History: Postoperatively, a review of procedure, anesthesia, and PACU medical records may be helpful in identifying potential exposures. Useful information may also be obtained from patient, family, or primary care physician interview.

B. Immediate laboratory studies

1. Plasma histamine: Reflects mast cell and basophil degranulation due to direct or IgE-mediated activation. Maximally elevated immediately, with a half-life of 20 minutes. Sensitivity 75% and specificity 51% in detecting anaphylaxis.

2. Serum tryptase: Reflects mast cell and basophil degranulation due to direct or IgE-mediated activation. Draw lab within 120 minutes; subsequent labs 1, 2, and 24 hours later for trending given potential for relapse. Tryptase is maximally elevated 30 minutes after initial reaction, with a half-life of 90 minutes. Sensitivity 64% and specificity 89% in detecting anaphylaxis.

C. Skin testing: Skin testing coupled with history is the mainstay of the diagnosis of an IgE-mediated reaction. Intradermal or skin-prick tests are usually carried out 4 to 6 weeks after a reaction because intracellular stocks of histamine and other mediators may still be lower than normal within 4 weeks of a reaction.

IX. **CLINICAL PEARLS**

A. Epinephrine is the drug of choice for anaphylaxis. Typical dosing includes:

1. Intramuscular: 10 μg/kg (max 0.5 mg) every 5 to 15 minutes as needed.

2. Intravenous: 5 to 10 μg bolus for mild hypotension or 100 to 500 μg for severe hypotension. Titration of infusion may also be used, starting at 1 to 5 μg/minute.

B. Epinephrine may cause arrhythmias, myocardial ischemia, or unwanted hypertension, especially at higher doses.

C. Studies in children and adults have demonstrated greater bioavailability of intramuscular epinephrine compared to subcutaneous epinephrine. Intramuscular concentrations are increased the fastest when delivered in the anterior thigh.

D. Although β_2-agonists assist with bronchodilation, they do not relieve airway edema or hypotension, which should be treated with epinephrine.

E. Antihistamines do not improve bronchoconstriction, airway edema, or hypotension. They merely treat pruritis, rash, and urticaria and are considered a secondary treatment.

F. Glucocorticoids are considered a secondary treatment for anaphylaxis, and there is minimal evidence that they attenuate delayed or longer term symptoms.

G. A passive straight leg raise shifts intravascular volume from the peripheral to central vascular compartments, thereby increasing venous return to the heart, end-diastolic filling pressure, and cardiac output.

H. In obstetric patients, left lateral uterine tilt >30 degrees is essential to avoid aortocaval compression from the gravid uterus.

I. Glucagon has been used to treat refractory hypotension in patients taking β-blockers, because β-blockade is thought to decrease the response to epinephrine. It is recommended this be given only in patients who are intubated because glucagon administration may cause gastrointestinal upset and emesis.

X. SUBSEQUENT CARE

Relapse of anaphylaxis symptoms may occur as late as 72 hours (median 11 hours) after initial symptoms. While this mechanism is not clearly understood, it may be explained by decreased plasma concentrations of anaphylaxis medications or a true immunologic phenomenon. Symptom relapse is reported to between 1% and 20% of patients. The level and duration of post-event monitoring is patient specific. It is determined by the severity of the underlying symptoms, level of supportive care available, and clinical impression. After a severe hypersensitivity reaction, close observation up to 72 hours in an intensive care unit is strongly recommended.

Subsequent outpatient follow-up with an allergist includes a thorough medical history of the patient to further evaluate for IgE-mediated reactions coupled with skin testing. Protocolized desensitization under a monitored setting may also be considered.

Suggested Readings

Ballantyne JC, Loach AB, Carr DB. Itching after epidural and spinal opiates. *Pain* 1988;33(2):149–160.

Campagna JD, Bond MC, Schabelman E, et al. The use of cephalosporins in penicillin allergic patients: a literature review. *J Emerg Med* 2012;42(5):612–620.

Greenberger PA, Ditto AM. Chapter 24: Anaphylaxis. *Allergy Asthma Proc* 2012;33(suppl 1):S80–S83.

Johansson SG, Bieber T, Dahl R, et al. Revised nomenclature for allergy for global use: report of the Nomenclature Review Committee of the World Allergy Organization, October 2003. *J Allergy Clin Immunol* 2004;113(5):832–836.

Lee S, Bellolio MF, Hess EP, et al. Time of onset and predictors of biphasic anaphylactic reactions: a systematic review and meta-analysis. *J Allergy Clin Immunol Pract* 2015;3(3):408–416.e2.

Mertes PM, Laxenaire MC. Anaphylactic and anaphylactoid reactions occurring during anaesthesia in France. Seventh epidemiologic survey (January 2001–December 2002). *Ann Fr Anesth Reanim* 2004;23(12):1133–1143.

Mertes PM, Laxenaire MC, Alla F. Anaphylactic and anaphylactoid reactions occurring during anesthesia in France in 1999–2000. *Anesthesiology* 2003;99(3):536–545.

Mertes PM, Malinovsky JM, Mouton-faivre C, et al. Anaphylaxis to dyes during the perioperative period: reports of 14 clinical cases. *J Allergy Clin Immunol* 2008;122(2):348–352.

Molina-infante J, Arias A, Vara-brenes D, et al. Propofol administration is safe in adult eosinophilic esophagitis patients sensitized to egg, soy, or peanut. *Allergy* 2014;69(3):388–394.

Murphy A, Campbell DE, Baines D, et al. Allergic reactions to propofol in egg-allergic children. *Anesth Analg* 2011;113(1):140–144.

Myers AL, Gaedigk A, Dai H, et al. Defining risk factors for red man syndrome in children and adults. *Pediatr Infect Dis J* 2012;31(5):464–468.

Nagel JE, Fuscaldo JT, Fireman P. Paraben allergy. *JAMA* 1977;237(15):1594–1595.

Saager L, Turan A, Egan C, et al. Incidence of intraoperative hypersensitivity reactions: a registry analysis. *Anesthesiology* 2015;122(3):551–559.

Sadleir PH, Russell T, Clarke RC, et al. Intraoperative anaphylaxis to sugammadex and a protocol for intradermal skin testing. *Anaesth Intensive Care* 2014;42(1):93–96.

Sampson HA, Muñoz-furlong A, Campbell RL, et al. Second symposium on the definition and management of anaphylaxis: summary report—second National Institute of Allergy and Infectious Disease/Food Allergy and Anaphylaxis Network Symposium. *Ann Emerg Med* 2006;47(4):373–380.

Sivagnanam S, Deleu D. Red man syndrome. *Crit Care* 2003;7(2):119–120.

Thomas M, Crawford I. Best evidence topic report. Glucagon infusion in refractory anaphylactic shock in patients on beta-blockers. *Emerg Med J* 2005;22(4):272–273.

Volcheck GW, Mertes PM. Local and general anesthetics immediate hypersensitivity reactions. *Immunol Allergy Clin North Am* 2014;34(3):525–546, viii.

Yip VL, Alfirevic A, Pirmohamed M. Genetics of immune-mediated adverse drug reactions: a comprehensive and clinical review. *Clin Rev Allergy Immunol* 2014;48(2–3):165–175.

Youssef N, Orlov D, Alie T, et al. What epidural opioid results in the best analgesia outcomes and fewest side effects after surgery?: A meta-analysis of randomized controlled trials. *Anesth Analg* 2014;119(4):965–977.

28

Transfusion Reactions

Adeola Sadik and Jarone Lee

I. TRANSFUSION REACTIONS

All types of transfusions carry the risk of causing subacute, acute, and delayed adverse events. Prompt recognition of a transfusion-related event may be difficult and even overlooked secondary to the patient's underlying illness. In order to accurately diagnose a transfusion reaction, a detailed assessment of the patient's vital signs prior to, during, and after transfusion must be examined in conjunction with any accompanying signs and symptoms (Table 28.1).

A. Epidemiology

According to the United States Food and Drug Administration (USFDA), from 2009 to 2013, transfusion-related acute lung injury (TRALI) caused the majority of transfusion-related deaths (38%), followed by transfusion-associated circulatory overload (TACO) (24%), and then acute hemolytic transfusion reactions (AHTRs) (total 22%: non-ABO and ABO incompatibilities at 15% and 7%, respectively). Transfusion-related infections accounted for 10% of transfusion-related fatalities, and anaphylaxis accounted for 5% of deaths. Other causes, such as transfusion-associated graft-versus-host disease (TA-GVHD) and hypotension, accounted for approximately 1% of transfusion-related deaths.

B. Noninfectious and Nonhemolytic Transfusion Reactions

1. Transfusion-related acute lung injury

TRALI is defined as new-onset acute lung injury within 4 to 6 hours of blood product transfusion. Patients usually present with acute hypoxemia, a PaO_2/FIO_2 ratio of less 300 mm Hg, and evidence of bilateral patchy infiltrates on chest radiography (without evidence of left atrial hypertension or other signs of left heart failure). TRALI is the most common cause of transfusion-related death, as documented by the USFDA. Case fatality estimates range from 5% to 25%. TRALI occurs when recipient neutrophils, located and sequestered within the lung, are activated by substances within donor blood products. These transfused substances can include anti–human neutrophil antibodies (HNAs), anti–human leukocyte antibodies (HLAs), and other mediators (cytokines and biologically active lipids and proteins) that bind to and cause the aggregation of the recipient's neutrophils in the pulmonary vasculature. The activated neutrophils release inflammatory mediators that increase the permeability of the pulmonary vasculature, causing pulmonary edema and lung injury.

Several known risk factors that increase the risk for TRALI include having undergone cardiac surgery, patients with hematologic malignancies (with whom treatment is being initiated), mechanical ventilation with high peak airway pressures, a history of smoking, chronic alcohol abuse, and high serum interleukin-8 levels. Signs and symptoms include dyspnea, an oxygen saturation of less than

TABLE 28.1	Types of Transfusion-related Reactions	
Reaction	**Signs and Symptoms**	**Treatment**
Allergic reaction	Hives, pruritus, wheezing, erythema	• Stop or slow rate of transfusion for 15–30 min • Give antihistamines • Monitor: hives (if only symptom), likely to resolve in less than 30 min and may resume transfusion • If isolated allergic reaction, unlikely to recur in future; no evidence for premedication • Give washed cells if repeated reactions
Anaphylaxis	Acute flushing, hypertension followed by hypotension, tachycardia, edema, bronchospasm, and shock, typically within minutes of initiating the transfusion	• ACLS, fluid resuscitation, initiation of vasopressors, if necessary • Epinephrine 0.3 mL of 1:1,000 solution SQ and methylprednisolone • Prevent by limiting future transfusions to IgA-deficient blood (ultrawashed or deglycerolized RBCs)
TRALI	Acute hypoxemia and noncardiogenic pulmonary edema May have fever and hypotension Some definitions: TRALI must occur within 6 h of last transfusion	• Resuscitation, supplemental oxygen, mechanical ventilation, and vasopressor support
TACO	Signs/symptoms are similar to that seen with TRALI, expect hypertension and volume overload	• Diuretics • Decrease subsequent transfusion rates and volumes, if possible
AHTR	Fever, chills, burning at IV site, flank pain, chest tightness, tachycardia, hypotension, hemoglobinuria, acute kidney injury, disseminated intravascular coagulation	• Intravenous fluid resuscitation • Diuretics • May require vasopressors
FNHTR	Fever (with a greater than 1 Celsius (C) change from pretransfusion temperature), chills, flushing, tachycardia Similar to AHTR, with less severe symptoms	• Treat symptoms with antipyretic • Monitor post-transfusion platelet count

TABLE 28.1	Types of Transfusion-related Reactions (*continued*)	
Reaction	**Signs and Symptoms**	**Treatment**
DHTR	Asymptomatic hematocrit decrease, flu-like illness, jaundice, unconjugated bilirubinemia	• Treatment rarely necessary • MUST identify the responsible antibody as a reference for future transfusions
Transfusion-associated GVHD	Fever, erythematous maculopapular rash, diarrhea, hepatomegaly, transaminitis, pancytopenia	• Majority of cases (>90%) are fatal, no proven treatment • Prevent by using irradiated products from related donors
Iron overload	Cirrhosis, endocrine failure, heart failure	• Chelation, decreases the amount of transfusions
Hyperkalemia	ECG changes, hyperkalemic cardiac arrest Occurrence decreases with fresh blood and/or washed RBCs	• Treat the hyperkalemia
Hypocalcemia	From citrate toxicity	• Treat if symptomatic
Hypothermia	Temperature below 35°C (95°F)	• Treat by warming blood

90%, cyanosis, hypotension, fever, chills, hypoxia, and a pulmonary artery pressure of less than 18 mm Hg.

TRALI can be difficult to distinguish from other causes of acute hypoxemia with noncardiogenic pulmonary edema, such as TACO and acute respiratory distress syndrome. As such, it is often a diagnosis of exclusion. The laboratory workup often includes a complete blood count with differential (to show evidence of neutropenia) and labs to exclude AHTRs. The mainstay of treatment of TRALI is respiratory support with lung protective mechanical ventilation and vasopressor support. About 80% of patients recover within 48 to 96 hours of onset of symptoms. Prevention of TRALI is aimed at identifying donors with antineutrophil and anti-HLA antibodies (such as childbearing female donors) and limiting future blood donations.

2. **Transfusion-associated circulatory overload**

TACO occurs when the volume of a transfused blood component cannot be effectively managed by the recipient, thus leading to progressive respiratory failure, hypoxemia, and dyspnea, along with evidence of right or left heart failure within 2 to 6 hours of blood component transfusion. TACO was the second leading cause of transfusion-related death in the United States from 2009 to 2013, as reported to the USFDA. TACO occurs as a result of the rapid infusion or a large volume of blood product transfusion in the setting of underlying cardiac, renal, and chronic pulmonary disease. It can often present in a similar fashion to TRALI and other causes of acute lung injury, and often proves to be difficult to distinguish between the two diagnoses. Symptoms may include dyspnea, an oxygen saturation of 90% or less, cyanosis, nonproductive cough, orthopnea, hypertension, tachycardia, left atrial hypertension, congestive heart failure, and evidence of myocardial ischemia with new-onset ST segment and T-wave changes on electrocardiography. Diagnosis involves monitoring for signs of volume overload and checking serum brain natriuretic peptide. Treatment frequently involves decreasing the infusion rate of subsequent transfusions and using diuretics with administration of blood products.

3. **Allergic reactions and anaphylaxis**

Post-transfusion allergic reactions are usually mild and are caused by IgE-mediated reactions to donor plasma proteins. These reactions are type 1 hypersensitivity reactions that lead to widespread mast cell activation and the systemic release of mediators of inflammation. They occur most often in patients who have received a prior blood component transfusion or in those who have been presensitized to an allergen within the donor blood product (typically serum proteins and medications). The allergic reaction can present with hives, erythema, pruritus, and wheezing. Treatment options involve slowing or stopping the transfusion, with concomitant administration of antihistamines or steroids. A subset of patients with IgA deficiency may have anti–IgA antibodies, which can react with the donor serum, and subsequently cause an anaphylactic reaction. Often, the IgA-deficient patient has not been sensitized to the responsible antigen by prior exposures. These patients typically have anti–IgA antibodies that develop naturally. Symptoms include dyspnea, bronchospasm, hypotension, sweating, flushing, nausea, vomiting, abdominal pain, chest pain, shock, and angioedema. Treatment is primarily supportive, focusing on the maintenance of hemodynamic stability and prevention of cardiovascular collapse with vasopressors, antihistamines, corticosteroids, respiratory support, and mechanical ventilation. IgA-deficient patients should be transfused with washed RBCs or blood products from IgA-deficient donors and with plasma-reduced platelets.

4. **Transfusion-associated dyspnea**

Transfusion-associated dyspnea is described as the acute onset of respiratory distress within 24 hours of blood component transfusion that cannot be diagnosed as TRALI, TACO, or a transfusion-associated allergic reaction.

5. **Alloantibodies**

There are more than 300 red blood cell (RBC) antigens. Almost all RBC transfusions will place the recipient at risk for the development of alloantibodies. However, not all RBC antigens have equal immunogenicity. The development of alloantibodies depends on the occurrence of the antigen, the propensity of the transfusion recipient to form antibodies, the number of transfusions that the recipient has been exposed to, and the antigen immunogenicity. Platelets also express HLAs and other antigens and may also induce the production of alloantibodies. Transfusion recipient sensitization may occur from prior transfusions, organ and nonorgan transplantation, and pregnancy, and may lead to a lack of an appropriate response to platelet transfusions. Using leukoreduced RBCs and platelets can reduce the occurrence of platelet alloantibody formation (Table 28.2).

6. **Post-transfusion purpura**

Post-transfusion purpura (PTP) is an acute and severe thrombocytopenia reaction that occurs within 2 to 14 days after blood product transfusion. PTP is caused by platelet alloantibodies in a previously sensitized recipient and is characterized by signs of severe thrombocytopenia including purpura, petechia, and evidence of bleeding.

TABLE 28.2	Types of Blood Products	
Blood Component	**Use**	**Indications**
Irradiated blood components	Gamma irradiation inactivates lymphocytes May prevent TA-GVHD	• Granulocyte transfusions • Directed donor transfusions from relatives • HLA-matched or crossmatched platelet transfusions • Recipients with Hodgkin's disease • Hematopoietic stem cell transplant recipients • Bone marrow transplant recipients • *May* be indicated for: non-Hodgkin's lymphoma, patients receiving chemotherapy/radiation for solid tumors
Saline-washed blood components	To prevent anaphylaxis in IgA-deficient patients Washing can remove antibodies and cytokines	• Febrile reactions not prevented by leukocyte reduction • Past anaphylactic transfusion reaction • IgA deficiency • Urticarial reaction
Leukocyte reduced RBCs and platelets	Leukocytes may cause febrile transfusion reactions, HLA/HNA alloimmunization, TRALI, decreased platelet responsiveness, CMV, HTLV, TA-GVHD, and immunomodulation	• Prevention of febrile reaction • Prevention of HLA/HNA alloimmunization • Heart transplant recipients • Bone marrow transplant recipients • Renal transplant recipients
CMV reduced	CMV infection in immunocompromised patients	• CMV negative donors

Platelet-specific antibodies must be detected for a true diagnosis of PTP to be made. Treatment includes intravenous immunoglobulins, plasmapheresis, exchange transfusions, and/or corticosteroids. However, most cases are self-limiting, and resolve within weeks of onset. Bleeding is treated with antigen-free platelets; plasma transfusions are often ineffective.

7. **Transfusion-associated graft-versus-host disease**

TA-GVHD is a rare and often fatal post-transfusion complication that takes place most commonly in immunocompromised patients (or in patients with comparable HLA profiles) in whom T-lymphocytes are transferred during blood product transfusion. The recipient is unable to mount an immune response against the foreign T-lymphocytes, leading to the proliferation of foreign T-lymphocytes in the host. The foreign T-lymphocytes then mount an immunogenic attack on host antigens. Signs and symptoms include a profound neutropenia, high fevers, an erythematous maculopapular rash, hepatocellular damage and hepatomegaly (as evidenced by elevated liver function tests [LFTs]), nausea and vomiting, diarrhea, cholestasis, and pancytopenia within 2 to 30 days after blood product transfusion. The diagnosis of TA-GVHD is often made clinically; however, biopsies from various host organs can show evidence of chimerism. Prevention is often the most effective treatment and occurs by irradiating all blood components for immunocompromised transfusion recipients or when the donor is first-degree relative (Table 28.2).

8. **Transfusion-related immunomodulation**

Blood transfusions may lead to post-transfusion immunomodulation in the recipient. The mechanisms of immunomodulation and immunosuppression are unclear. However, possible evidence for the occurrence can be seen in postrenal transplantation patients in whom improved organ survival occurs. Transfusion recipients have also been noted to have an increased vulnerability to transfusion-related infections. Currently, no treatment exists, and prevention is aimed at the avoidance of unnecessary transfusions.

C. **Hemolytic Transfusion Reactions**

1. **Acute hemolytic transfusion reaction**

An AHTR occurs when immunologically incompatible RBCs are transfused to a patient, causing recipient antibodies to scale an attack against donor RBC antigens. This can lead to acute (within 24 hours of blood component administration) intravascular hemolysis and other severe complications. AHTRs were the fourth leading cause of transfusion-related fatalities from 2009 to 2013. Non-ABO incompatibility (usually due to sensitization from a prior exposure) caused more fatalities than ABO incompatibility during this time period. AHTRs are usually caused by processing errors that can occur at any point from the collection of blood to the processing and administration of blood products. The clinical signs and symptoms associated with AHTRs occur as a result of the widespread immunologic response, activation of the clotting cascade, and the release of vasoactive substances that lead to tissue hypoperfusion, ischemia, and end-organ failure. The main risk factor for AHTRs involves a failure in the often rigid protocols in place in many clinical setting for the administration of blood and blood products. Signs and symptoms vary in severity and can include subclinical hemolysis to fever, chills, nausea, vomiting, dyspnea, hypotension, disseminated intravascular coagulation (DIC), hemoglobinuria, chest and abdominal pain, renal failure leading to oliguria and anemia. Anesthetized patients may initially demonstrate nonspecific signs such a tachycardia, hypotension, fever, and hemoglobinuria, with evidence of red/brown urine. The severity of symptoms is directly related to the volume of the transfusion. This necessitates the provider to recognize the signs and symptoms early, and stop the transfusion appropriately. The diagnosis of AHTRs usually involves the provider searching for laboratory evidence of hemolysis (elevated lactate dehydrogenase [LDH], decreased haptoglobin, anemia, and direct antiglobulin testing) and evidence of hemoglobinuria, renal failure, and DIC. The patient's blood and the donor blood should be sent for repeat cross-matching to obtain the correct ABO classification. Management of severe AHTRs involves supportive care with mechanical ventilation, vasopressor support, intravenous fluids, diuretics to maintain sufficient blood pressure, renal perfusion pressure, and urine output. Additionally, ongoing evidence of hemolysis should be monitored and early signs of DIC should be aggressively treated with coagulation factor repletion and compatible RBC transfusion.

2. **Delayed hemolytic transfusion reaction**

   A delayed hemolytic transfusion reaction (DHTR) occurs when the antibodies to RBC antigens develop between 24 hours and 10 days (but can occur up to 28 days) after blood component transfusion, leading to clinical or subclinical evidence of hemolysis. DHTRs usually occur after a patient has been exposed to RBC antigens (usually of the non-ABO variety: Kidd, Kell, Duffy, Rh, and MNS) commonly from a previous blood transfusion or pregnancy, and an immunologic response is mounted. When a reexposure occurs, a large-scale immune response ensues, leading to hemolysis. Signs and symptoms are usually milder than in AHTRs, and may include a mild anemia, and elevated indirect bilirubin and LDH. DHTR-associated hemolysis is usually extravascular. Prevention is established by limiting all future transfusions to antigen-free blood.

3. **Delayed serologic transfusion reaction**

   A delayed serologic transfusion reaction takes place when a transfusion recipient develops antibodies against RBC antigens from 24 hours to 28 days after blood transfusion without clinical or laboratory evidence of hemolysis.

D. **Nonhemolytic Transfusion Reactions**

1. **Febrile nonhemolytic transfusion reaction**

   Febrile nonhemolytic transfusion reactions (FNHTRs) are characterized by a transfusion recipient temperature of 38°C (100.4°F) or an increase in temperature of 1°C (1.8°F) from the pretransfusion temperature, with or without chills/rigors, during blood product transfusion or within 4 hours after the end of the transfusion that is not related to the patient's underlying condition. FNHTRs occur as a result of the transfusion of blood product cytokines or because of recipient HLAs, HNAs, and platelet antigens that stimulate endogenous cytokine release. FNHTRs are a diagnosis of exclusion, because fever is a common sign with many transfusion reactions. The use of leukoreduced RBCs and platelets significantly decreases the occurrence of FNHTRs. If a FNHTR occurs despite the use of leukoreduced blood products, the transfusion recipient should be given saline washed products and pretreatment with an antipyretic for all future transfusions (Table 28.2).

E. **Infectious Transfusion Reactions**

1. **Transfusion-transmitted infection**

   Transfusion-transmitted infections (TTIs) (Table 28.3) occur when a pathogen is seeded into a blood product at any step in the production process and can be donor transmitted or, more commonly, due to environmental contamination (taking place at any point from phlebotomy to storage). Bacterial infections occur most commonly from platelet transfusions, because of their storage at room temperature. According to data from the USFDA, *Staphylococcus aureus* has accounted for most of the TTI-related fatalities in the past 5 years. However, *Yersinia enterocolitica* for packed RBCs, and *Staphylococcus epidermidis* for platelets are also common infections. The most common parasitic RBC TTI is *Babesia microti*, which often occurs in immunocompromised

TABLE 28.3	Transfusion Transmitted Infections

Bacteria (Environmental or Donor Transmitted)

- *Staphylococcus aureus* (methicillin-sensitive and resistant)
- *Escherichia coli*
- *Serratia marcescens*
- *Staphylococcus epidermidis*
- *Morganella morganii*
- *Streptococcus viridans*
- *Streptococcus pneumoniae*
- *Staphylococcus warneri*
- *Yersinia enterocolitica*
- *Klebsiella pneumoniae*

Parasites

- *Babesia microti* (Babesiosis)
- Malaria
- *Trypanosoma cruzi* (Chagas disease)
- *Toxoplasma gondii* (Toxoplasmosis)

Viruses

- Hepatitis A
- Hepatitis B
- Hepatitis C
- Hepatitis delta agent
- HIV-1 and -2
- GB virus C (hepatitis G)
- HTLV-1 and -2
- Epstein–Barr virus
- Cytomegalovirus
- West Nile virus
- Parvovirus B19

Spirochetes and Prions

- *Borrelia burgdorferi* (Lyme disease)
- *Treponema pallidum* (Syphilis)
- Variant Creutzfeldt–Jakob disease (Mad cow disease)

and asplenic patients. Current screening practices (obtained from standards created by the American Association of Blood Banks) have reduced (but have not eliminated) the incidence of donor TTIs. Current practice includes screening for hepatitis B virus, hepatitis C virus, HIV-1 and -2, human T-lymphotropic virus types I and II, *Trypanosoma cruzi* (Chagas disease), and West Nile virus. Signs and symptoms can include high fever, chills and rigors, and hypotension shortly after starting a transfusion. The diagnosis of TTIs is often made by Gram stain and culture of the offending blood product and the recipient. Treatment involves using antimicrobial drugs (if available), and supportive treatment of bacteremia and sepsis.

F. Approach to a Suspected Transfusion Reaction

1. Stop the transfusion immediately.
2. Check and record all vital signs.
3. If evidence of cardiovascular collapse, begin cardiopulmonary resuscitation and begin volume resuscitation and vasopressor support, if indicated.
4. Ensure that the patient's identity (name, date of birth, medical record number) matches that on the transfused blood product.
5. Do not discard the transfused blood product.
6. Notify the hospital blood bank about the transfusion reaction and begin the hospital-mandated documentation process.
7. Obtain blood and urine samples from the recipient.
8. Send the transfused blood product for repeat cross-matching.

Suggested Readings

Alter HJ, Klein HG. The hazards of blood transfusion in historical perspective. *Blood* 2008;112(7):2617–2626.

Brecher ME, Blajchman MA, Yomtovian R, et al. Addressing the risk of bacterial contamination of platelets within the United States: a history to help illuminate the future. *Transfusion* 2013;53(1):221–231.

Centers for Disease Control and Prevention. *National Healthcare Safety Network Biovigilance Component Hemovigilance Module Surveillance Protocol.* Version 2.1.3. Atlanta, GA: National Center for Emergency and Zoonotic Infections Diseases; 2014. Available at: http://www.cdc.gov/nhsn/PDFs/hemovigModuleProtocol_current .pdf. Accessed February 5, 2015.

Dasararaju R, Marques MB. Adverse effects of transfusion. *Cancer Control* 2015;22(1):16–25.

Dean L. Chapter 3, Blood transfusions and the immune system. In: *Blood Groups and Red Cell Antigens* [Internet]. Bethesda, MD: National Center for Biotechnology Information (US); 2005.

Ezidiegwu CN, Lauenstein KJ, Rosales LG, et al. Febrile nonhemolytic transfusion reactions. Management by premedication and cost implications in adult patients. *Arch Pathol Lab Med* 2004;128(9):991–995.

Geiger TL, Howard SC. Acetaminophen and diphenhydramine premedication for allergic and febrile nonhemolytic transfusion reactions: good prophylaxis or bad practice? *Transfus Med Rev* 2007;21(1):1–12.

Goodnough LT. Risks of blood transfusion. *Crit Care Med* 2003;31(Suppl 12):S678–S686.

Heal JM, Phipps RP, Blumberg N. One big unhappy family: transfusion alloimmunization, thrombosis, and immune modulation/inflammation. *Transfusion* 2009;49(6):1032–1036.

Kleinman S, Caulfield T, Chan P, et al. Toward an understanding of transfusion-related acute lung injury: statement of a consensus panel. *Transfusion* 2004;44(12):1774–1789.

Middelburg RA, Bom JG. Transfusion-related acute lung injury not a two-hit, but a multicausal model. *Transfusion* 2015;55(5):953–960. doi:10.1111/trf.12966.

Perrotta PL, Snyder EL. Non-infectious complications of transfusion therapy. *Blood Rev* 2001;15(2):69–83.

Refaai MA, Blumberg N. Transfusion immunomodulation from a clinical perspective: an update. *Expert Rev Hematol* 2013;6(6):653–663.

Tormey CA, Stack G. Limiting the extent of a delayed hemolytic transfusion reaction with automated red blood cell exchange. *Arch Pathol Lab Med* 2013;137(6):861–864.

Toy P, Popovsky MA, Abraham E, et al. Transfusion-related acute lung injury: definition and review. *Crit Care Med* 2005;33(4):721–726.

US Food and Drug Administration. Guidance for industry: circular of information for the use of human blood and blood components. Available at: http://www.fda.gov /biologicsbloodvaccines/guidancecomplianceregulatoryinformation/guidances /blood/ucm364565.htm. Accessed February 18, 2015.

US Food and Drug Administration. Transfusion/donation fatalities. Available at: http://www.fda.gov/BiologicsBloodVaccines/SafetyAvailability/ReportaProblem /TransfusionDonationFatalities/default.htm Accessed March 5, 2015.

Vamvakaa EC. Pneumonia as a complication of blood product transfusion in the critically ill: transfusion-related immunomodulation (TRM). *Crit Care Med* 2006;34(5 Suppl):S151–S159.

Vlaar AP, Juffermans NP. Transfusion-related acute lung injury: a clinical review. *Lancet* 2013;382(9896):984–994.

Young C, Chawla A, Berardi V, et al; Babesia Testing Investigational Containment Study Group. Preventing transfusion-transmitted babesiosis: preliminary experience of the first laboratory-based blood donor screening program. *Transfusion* 2012;52(7):1523–1529.

Perioperative Injuries (Ocular, Oropharyngeal, Dental, Nerve, Extravasation)

Bryan Simmons and Edward A. Bittner

Ocular, oropharyngeal, dental, nerve, and extravasation injuries represent a notable source of perioperative complications that can be debilitating. Even minor postoperative complications are important to patients, and better efforts to prevent and treat such complications should lead to improved postoperative recovery and patient satisfaction.

I. **Perioperative Ocular Injury** can affect the anterior chamber of the eye (cornea and conjunctiva) or the posterior chamber of the eye, its blood supply, and the optic nerve. Severity ranges from transient blurring of vision to irreversible blindness. Transient blurring of vision can be attributed to cycloplegia from anticholinergic medications, use of ocular lubricants, excessive corneal drying, or a corneal abrasion. The most common perioperative ocular injury is corneal abrasion, which typically does not result in permanent visual changes. However, injuries affecting the posterior chamber, the optic nerve, and its blood supply, such as **Ischemic Optic Neuropathy (ION)** or **Central Retinal Artery Occlusion (CRAO)**, usually result in some degree of permanent visual changes or blindness. In an ASA closed claims report, ocular injury accounted for 3% of all anesthetic claims.

A. **Corneal Abrasions**

Corneal abrasions occur due to disruption of the corneal epithelium and underlying corneal layers.

1. **Epidemiology**

a. **Incidence.** Corneal abrasion is the most common ocular injury in the perioperative period, with reported incidences ranging from 0.17% to 44%. In an ASA closed claims report, corneal abrasions accounted for 1.2% of all claims and 35% of eye injury claims.

b. **Risk factors** include:

1. Patient-related risk factors: advanced age
2. Surgical-related risk factors: Trendelenburg and prone positioning, large-volume blood loss, urologic surgery
3. Anesthesia-related risk factors: general anesthesia, greater length of PACU stay, use of oxygen during transport/recovery

2. **Pathophysiology**

The cornea forms the anterior portion of the globe and is composed of five layers. The outermost layer is a delicate epithelium that is continuous with the conjunctiva. The cornea is protected by a tear film that functions to prevent evaporation, lubricate the eyelids, supply dissolved oxygen to the cornea, irrigate the cornea of debris, and supply immunologic factors to the corneal surface. This protective film is regenerated by blinking. Corneal abrasions occur when the corneal epithelium and underlying layers are damaged. Mechanisms of injury include direct trauma, chemical injury, corneal drying resulting from failure of the eyelids to close properly (lagophthalmos), and pressure on the globe leading to decreased oxygen delivery and corneal edema, which in turn leads to desquamation of the corneal epithelium. General anesthesia decreases tear production and normal protective reflexes, which further predispose patients to corneal abrasions.

3. **Clinical significance**

The corneal epithelium is self-regenerating, and the majority of corneal abrasions resolve within days to weeks without long-term sequelae. It is important to avoid secondary infection of the compromised cornea, because these can lead to permanent corneal ulceration. In an ASA closed claims analysis, corneal abrasions were associated with fewer permanent injuries (16%) and lower median claim payments than other ocular injuries.

4. **Signs/symptoms** include eye pain, blurry vision, increased tear production, eye redness, photophobia, excessive squinting, and foreign body sensation.

5. **Diagnosis** is based on clinical history, symptoms, and uptake of fluorescein dye by the corneal epithelium on slit-lamp examination.

6. **Management** consists of a combination of artificial tears and antibiotic ointment (erythromycin or bacitracin eye ointment QID × 48 hours). Ophthalmology consultation should be considered, particularly if symptoms do not resolve within 24 hours.

7. **Prevention**

Strategies to prevent corneal abrasions include careful covering of the eyes (with tape or eye patches) after induction of anesthesia, mindfulness of dangling objects over the patients' face, and attention to patients emerging and recovering from anesthesia.

8. **Outcome**

In the majority of cases, corneal abrasions are not permanent injuries. In two retrospective studies, there were no cases of permanent injury resulting from perioperative corneal abrasions; however, of the corneal abrasions submitted to the ASA closed claims database, 16% resulted in permanent injuries.

9. **Subsequent care**

If the patient is asymptomatic after 48 hours, there is typically no follow-up required; however, if symptoms persist, the patient should follow up with an ophthalmologist.

B. **Postoperative Visual Loss**

1. **Overall incidence**

In retrospective studies, the overall incidence of postoperative visual loss (POVL) following nonocular surgery has ranged from 1 in 60,000 to 1 in 125,000. Spine and cardiac surgery are associated with higher incidence of POVL.

2. **Ischemic optic neuropathy**

a. **Incidence.** In retrospective studies, the incidence of ION following spine surgery has ranged from 0.028% to 0.1%, whereas ION following cardiac surgery has varied between 0.06% and 1.3%.

b. **Risk factors.** In prone spine surgery, factors found to confer higher risk of ION include male gender, obesity, anesthesia duration, large-volume blood loss, and low ratio of colloid to crystalloid fluid resuscitation. In cardiac surgery, risk factors include longer cardiopulmonary bypass times, low postoperative hemoglobin, transfusion of RBC or non-RBC blood components, and severe vascular disease.

c. **Pathophysiology.** There are two types of ION—anterior ION (AION) and posterior ION (PION). AION is more common among cardiac surgery, whereas PION is more common following spine surgery.

ION is thought to be caused by a decrease in O_2 delivery to the optic nerve because of hypoperfusion or embolism. The anterior optic nerve derives its blood supply primarily from the posterior ciliary arteries, whereas the posterior optic nerve is supplied by penetrating pial arteries and branches of the central retinal artery. Ischemic insult to the optic nerve initially causes optic nerve edema and later atrophy, leading to visual loss.

d. **Clinical significance.** Roughly 30% of patients will show some improvement following diagnosis, but ION usually results in some degree of permanent visual loss.

e. **Signs/symptoms.** Hallmark symptom of ION is painless visual loss.
   1. AION—Symptom onset may not be evident until more than 24 hours postoperatively. Signs/symptoms of AION include altitudinal visual field deficit, central scotoma, blindness, and afferent pupil defect or nonreactive pupils with bilateral symptoms in more than half of the cases.
   2. PION—Symptom onset is typically within 24 hours postoperatively. Signs/symptoms include blindness, altitudinal visual field deficit, central scotoma, afferent pupil defect or nonreactive pupils with bilateral involvement in two-thirds of the cases.

f. **Workup.** Ophthalmology consultation should be sought for anyone with postoperative visual changes.
   1. **Fundoscopic examination.** With AION, initial fundoscopic exam reveals optic disc edema that progresses to disc pallor and atrophy within 2 to 3 weeks. In PION, the optic disc is normal, with disc pallor and atrophy becoming evident in 6 to 8 weeks.
   2. Fluorescein fundus angiography is used to evaluate the circulation of the retina and choroid. If preformed shortly after symptom onset, this examination reveals a filling defect in the prelaminary region in AION, but is normal in PION.

g. **Management.** There is no proven treatment for ION; however, advocated treatments have included diuretics (mannitol, furosemide, and acetazolamide), high-dose steroids, surgical optic nerve decompression (in AION), and correction of hypotension and anemia.

h. **Prevention.** The ASA Task Force on Perioperative Visual Loss with Spine Surgery published an updated Practice Advisory in 2012. Advisory statements include the following:
   1. Blood pressure should be monitored continually in high-risk patients, and deliberate hypotension be used on a case-by-case basis.
   2. Colloids should be used along with crystalloids in patients with substantial blood loss.
   3. Direct pressure on the eye should be avoided.
   4. The patient's head should be positioned at or above the level of the heart when possible.
   5. Consideration should be given to staged spine surgeries to minimize time in the prone position.

i. **Outcomes.** Following initial diagnosis of AION, roughly 50% of patients have no improvement or worsening of visual symptoms, whereas 30% improve. In PION, results are similar: roughly 45% of patients have no improvement and 30% improve; however, PION is typically associated with more severe visual loss upon diagnosis.

3. **Retinal artery occlusion**
   a. **Epidemiology**
      1. **Incidence.** The overall incidence of retinal artery occlusion (RAO) is unclear; however, it seems to be highest in cardiac,

lower extremity joint, and spine fusion surgeries, with incidences of 0.06%, 0.009%, and 0.007%, respectively.

2. **Risk factors.** Because of limited available data, no firm risk factors have been established; however, retinal vascular occlusion has been associated with increasing age, male gender, blood transfusion, use of a horseshoe headrest, and anemia as well as cardiac, orthopedic, and spinal surgery.

3. **Pathophysiology.** Retinal vascular occlusion encompasses CRAO, which decreases blood supply to the entire retina, and branch retinal artery occlusion (BRAO), which decreases blood supply to only a portion of the retina. Mechanisms that have been described include: decreased arterial supply to the retina, retinal artery embolism, external compression of the eye, impaired venous drainage of the retina, and arterial thrombosis. The most common cause is thought to be external compression because of poor intraoperative positioning, which increases intraocular pressure and subsequently occludes the arterial circulation.

4. **Signs/symptoms.** Symptoms include painless visual loss, blindness (CRAO) or scotoma with intact peripheral vision (BRAO), and abnormal pupillary reactivity. Fundoscopic exam reveals a normal optic disc initially that later becomes atrophic and whitening of the retina with a cherry red macula.

5. **Workup.** Urgent ophthalmology consultation should be sought if RAO is suspected.

6. **Management.** No treatment has proven effective for RAO. Advocated treatments include acetazolamide or mannitol, local hypothermia, ocular massage, inhaled CO_2 for retinal artery vasodilation, hyperbaric oxygen therapy, and systemic as well as localized thrombolysis.

b. **Prevention.**
   1. See Prevention of ION above.
   2. Avoid external compression on the orbit and the horseshoe headrest.
   3. Frequent checking of eyes during prone surgery.

c. **Outcome.** There are no outcome data available for perioperative RAO, but most cases result in permanent visual loss.

4. **Cortical blindness** refers to infarction of the parietal–occipital areas of the cortex, responsible for reception and integration of visual input, resulting in visual loss.

a. **Epidemiology**
   1. **Incidence.** In one retrospective study analyzing the eight most commonly performed surgeries in the United States, the incidence of cortical blindness was 0.0038%, occurring most commonly among spinal fusion, cardiac, and hip surgery. In this study, cortical blindness was more common among patients less than 18 years of age. Other retrospective and prospective studies of cortical blindness following cardiac surgery have reported incidences between 0.2% and 5%.

   2. **Risk factors**
      a. No concrete risk factors have been established, but associated factors have included those that put patients at risk of stroke: age, diabetes, prior CVA/TIA, history of CAD and previous CABG, and history of vascular disease.
      b. Surgical and anesthetic-associated factors include cardiac, hip, and spine surgery (see above) as well as cardiopulmonary bypass, hypotension, anemia, and hemodilution.

3. **Pathophysiology.** Cortical blindness results from infarction of the parietal–occipital areas of the cortex, which ultimately occurs due to decreased O_2 delivery and neuronal cell death. Mechanisms include hypoperfusion (global ischemia, cardiac arrest, hemorrhage, local ischemia, and watershed infarctions) as well as thrombotic or embolic events, intracranial hypertension, and vasospasm. In cardiac surgery, the major culprit of cortical blindness is thought to be embolism, particularly from aortic atherosclerosis. Paradoxical emboli have been described as a source of cortical blindness in patients with congenital heart disease, allowing a right-to-left shunt.

4. **Clinical significance.** Cortical blindness is frequently accompanied by other neurologic deficits. Following cardiac surgery, CNS dysfunction such as stroke (including cortical blindness) increases ICU length of stay and perioperative mortality.

5. **Signs/symptoms.** Cortical blindness is associated with
   a. Painless visual loss with an intact pupillary response to light, which indicates that lesion is distal to the optic chiasm (and the pathways of the light reflex).
   b. An unremarkable fundoscopic exam (normal optic disc, retina, macula, etc.)
   c. Lack of response to visual threat
   d. Normal eye movement
   e. Depending upon the location of the lesion, the patient may have complete blindness (rare), which necessitates infarction of the bilateral parietal–occipital cortex, or unilateral blindness produces homonymous hemianopia.
   f. Often accompanied by other neurologic deficits (other areas of cortex affected by the stroke)

6. **Workup.** Radiologic imaging with CT or MRI reveals the area of infarction. Ophthalmology and/or neurology consultation should be obtained.

7. **Management.** Visual recovery occurs over time. Treatment is supportive and aimed at minimizing stroke and cardiovascular risk factors as well as further neurologic insults.

8. **Prevention.** To date, there have not been any interventions that have been shown to decrease the incidence or severity of cortical blindness. Maintaining adequate perfusion pressure should avoid periods of hypoperfusion. The majority of research has focused on preventing embolic events during cardiac surgery with decreased manipulation of the aorta, transcranial Doppler monitoring, and off-pump CABG.

9. **Outcome.** Improvement in visual acuity has been reported in a number of case reports of cortical blindness. Although the recovery is protracted, visual acuity improves in roughly 60% of cases.

II. **Perioperative Oropharyngeal Injury** typically involves the lips, tongue, nasal cavity, pharynx, larynx, esophagus, or temporomandibular joint (TMJ).
A. **Epidemiology**
   1. **Incidence**
   In an ASA closed claims report, 6% of claims in the database were for injury to airway structures including the larynx, pharynx, esophagus, trachea, TMJ, and nose. According to data obtained from the National Surgical Quality Improvement Program (NSQIP), the incidence of airway injury (including dental injury) was 0.2%. The most common injuries were lip laceration/hematoma, tooth injury, tongue laceration, pharyngeal laceration, and laryngeal laceration.

2. **Risk factors**
   a. Risk factors for airway injury found on analysis of the NSQIP database include Mallampati classes III and IV and age greater than 80.
   b. Risk factors specific to pharngyoesophageal perforation include female gender, difficult intubation, and age greater than 60.

B. **Common Airway Injuries During Anesthesia by Location**
1. **Nasal cavity**
   a. Nasotracheal intubation may cause soft tissue injury including mucosal abrasions or lacerations, avulsion of turbinates, or posterior pharyngeal lacerations. Epistaxis from nasotracheal intubation ranges from 29% to 96%, which is usually self-limited, but life-threatening bleeding has been reported.
   b. Prolonged nasotracheal intubation can result in mucosal ischemia, ulceration, necrosis, and sinusitis.
   c. **Prevention**
      1. Ideally, the most patent nostril should be used for nasotracheal intubation to limit complications. Digital manipulation or review of radiographic imaging can help identify the most patent nostril.
      2. Use of lubricants and nasal decongestants (oxymetazoline, cocaine, phenylephrine, etc.) is recommended.
   d. **Management**
      1. Small mucosal abrasions, lacerations, and hematomas usually resolve with conservative treatment (nasal pressure).
      2. Large hematomas and turbinate avulsions require otolaryngology consultation and evaluation.
      3. Nasopharyngeal lacerations should be closely followed for the development of retropharyngeal hematoma or abscess formation.

2. **Pharyngoesophageal perforation**
   a. **Incidence.** The incidence of pharyngeal or esophageal perforation as a complication of anesthesia is unknown; however, in an ASA closed claims analysis of airway injury, pharyngeal perforation accounted for 7% of all airway injury claims, roughly half of which were associated with difficult intubation. Esophageal perforation accounted for 16% of all airway claims.
   b. **Risk factors.** In the ASA closed claims analysis, risk factors associated with pharyngoesophageal perforation include difficult intubation, age over 60, and female gender.
   c. **Clinical significance.** In the closed claims database, 23% of patients filing claims for pharyngoesophageal perforation died. Other sources have reported overall mortality of esophageal perforation to be as high as 25%. Infectious sequelae (mediastinitis, retropharyngeal abscess, etc.) developed in 65% of cases. A delay in diagnosis is associated with development of late infectious complications. Retropharyngeal abscess arising from pharyngeal perforation can quickly progress to airway collapse.
   d. Reported mechanisms by which pharyngoesophageal perforation occurs during anesthesia include intubation, orogastric and nasogastric tube placement, combitube placement, and transesophageal echocardiography.
   e. **Symptoms** of pharyngoesophageal perforation include sore throat, dysphagia, chest pain, cough, dyspnea, and fever. **Signs** may include subcutaneous emphysema, pneumomediastinum, or pneumothorax, particularly with positive-pressure mask ventilation.

f. **Diagnosis** of pharyngoesophageal perforation requires a high level of suspicion. Severe and unexplained throat pain, deep cervical pain, or chest pain following difficult intubation should prompt a workup for pharyngoesophageal perforation. Contrast esophagography is the gold standard by which esophageal perforation is diagnosed; however, other helpful studies include lateral neck x-ray, chest x-ray, computed tomography, and flexible esophagoscopy.

g. **Treatment** includes operative and nonoperative management. Surgical consultation should be obtained once esophageal perforation is suspected. Contained ruptures can be managed nonoperatively with broad spectrum antibiotics, whereas uncontained ruptures require broad spectrum in addition to drainage or surgical repair.

3. **Larynx**

a. **Hoarseness**

1. Hoarseness as well as vocal fatigue, sore throat, or dysphagia can occur in up to 97% of intubations. Anesthesia parameters most commonly associated with the development of these symptoms include endotracheal cuff volume and pressure as well as number of intubation attempts. Although these symptoms were worse 2 hours postoperatively, nearly all of these symptoms resolve within 24 to 72 hours.

2. Management of postoperative hoarseness is primarily supportive; however, when symptoms persist or progress, more serious laryngeal injury should be suspected.

b. **Laryngeal injury**

1. The incidence of vocal cord injury has been reported to occur as frequently as 69% following short-term (<5 hours) general anesthesia with endotracheal intubation. The most common injuries include vocal cord paralysis, vocal cord hematomas and granulomas, interarytenoid adhesions, and arytenoid luxation.

2. **Vocal cord paralysis**

a. Intubations resulting in vocal cord paralysis range from 0.033% to 0.07%.

b. Symptoms include increased vocal effort, dysphonia, dysphagia, and aspiration.

c. Vocal cord paralysis due to endotracheal intubation is related to compression of the internal branch of the recurrent laryngeal nerve as it enters the larynx between the cricoid and thyroid cartilages near the cricoarytenoid joint. If the endotracheal tube (ETT) cuff sits too high and its pressure exceeds capillary perfusion pressure, blood flow is compromised, resulting in nerve dysfunction. Paralyzed vocal cord is usually found in the paramedian position. Left vocal cord paralysis is more common than right-sided paralysis; this is thought to be due to intubations being performed from the right side of the patient, with the trajectory of the ETT going from right to left favoring left-sided compression of the recurrent laryngeal nerve.

d. **Management.** When vocal cord paralysis is suspected, otolaryngology consultation and examination should be sought. Flexible laryngoscopy confirms the diagnosis. Physical examination of other cranial nerves should be normal.

e. **Outcome.** Patient may recover spontaneously; however, recovery is unlikely if no motion is appreciated within 6 to 12 months. Medialization of immobile vocal cords in the

paramedian and lateral positions can be performed to promote glottic sufficiency; this is usually not required of immobile vocal cords in the midline position. Roughly 35% of
patients with unilateral vocal cord paralysis will recover.

3. **Arytenoid dislocation**
   a. **Incidence.** The incidence of arytenoid dislocation is unknown;
   however, in an ASA closed claims analysis, arytenoid dislocation accounted for 2.6% claims filed for airway injury.
   b. **Anatomy.** The arytenoid cartilages, which lie directly posterior
   to the thyroid cartilage, articulate with the superior, posterior
   portion of the cricoid cartilage. The vocal process of both the
   arytenoids gives rise to the posterior vocal ligaments.
   c. **Pathophysiology.** The mechanism of injury is different for anterior and posterior arytenoid dislocation. Anterior dislocation
   is due to anteriorly directed pressure on the posterior portion
   of the arytenoids, usually from a laryngoscope or sometimes
   an ETT. Posterior dislocation is thought to occur during extubation of an incompletely deflated ETT cuff.
   d. Symptoms of arytenoid dislocation include hoarseness,
   breathiness, and vocal fatigue. Examination of the vocal cords
   upon direct laryngoscopy will reveal unilateral vocal cord immobility similar to unilateral vocal cord paralysis.
   e. Workup includes otolaryngology consultation for differentia-
   tion between vocal cord paralysis and arytenoid dislocation.
   Treatment usually consists of endoscopic reduction of the
   dislocation.

4. **TMJ disarticulation**
   a. Disarticulation of the TMJ most commonly occurs due to scissoring of the patient's mouth open for direct laryngoscopy. This
   results in the mandible being "locked" in an open position, with
   the mandibular condyle sliding anterior to the articulating
   surface.
   b. **Management.** Reinsertion of the mandibular condyles into their
   natural position can be done while the patient is under general
   anesthesia. While facing the patient, the provider grips the patient's mandible by placing his/her thumbs in the patient's mouth
   along the mandibular molars. Bilateral pressure is directed inferior and then posterior to return the mandibular condyles to their
   natural position.
   c. **Prevention.** Unnecessary vigorous scissoring of the mouth should
   be avoided, particularly in patients with TMJ pathology.

C. **Clinical Significance**
Analysis from the NSQIP data revealed that airway injury was not associated with increased 30-day mortality or hospital length of stay. In
the ASA closed claims analysis, airway injury tended to be less severe
and was associated with a lower median settlement when compared
to other injuries sustained under anesthesia. Most airway injuries were
temporary or nondisabling, with only 8% of airway injuries resulting in
death; however, 23% of patients filing claims for pharnygoesophageal
perforation died.

III. **PERIOPERATIVE DENTAL INJURY**
A. **Epidemiology**
   1. **Incidence**
   Perioperative dental injury occurring under general anesthesia is
   among the most common perioperative anesthetic injury. In retrospective studies, the incidence varies from 0.02% to 0.1%, whereas

small prospective studies have suggested an incidence as high as 25% during general endotracheal anesthetics.

2. **Risk factors**
   a. Patient-related risk factors: age and preexisting poor dental condition.
   b. Anesthesia-related risk factors: general anesthesia with intubation, number of intubation attempts, and increased difficulty of laryngoscopy and intubation.

B. **Anatomy**
   1. Adults have 32 teeth—4 central incisors, 4 lateral incisors, 4 canines, 8 premolars, and up to 12 molars.
   2. Every tooth has two parts:
      a. Crown—composed of three layers: enamel (outer), dentin (middle), and pulp (inner).
      b. Root—composed of three layers: cementum (outer), dentin (middle), and pulp (inner).

C. **Nomenclature—Universal Numbering System**
   1. Each tooth is assigned a number (1 to 32).
   2. Numbering starts with the right posterior maxillary molar and proceeds in a clockwise fashion along the maxillary dentition. Numbering of the mandibular dentition continues in a clockwise fashion starting with the third left mandibular molar (#17).
   3. Dentition is separated into four quadrants—two maxillary (upper) and two mandibular (lower).
   4. Each quadrant contains one central incisor, one lateral incisor, one canine, two premolars, and up to three molars.

D. **Pathophysiology**
   1. Preexisting dental disease, such as dental caries or periodontitis, compromises the natural structure of the dentition, making it more vulnerable to injury. This has shown to increase the risk of perioperative dental injury up to 3.4 fold.
   2. Types of dental injury
      a. Fracture refers to a crack in tooth that can involve just the enamel (Ellis Type I) or extend into the dentin (Ellis Type II), or pulp (Ellis Type III).
      b. Displacement (subluxation) refers to loosening of the tooth without complete avulsion.
      c. Avulsion denotes complete extraction of the tooth.
   3. The most common type of injury is enamel (Ellis Type I) fracture.
   4. The most common location is the upper incisors.

E. **Clinical Significance**
   Dental injury is the most common medicolegal complaint against anesthesiologists.

F. **Signs/Symptoms**
   Large fractures, obvious displacement, and avulsed teeth are usually obvious and found prior to the conclusion of the anesthetic. Smaller fractures may go unnoticed until after discharge. If fractures include the dentin or pulp (Type II or III), patients will typically complain of cold or pressure sensitivity. Smaller enamel fractures may be found on closer inspection by the patient or provider.

G. **Management**
   1. Injury location and severity should be documented immediately.
   2. Dental consultation should be sought as early as feasible.
   3. In the case of avulsion, the tooth should be retrieved. If the location of the tooth is unknown, a chest radiograph should be obtained to determine whether the tooth was aspirated.

4. If a tooth has been completely avulsed from its socket, it should be stored in cold normal saline or fresh milk until it can be reimplanted. Success rates approach 90% if reimplanted within 30 minutes.

H. Prevention

1. The preoperative dental assessment is thought to be the most important factor in preventing perioperative dental trauma.

2. Mouthguards have been advocated; however, similar incidences of dental injury occur with or without the use of mouthguards for intubation (0.062% vs. 0.063%).

3. Modifications of laryngoscopy blades have been advocated, but never formally evaluated in any studies.

4. Soft bite block should be placed between the molars, and oral airways should not be used as bite blocks, as these have also been attributed to dental trauma.

I. Subsequent Care

The patient should follow up with a dentist for subsequent care. Documentation of the dental injury and educating the patient to notify anesthesia providers of prior dental injury will allow preanesthetic planning in order to avoid future dental injury.

IV. PERIOPERATIVE NERVE INJURY

A. Epidemiology

1. **Incidence**

The incidence of perioperative nerve injury in retrospective studies has ranged from 0.03% to 0.14%. Perioperative nerve injury remains the second most frequent cause for claims in the ASA closed claims database, accounting for 16% of claims. The most frequent site of peripheral nerve injury was the ulnar nerve, brachial plexus, lumbosacral nerve root, and spinal cord. The incidence of perioperative peripheral nerve injuries has changed over time, with ulnar nerve and brachial plexus injury decreasing and spinal cord injury increasing.

2. **Risk factors**

Patient-related risk factors include hypertension, tobacco use, and diabetes mellitus. General and epidural anesthesia are risk factors for perioperative nerve injury, whereas spinal anesthesia and peripheral nerve blocks were not found to be risk factors. Surgical risk factors include patients undergoing neuro-, cardiac, general, or orthopedic surgery. Risk factors found for ulnar neuropathy include male gender, length of hospital stay longer than 14 days, and very thin as well as obese body habitus.

B. Pathophysiology

Mechanisms of peripheral nerve injury include:

1. Blunt trauma (e.g., needle placement during nerve block, surgical transection)

2. Toxic injury (e.g., anesthetic or other agent injected near the nerve)

3. Compressive injury (e.g., prolonged tourniquet use, poorly padded patient positions)

4. Stretch injury (e.g., prolonged traction or poor positioning)

5. Ischemic injury (e.g., prolonged tourniquet use, vasoconstrictors in anesthetic agent)

C. Common Perioperative Nerve Injuries

1. **Position-related nerve injuries**

a. **Ulnar neuropathy.** The etiology of perioperative ulnar nerve injury is multifactorial and incompletely understood; however, it is thought to be due in part to hyperflexion of the elbow and compression of the ulnar nerve as it courses over the medial epicondyle of the humerus. In the ASA closed claims study, only 9% of ulnar nerve injuries had a clear source of injury.

b. Brachial plexus neuropathy has been attributed to both compression and stretch injury, specifically intraoperative abduction of the arm greater than 90 degrees, lateral rotation of the head, use of shoulder braces during Trendelenburg positioning, and sternal retraction for internal mammary artery dissection. In cardiac surgery, brachial plexus injury has also been attributed to internal jugular vein cannulation prior to widespread use of ultrasound.

c. Sciatic neuropathy is most often associated with the lithotomy position. As it courses over the fibular head, the common peroneal nerve can be compressed and injured by the leg supports. Other branches of the sciatic nerve can be stretched by hyperflexion of the hips or extension of the knees.

2. **Regional anesthesia-related nerve injury**

In an ASA closed claims analysis, nerve injury was the most common complication, accounting for 51% of claims associated with peripheral nerve blocks. Nerves most commonly injured by regional anesthesia (in descending order) include the brachial plexus, median nerve, ulnar nerve, spinal cord, and phrenic nerve. The three most common blocks associated with nerve injury include interscalene, axillary, and intravenous regional anesthesia. In a separate prospective study, the incidence of nerve injury following peripheral nerve block was 0.04%. Proposed mechanisms include needle trauma to the spinal cord or peripheral nerve, intraneural injection, infection, and hematoma.

D. **Signs/Symptoms**

Symptoms include numbness, paresthesia, motor weakness, or persistent pain in the distribution of a peripheral nerve. The onset of symptoms may be delayed anywhere from 1 to 28 days postoperatively. Signs may include an inability to oppose the fifth finger (ulnar nerve injury), upper extremity weakness corresponding to a particular nerve root (brachial plexus injury), or foot drop with an inability to dorsiflex the toes (common peroneal nerve injury).

E. **Workup**

Once a postoperative peripheral nerve injury is suspected, documentation of the symptoms and physical examination is crucial. It is also important to determine any preexisting nerve problem. The goal of the physical examination is to determine if the process is affecting a single nerve, multiple nerves, a plexus, or the CNS. Additional studies include neurophysiology testing (electromyography and nerve conduction studies) and imaging (preferably MRI). Neurology consultation for further evaluation is recommended.

F. **Management**

Most peripheral nerve injuries are transient and resolve without treatment. For cases where reinnervation or clinical improvement is not apparent over a period of weeks to months, referral to a peripheral nerve surgeon may be appropriate.

G. **Prevention**

The ASA published a Practice Advisory for the Prevention of Perioperative Peripheral Neuropathies in 2000 that was updated in 2011. Highlights of the practice advisory are emphasized below:

1. The upper extremity should not be abducted greater than 90 degrees in the supine position.

2. In the supine position, the upper extremities should be supinated (or in neutral position) and pressure on the postcondylar groove limited to decrease ulnar neuropathy. When arms are tucked, neutral arm positioning is recommended.

3. To limit neuropathies of the sciatic nerves and its branches, the degree of flexion and extension of both the hips and knees should be considered when positioning the patient.

4. Prolonged pressure on the peroneal nerve at the fibular head should be avoided.

5. In the lateral position, chest rolls can decrease the risk of upper extremity neuropathy.

6. The use of shoulder braces in steep Trendelenburg positioning may increase the risk of brachial plexus nerve injuries.

7. Periodic perioperative assessments of patient positioning should be performed.

H. Outcomes

1. Position-related nerve injury

a. In the ASA closed claims analysis of all nerve injury claims (for all types of anesthetics), 23% resulted in permanent injury. In cases of postoperative ulnar neuropathy, 59% of patients regained complete motor and sensory function.

b. In cases of postoperative lower extremity neuropathy in patients in the lithotomy position, 93% of patients regained complete motor and sensory function.

2. Regional anesthesia-related nerve injury

In the ASA closed claims analysis examining nerve injury following peripheral nerve blocks, 68% resulted in temporary or nondisabling injury.

V. EXTRAVASATION INJURY

Extravasation injury is defined as damage from unintentional injection or leakage of solutions from a vessel into surrounding tissue spaces during intravenous infusion. The damage can extend to involve nerves, tendons, and joints and can continue for months after the initial insult. If treatment is delayed, surgical debridement, skin grafting, and even amputation may be the unfortunate consequences of such an injury. A compartment syndrome may result from extravasation of fluid into an extremity. If the amount of extravasated fluid is sufficiently large, blood flow to the distal portion of the extremity may be compromised with resulting tissue ischemia.

A. Epidemiology

1. Incidence

Extravasation of fluid is common in the perioperative setting. Most of the available data on extravasation are related to peripheral intravenous lines; however, extravasation with central venous lines does occur. For central venous catheters, extravasation is less frequent but potentially more dangerous because of the vulnerable anatomical structures and because extravasation might easily escape attention.

An ASA closed claims analysis found that 2% of the claims were related to peripheral vascular catheterization and half of these resulted from the extravasation of drugs or fluid. IV claims involved a larger proportion of cardiac surgery procedures during which arms were tucked.

2. Risk factors

Risk factors may be patient, agent, or provider related and often involve a combination of factors. Patient-related risk factors include preexisting cutaneous, vascular, or lymphatic pathology and abnormal anatomy (e.g., fragile, mobile veins or poor nutrition). In addition, altered mental status or anesthetic effects may impede the patient's ability to report any sensation at the infusion site. Agent-related risk factors include the toxicity of drug, the amount of agent extravasated, the infusion pressure, and duration of tissue exposure. Provider-related factors include decreased vigilance or awareness of health care professionals.

3. **Anatomy**

Sites most often implicated in extravasation injuries include the dorsum of the hand and foot, ankle, antecubital fossa, and near joints or joint spaces where there is little soft tissue protection for underlying structures. Limbs with local vascular problems such as lymphedema may have reduced venous flow, causing pooling and potential leakage of infused fluids around the site of cannulation.

4. **Nomenclature**

Agents and solutions that can cause tissue destruction are called vesicants.

5. **Pathophysiology**

With extravasation injuries, the degree of cellular injury is determined by the volume of the infiltrating solution and physicochemical characteristics, such as pH, osmolarity, and degree of dissociability (pKa). Infiltration of vasopressors such as epinephrine can produce local vasoconstriction and tissue ischemia, and in contrast, vasodilators may exacerbate the effects of extravasation by increasing local blood flow and enlarging the area of injury. Parenteral alimentation fluids, alkaline solutions such as thiopental, and hyperosmolar or concentrated electrolyte solutions (antibiotics, calcium, potassium, and sodium bicarbonate solutions) also have the potential to cause severe tissue necrosis when extravasation occurs.

6. **Signs/symptoms**

a. The full effect of the extravasation injury is often not immediately apparent but may evolve over days or weeks. Early symptoms of a vesicant extravasation include local pain, erythema, burning, pruritus, swelling, blanching, blistering, and discoloration of the skin. Pain is often the most useful symptom to alert the clinician to the possibility of a complication. Later symptoms include local blistering (indicative of at least a partial thickness skin injury), mottling/darkening of skin, induration, and ulceration. The resultant area of damage is often considerably larger than the initial physical appearance at the time of extravasation.

b. A lack of blood return from a cannula is commonly quoted as a sign that extravasation has occurred. However, this may be misleading because the act of attempting to draw back blood can move the cannula back into the vein while a hole remains in the vein wall. Alternatively, the bevel of the needle can puncture the vein wall during catheter insertion, allowing drug to escape into the tissue, whereas the lumen of the needle may still remain in the blood vessel and allow adequate blood return.

7. **Management**

a. After an extravasation has occurred, a systematic approach may help to prevent extensive tissue injury. Infusion of drugs through the line must be stopped immediately. Knowledge of the causative agent is crucial, including the amount, the particular region, and the length of contact with the extravasated agent all affecting potential corrective procedures.

b. Conservative measures such as elevating the involved extremity or applying heat or cold have not been shown to be beneficial, although early aspiration of the intravenous cannula and flushing with saline may be useful. In the case of extravasation of vasopressors, early infiltration with phentolamine may be effective.

c. To evaluate the extent of deep tissue damage, magnetic resonance imaging (T1- and T2-weighted images) may be helpful.

d. The indications for surgery in an extravasation injury patient include full-thickness skin necrosis, chronic ulcer, and persistent pain.

e. If the amount of extravasated fluid is sufficiently large, blood flow to the distal portion of the extremity may be compromised with resulting tissue ischemia. Untreated ischemia may result in reversible changes in nerve function within 30 minutes and irreversible changes after 12 to 24 hours. Measurement of elevated compartment pressures in conjunction with the clinical examination is used to make the diagnosis of compartment syndrome. Fasciotomy may be required for perfusion to the compromised extremity.

8. **Prevention**

a. Measures to prevent extravasation include careful insertion of peripheral venous cannula, flushing with sterile saline to ensure patency, and fastening it securely where it is always in view for regular inspection.

b. Hyperosmolar fluids, acidic or alkaline solutions, or infusates with irritant or vesicant properties should be given through central venous lines, if possible, or should be diluted appropriately.

c. When a central venous catheter is used, all vesicants should be administered through the most distal port of this line.

9. **Subsequent care**

Local necrosis may heal with conservative management, leaving minimal long-term sequelae, or may progress to significant eschar formation and tissue ulceration that ultimately require surgical debridement and skin grafting.

Suggested Readings

Apfelbaum J, Roth S, Connis R, et al. Practice advisory for perioperative visual loss associated with spine surgery: an updated report by the American Society of Anesthesiologists Task Force of Perioperative Visual Loss. *Anesthesiology* 2012;116:274–285.

ASA Task Force on Prevention of Perioperative Peripheral Neuropathies. Practice advisory for the prevention of perioperative peripheral neuropathies. *Anesthesiology* 2011;114:741–754.

Lee L, Roth S, Todd M, et al. Risk factors associated with ischemic optic neuropathy after spinal fusion surgery. *Anesthesiology* 2012;116:15–24.

Schummer W, Schummer C, Bayer O, et al. Extravasation injury in the perioperative setting. *Anesth Analg* 2005;100:722–727.

Special Considerations

SECTION III

Special Considerations

Pediatric Postanesthesia Care Unit

Ashlee Holman and Erik Shank

OVERVIEW

Transport from the Operating Room to Arrival in the Postanesthesia Care Unit

The pediatric postanesthesia care unit (PACU) is a unique setting in which physicians and nurses must be prepared to deal with children in various stages of anesthetic emergence *after* surgery or therapeutic/diagnostic procedures. Pediatric patients may arrive in the PACU fully anesthetized (e.g., after deep extubation in the operating room [OR]), at an intermediate stage of early or late emergence, or fully awake. They may arrive endotracheally intubated, with a laryngeal mask airway (LMA) in place, extubated with an oral airway, or with a natural airway.

Transport of the patient from the OR to the PACU must be performed by an experienced team that includes an expertly trained pediatric anesthesiologist. Focus should be directed at cardiopulmonary stability while maintaining a patent airway. Children may be transported in the lateral position to decrease risk of airway obstruction by the tongue and to maximize oropharyngeal volume. An oral airway placed in the OR and left for transport may also be helpful in maintaining a patent airway. Supplemental oxygen via mask or nasal cannula should be initiated prior to leaving the OR. Utilization of continuous pulse oximetry and a precordial stethoscope is recommended.

The patient should be in stable condition before leaving the OR. All monitors used for the procedure (pulse oximetry, blood pressure cuff, electrocardiograph [ECG] leads, etc.) should remain in place during transport, and the specific face mask and oral airway used during the case should always accompany each pediatric patient to the PACU. A transport pack containing laryngoscopes, endotracheal (ET) tubes, and resuscitation/intubation medications should be present for transport of potentially unstable and/or intubated patients.

The goal of the anesthesiologist is to facilitate safe and seamless transition of care to the PACU staff upon arrival in the recovery unit. The patient should not be stimulated during this time unless absolutely necessary. Monitors are left in place from the OR so as to be reconnected quickly and unobtrusively in the PACU and to minimize stimulation of the patient. Initial attention should focus on airway patency, adequacy of ventilation, oxygen saturation, heart rate (HR), blood pressure, and temperature. Supplemental oxygen should be continued if needed.

The handoff to the PACU staff by the anesthesiologist should include verification of patient identity and a standardized report detailing the patient's age, weight, allergies to medication, past medical history, medications, operative procedure, intraoperative issues, anesthetic technique and agents, intraoperative medications, intravenous (IV) access, estimated blood loss, fluid replacement, and urine output. Specific circumstances, such as family dynamics, the child's emotional status, developmental delay, or language barrier, should also be discussed.

Monitoring of vital signs and patient status should be continued throughout the patient's stay in the PACU. Vital signs should be measured and recorded at least every 15 minutes after arrival until the patient is discharged. Parents or caregivers should be allowed into the recovery room as soon as the child is settled and determined to be stable with regard to cardiovascular and respiratory status. Adequate lighting should be provided to ensure the ability to assess the child's condition from the doorway.

The anesthesiologist on staff in the PACU should be alerted immediately if any issue arises with the patient. The following section will discuss common problems and situations pertinent to the care of infants and children in the PACU.

SPECIFIC CONCERNS AND CONSIDERATIONS

Hypoxemia

Hypoxemia in children may result from causes similar to those in adult patients and may be broadly categorized as hypoxemia secondary to low inspired fraction of oxygen (FiO_2), hypoventilation, cardiac shunt, ventilation–perfusion mismatch, and diffusion hypoxia. In the pediatric patient, hypoxia occurs more rapidly than in adults, secondary to increased oxygen consumption, decreased functional residual capacity (FRC), increased airway resistance, increased chest wall compliance (resulting in poor maintenance of negative intrathoracic pressure, thus leading to functional airway closure), and increased work of breathing.

Hypoventilation and airway obstruction are the most common causes of hypoxemia for pediatric patients in the PACU.

Hypoventilation

In review, minute ventilation (MV) equals tidal volume (TV) multiplied by respiratory rate (RR). A decrease in TV or RR will result in decreased MV and subsequent hypoventilation. Causes of hypoventilation include a decrease in ventilatory drive, insufficient muscle strength, or other mechanical reasons.

Volatile anesthetics, opioids, benzodiazepines, and other sedating medications decrease the ventilatory drive in the pediatric patient. This effect is more profound in infants with apnea of prematurity, former preterm infants less than 55 weeks of age, children with central nervous system (CNS) injuries, morbidly obese children, and children with obstructive sleep apnea. If opioid overdose is suspected (slow RR, large TV), naloxone 0.5 to 1 μg/kg IV, administered in incremental doses, may reverse respiratory depression without precipitating pain or anxiety. Flumazenil 0.01 to 0.02 mg/kg IV may reverse benzodiazepine-induced respiratory depression.

Muscular weakness may result from inadequate reversal of neuromuscular-blocking agents or preexistent neuromuscular disease (muscular dystrophy, myasthenia gravis, etc.). Inability to lift extremities, perform a sustained head lift, paradoxic chest wall movement, or demonstration of residual neuromuscular blockade via peripheral nerve stimulator should be managed with administration of supplemental reversal agents. In children with preexisting neuromuscular disease, supplemental ventilatory support may need to be considered.

Mechanical causes of hypoventilation include airway obstruction, splinting secondary to pain, restriction from casts or bandages, or abdominal distention due to procedural insufflation or gastric air from positive-pressure ventilation (PPV) via mask airway.

Airway Obstruction

The most common and serious pediatric respiratory problem in the PACU is airway obstruction. This is a broad classification of complications that encompass upper airway obstruction, laryngospasm, and bronchospasm. Inspiratory stridor, paradoxic chest wall motion, and intercostal and tracheal retractions are common findings in upper airway obstruction and laryngospasm. Retractions, expiratory wheezing, and prolonged expiratory period may be observed in bronchospasm. Children with current upper respiratory infections (URIs) or those recovering from URIs are more prone to desaturation secondary to laryngospasm or bronchospasm, likely as a result of airway hyperreactivity and increased secretions.

Infants and children are more susceptible than adults to upper airway obstruction because of several anatomic differences (Fig. 30.1). These differences include presence of enlarged tonsils, a larger tongue in proportion to the rest of the oral cavity, a more cephalad larynx, and smaller distance between the tongue and glottis, resulting in easier obstruction.

Initial interventions should include stimulation of the child, repositioning to improve airway patency, suctioning of secretions, and, if needed, insertion of an oral or nasal airway or application of jaw thrust. Care must be taken in placing a nasal airway because resultant intranasal bleeding can further aggravate obstruction. If the airway is not recovered with these interventions, tracheal intubation should be considered.

Laryngospasm is defined as glottic closure due to reflex contraction of the laryngeal muscles and may be categorized as complete (silent chest movement with no ventilation possible) or partial (chest movement accompanied by "crowing" stridor with marginal ventilation possible). It occurs because of an anesthetic-induced depression of CNS inhibition of the glottic reflexes accompanied by stimulation at an inadequate depth of anesthesia. The incidence of laryngospasm is 17/1,000 in children up to 9 years of age and increases to 96/1,000 in children with URIs within 6 weeks of the anesthetic.

Immediate treatment involves administration of 100% FiO_2, firm jaw thrust, and application of positive airway pressure (Fig. 30.2). If laryngospasm cannot be broken with these measures, pharmacologic treatment should be

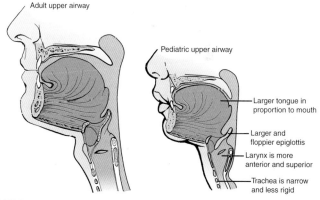

Adult upper airway

Pediatric upper airway

Larger tongue in proportion to mouth

Larger and floppier epiglottis

Larynx is more anterior and superior

Trachea is narrow and less rigid

FIGURE 30.1 Differences between the adult and pediatric airway. (From Berg SM, Bittner EA, Zhao KH. *Anesthesia Review: Blasting the Boards.* Philadelphia, PA: Wolters Kluwer; 2016.)

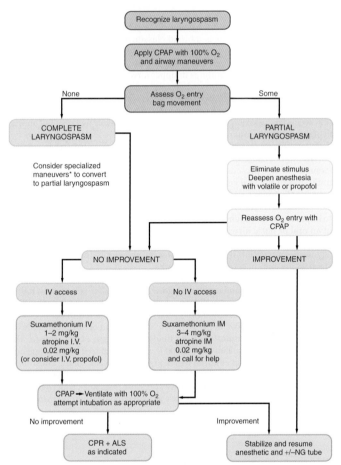

FIGURE 30.2 Laryngospasm treatment algorithm. *Specialized maneuvers: 1. Pressure in laryngospasm notch and 2. Pull mandible forward. (From Hampson-Evans D, Morgan P, Farrar M. Pediatric laryngospasm. *Paediatr Anaesth* 2008;18:303–307, with permission.)

considered early. Succinylcholine 1 to 2 mg/kg IV or 2 to 4 mg/kg IM along with atropine 0.02 mg/kg IV/IM, to prevent succinylcholine-induced bradycardia, is the gold standard for treatment of complete laryngospasm. Propofol has been used to treat partial laryngospasm but should not delay administration of succinylcholine if oxygenation worsens or if bradycardia develops. Intubation may be required to reoxygenate the child or if laryngospasm recurs after treatment. Post-laryngospasm, children should be observed for 2 to 3 hours to monitor for potential sequelae (e.g., negative-pressure pulmonary edema).

Postintubation croup or subglottic edema are complications that can arise in the PACU. These conditions are more common in children with a history of croup and previous prolonged intubation and are thought to develop secondary to edema from tight-fitting ET tubes, traumatic intubation, large volume shifts, and long surgical procedures. Treatment includes humidified oxygen and nebulized racemic epinephrine (0.5 mL in 3 mL normal saline over 10 minutes). Dexamethasone 0.5 mg/kg IV should be administered if it was not already given intraoperatively. Heliox (70%:30% helium/oxygen) may offer improved ventilation because of decreased airway resistance. The definitive treatment for ongoing severe respiratory compromise secondary to subglottic edema is tracheal intubation with a smaller ET tube than what was originally used intraoperatively.

Lower airway diseases such as asthma, secondhand cigarette smoke exposure, and airway manipulation are associated with a higher risk of perioperative bronchospasm in the pediatric patient. First-line treatment in the PACU includes administration of 100% FiO_2, short-acting inhaled β-agonists (e.g., albuterol nebulizer 0.05 to 0.15 mg/kg/dose in infants and 2.5 mg/dose for older children), and inhaled anticholinergic agents. Epinephrine 5 to 10 μg/kg IV bolus followed by 0.1 to 0.5 μg/kg/minute continuous infusion may be initiated in severe bronchospasm. Methylprednisolone 0.5 to 1 mg/kg IV or hydrocortisone 2 to 4 mg/kg IV should be administered but will not help in the acute period. IV magnesium 50 mg/kg and/or reinduction of anesthesia with sevoflurane should be considered in severe refractory bronchospasm. Emergent intubation may be required in children at high risk for respiratory arrest.

CARDIOVASCULAR INSTABILITY

Arrhythmias

As in the adult patient, the pediatric patient may also exhibit cardiac rhythm disturbances in the postoperative period. Most concerning in the pediatric PACU is bradycardia, which is significant because of the resultant decrease in cardiac output (CO). In review, CO is equal to HR multiplied by stroke volume (SV). As opposed to adults, small infants and children are unable to compensate for a decrease in CO by increasing SV because of their relatively stiff ventricles and diminished contractile ability. CO is therefore dependent on maintenance of an adequate HR (Table 30.1).

The most common cause of bradycardia in infants and children is hypoxemia until proven otherwise. Other secondary causes of bradycardia include medication effect, vagal stimulation, high neuraxial blockade, and increased intracranial pressure. Treatment should include immediate administration of 100% FiO_2, ensuring a patent airway, and assisting ventilation if necessary, followed by identifying and correcting the underlying problem. Atropine 0.02 mg/kg IV should be administered if oxygen supplementation does not correct the bradycardia. Epinephrine 2 to 10 μg/kg IV may also be needed. If there is no response, cardiopulmonary resuscitation (CPR), including chest

TABLE 30.1	Normal Ranges of Pediatric Heart Rate
Age	**Heart Rate (beats/min)**
Premature	120–170
0–3 months	100–150
3–6 months	90–120
6–12 months	80–120
1–3 years	70–110
3–6 years	65–110
6–12 years	60–95
>12 years	55–85

compressions for HR <60 beats/minute, should be initiated and is outlined in the following section.

Tachycardia in the pediatric patient may signify pain, anxiety, distended bladder, medication effect, or emergence delirium (ED), or may be an indicator of a more severe underlying process such as hypoxemia, hypercarbia, hypovolemia, developing sepsis, or previously unrecognized congenital heart disease or conduction abnormality.

Premature atrial or ventricular beats are uncommon in children and may warrant further investigation and cardiology consultation.

Hypotension/Hypertension

The normal blood pressure range for the pediatric patient depends on the age of the patient (Table 30.2).

The most common cause of hypotension in children is hypovolemia, usually as a result of inadequate intraoperative fluid resuscitation or ongoing blood loss. Other common signs of hypovolemia in children include dry mucus membranes, poor skin turgor, and urine output <0.5 mL/kg/hour. Hypovolemia should be initially treated with an isotonic crystalloid bolus of 10 to 20 mL/kg. Packed red blood cells (PRBCs) 4 mL/kg may be administered if anemia is suspected.

Other causes of hypotension in the pediatric patient may be categorized similarly to the adult patient as decreased preload (PPV, pneumothorax, cardiac tamponade, inferior vena cava compression), decreased afterload (vasodilation, medication effect, sepsis, sympathetic blockade from regional anesthesia), or pump failure (dysrhythmias, decreased inotropy, medication effect, sepsis, congestive heart failure, or hypothermia). Rare causes include anaphylaxis, transfusion reaction, severe liver failure, or adrenal insufficiency. Evaluation should include a full survey of infusion lines to assess for kinking or infiltration.

Hypertension is less common in the pediatric patient and is often caused by incorrect blood pressure measurement or pain. Other causes include hypervolemia, distended bladder, hypoxemia, hypercarbia, ED, increased intracranial pressure, medication effect, preexisting hypertension, or, rarely, malignant hyperthermia, undiagnosed coarctation, or pheochromocytoma. Treatment with antihypertensive agents is rarely required.

PEDIATRIC ADVANCED LIFE SUPPORT (PALS)

Cardiac arrest in children most commonly occurs as a result of noncardiac conditions, with respiratory insufficiency identified as the primary cause in

TABLE 30.2	Normal Ranges of Pediatric Blood Pressure	
	Blood Pressure (mm Hg)	
Age	**Systolic**	**Diastolic**
Premature	55–75	35–45
0–3 months	65–85	45–55
3–6 months	70–90	50–65
6–12 months	80–100	55–65
1–3 years	90–105	55–70
3–6 years	95–110	60–75
6–12 years	100–120	60–75
>12 years	110–135	65–85

TABLE 30.3	Reversible Causes of Cardiac Arrest	
6 H's	**5 T's**
Hypovolemia	Tension pneumothorax
Hypoxia	Tamponade, cardiac
Hydrogen ion (acidosis)	Toxins
Hypoglycemia	Thrombosis, pulmonary
Hypokalemia/Hyperkalemia	Thrombosis, coronary
Hypothermia	

over 50% of cases. In 2016, the American Heart Association (AHA) produced updated guidelines for CPR in infants and children.

Rapid identification of cardiac arrest and initiation of CPR is integral in maximizing the chance for successful resuscitation. Reversible causes (6 H's and 5 T's) must be evaluated and treated appropriately (Table 30.3).

Providing quality chest compressions is of utmost importance, with the provider's focus centering on ensuring an adequate rate (100–120 compressions/minute) and chest wall depression (1/3 the anterior–posterior diameter of the chest) while allowing time for complete chest wall recoil. Interruptions in chest compressions should be minimized.

Neonates (<4 weeks of age) and infants (<6 months of age) may be small enough to allow use of the two-thumb-encircling technique for chest compressions, described as using both thumbs to depress the sternum while the remaining fingers encircle the child's back allowing for circumferential squeezing of the chest. In older infants and children, the sternum can be compressed with two fingers or 1 to 2 hands, depending on the size of the child.

For mask ventilation, the provider should follow a 30:2 (for one provider) or 15:2 (for two providers) compression-to-ventilation ratio; if an advanced airway is in place, 8 to 10 breaths/minute with continuous compressions are appropriate. Attention should be directed at maintaining proper head positioning and relief of upper airway obstruction as well as ensuring adequate chest movement. ET intubation should be attempted as soon as possible.

Defibrillation should occur immediately if the cardiac rhythm is identified as ventricular fibrillation (VF) or pulseless ventricular tachycardia (pVT). Shock energy should be delivered as 2 J/kg for the first shock, 4 J/kg for the second shock, and >4 J/kg up to a maximum of 10 J/kg or adult dose for subsequent shocks. Synchronized cardioversion for unstable supraventricular tachycardia (SVT) or ventricular tachycardia (VT) should begin with 0.5 to 1 J/kg and may then be increased to 2 J/kg if ineffective.

IV or intraosseous (IO) access should be obtained expeditiously. Medication therapy for asystole or pulseless electrical activity (PEA) arrest includes epinephrine IV/IO 10 μg/kg (or 0.1 mL/kg of the code concentration 1:10,000), repeated every 3–5 minutes. ET epinephrine dosing is 100 μg/kg. Amiodarone may be administered in VF/pVT at a bolus dose of 5 mg/kg IV, repeated up to 2 times.

In the case of symptomatic bradycardia (HR <60 beats/minute with poor perfusion), epinephrine 0.01 mg/kg IV or atropine 0.02 mg/kg IV may be administered along with initiation of chest compressions and consideration of transthoracic or transvenous pacing.

For SVT (in infants, HR >220 beats/minute and in children, HR >180 beats/minute), vagal maneuvers should be performed without delay followed by administration of adenosine 0.1 mg/kg IV (maximum 6 mg) for the first dose and 0.2 mg/kg IV (maximum 12 mg) for the second dose prior to cardioversion. Amiodarone infusion (5 mg/kg IV over 30 to 60 minutes) or procainamide infusion (15 mg/kg IV over 30 to 60 minutes) may be initiated for VT in consultation with a cardiologist.

NEONATAL RESUSCITATION

In 2016, the American Academy of Pediatrics and the AHA published updated guidelines for neonatal resuscitation. These guidelines were developed primarily for newborns transitioning from intrauterine to extrauterine life; however, these recommendations are also applicable to neonates and small infants who may require resuscitation within the first few months of life and who may undergo procedures requiring perioperative care.

Rapid assessment of the newborn should include a concise evaluation based on the following: (1) Was the baby born at term? (2) Is the baby crying or breathing? and (3) Is there good muscle tone? If the answer is "no" to any of these three questions, initial steps in stabilization should include stimulation, clearing the airway, and providing warmth. Pulse oximetry and application of continuous positive airway pressure (CPAP) may be considered for labored breathing or cyanosis if the HR >100 beats/minute. Resuscitation should begin with air or blended oxygen; however, FiO_2 may be increased as needed.

Preliminary evaluation and initiation of ventilatory support should be completed within 60 seconds. If apnea is present, breathing is labored or gasping, or HR <100 beats/minute, PPV should be initiated at a rate of 40 to 60 breaths/minute with inflation pressures of 20 cm H_2O. More aggressive ventilation may be required (positive pressures up to 40 cm H_2O), and observed chest rise should determine the ultimate ventilatory pressure applied. For HR <60 beats/minute, chest compressions via the two-thumb-encircling technique should be delivered to the lower sternum with a depth of one-third the anterior–posterior diameter of the chest. Coordination of compressions with PPV is essential. If adequate chest rise cannot be appreciated, a secure airway, namely tracheal intubation, must be established.

Epinephrine 10 to 30 μg/kg IV or 50 to 100 μg/kg ET should be administered if the HR remains <60 beats/minute despite adequate ventilation with 100% oxygen and chest compressions. Volume expansion with a 10 mL/kg bolus of isotonic crystalloid solution may also be necessary.

Emergence Delirium

ED occurs in 10% to 20% of children. It may be manifested by uncooperativeness, irritability, thrashing, kicking, inconsolable crying, and screaming and may also include severe disorientation and the inability to recognize common objects or caregivers. ED generally occurs within the first 30 minutes of recovery from anesthesia, is self-limited (between 5 to 15 minutes), and may resolve spontaneously. The Pediatric Anesthesia Emergence Delirium (PAED) Scale is a validated tool that may be useful in evaluating emergence behaviors in children (Table 30.4).

Children between the ages of 2 to 5 years are at highest risk. Preoperative anxiety is also associated with increased risk of ED. Anesthetic-and procedure-related factors that may contribute to ED include rapid emergence from anesthesia, use of less soluble volatile anesthetics like sevoflurane or desflurane, painful procedures, and having undergone certain procedures such as tonsillectomy, thyroid surgery, dental surgery, and surgery involving the eyes and ears.

Strategies for managing ED can be divided into two categories: prevention and treatment. Adequate pain control is of utmost importance in the prevention as well as in the treatment of ED. Opioids, ketorolac, ketamine, clonidine, acetaminophen, and regional anesthesia have all been shown to decrease the incidence of ED as well as eliminate pain as a source of agitation.

TABLE 30.4	Pediatric Anesthesia Emergence Delirium (PAED) Scale				
	0	**1**	**2**	**3**	**4**
Child makes eye contact with caregiver	Extremely	Very much	Quite a bit	Just a little	Not at all
Child's actions are purposeful	Extremely	Very much	Quite a bit	Just a little	Not at all
Child is aware of his or her surroundings	Extremely	Very much	Quite a bit	Just a little	Not at all
Child is restless	Not at all	Just a little	Quite a bit	Very much	Extremely
Child is inconsolable	Not at all	Just a little	Quite a bit	Very much	Extremely

(Modified from Sikich N, Lerman J. Development and psychometric evaluation of the pediatric anesthesia emergence delirium scale. *Anesthesiology* 2004;100:1138–1145.)

Dexmedetomidine administered intraoperatively prior to emergence has also been effective in preventing ED. Use of midazolam is controversial, because it may result in unintentional paradoxic hyperactivity.

In the PACU, rescue treatment should be aimed at relieving pain and providing light sedation. This can include the use of medications such as fentanyl 1 to 2 μg/kg IV, propofol 0.5 to 1.0 mg/kg IV, midazolam 0.02 to 0.10 mg/kg IV, and dexmedetomidine 0.5 μg/kg IV. In addition, reuniting children with their parents early in the postoperative period, as well as leaving agitated children undisturbed or being held by a parent, may decrease the duration of delirium. Protecting the child from self-injury and damage to the surgical site should remain a top priority, and physical restraint may be necessary. Explaining to parents that this is a common, self-limited condition and that their child is not in danger may be useful because ED can be very upsetting to parents and caregivers.

PAIN

Evaluation of postoperative pain in the PACU should begin with the use of a pain scale that has been validated for assessment in children. The Wong–Baker FACES Pain Scale may be used in children who are verbal and developmentally appropriate (Fig. 30.3). Young children, nonverbal children, or developmentally delayed children may be assessed with the Face, Legs, Activity, Cry, Consolability (FLACC) Scale (Table 30.5).

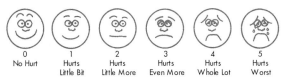

0	1	2	3	4	5
No Hurt	Hurts Little Bit	Hurts Little More	Hurts Even More	Hurts Whole Lot	Hurts Worst

FIGURE 30.3 Wong-Baker FACES Pain Scale. (From Wong-Baker FACES Foundation. Wong-Baker FACES Pain Rating Scale. 2016. Retrieved May 2016, with permission from http://www.WongBakerFACES.org. Originally published in Whaley & Wong's Nursing Care of Infants and Children. © Elsevier Inc.)

Revised FLACC Scale for Pain Assessment

Revised FLACC Scale for Pain Assessment in the Cognitively Impaired

	0	1	2
Face	No particular expression or smile	Occasional grimace/frown, withdrawn or disinterested (*appears sad or worried*)	Consistent grimace or frown, frequent/constant quivering chin, clenched jaw (*distressed-looking face, expression of fright or panic*)
Legs	Normal position or relaxed	Uneasy, restless, tense (*occasional tremors*)	Kicking or legs drawn up (*marked increase in spasticity, constant tremors, or jerking*)
Activity	Lying quietly, normal position, moves easily	Squirming, shifting back and forth, tense (*mildly agitated, shallow, splinting respirations with intermittent sighs*)	Arched, rigid, or jerking (*severe agitation, headbanging, shivering, breath holding, gasping, or sharp intake of breath, severe splinting*)
Cry	No cry	Moans or whimpers, occasional complaint (*occasional verbal outburst or grunt*)	Crying steadily, screams or sobs, frequent complaints (*repeated outbursts, constant grunting*)
Consolability	Content, relaxed	Reassured by occasional touching, hugging, or "talking to," distractible	Difficult to console or comfort (*pushing away caregiver, resisting care or comfort measures*)

Common Analgesic Medications

As with the adult patient, a multimodal approach should be initiated early in children. Options for pain control in the PACU include opioids, nonopioid analgesics such as acetaminophen, nonsteroidal anti-inflammatory drugs (NSAIDs), ketamine, and α_2-agonists, and neuraxial/regional anesthesia.

Acetaminophen may be given by multiple routes, including orally (PO), IV, and per rectum (PR). Dosing is 15 mg/kg PO, 7.5 mg/kg IV (in children 2 months to 2 years) or 15 mg/kg IV (in children >2 years), and up to 40 mg/kg PR. NSAIDs, such as ibuprofen 10 mg/kg PO or ketorolac 0.5 mg/kg IV, are useful medications but should be used cautiously in patients at high-risk for bleeding complications or those with renal insufficiency. Ketamine 0.25 to 1 mg/kg IV may be considered for refractory pain.

α_2-Agonists, such as clonidine and dexmedetomidine, are also effective in treatment of pain and reducing postoperative opioid consumption. Dosing for clonidine is 0.5 to 1 μg/kg IV, 4 to 5 μg/kg PO/PR, and 1 to 2 μg/kg neuraxial. Dexmedetomidine may be administered PO, intranasally (IN), or IV. Dosing is 2.5 to 4 μg/kg PO and 1 to 2 μg/kg IN. IV dosing includes a loading dose of 0.5 to 1 μg/kg over 10 to 20 minutes followed by a continuous infusion rate of 0.2 to 1 μg/kg/hour. Bradycardia may develop with these medications, so pretreatment with glycopyrrolate or atropine may be necessary.

Opioids are indicated after moderately to severely painful procedures. Dosing should be based on age, weight, physiologic development, underlying medical/surgical conditions, coadministered medications, prior history of opioid exposure, and severity of pain. If the patient is able to take oral medication, oxycodone 0.1 mg/kg PO may be considered. If the patient is unable to tolerate oral medication, fentanyl 0.5 to 2 μg/kg IV is effective for rapid, short-acting pain relief. Longer-acting opioids, such as morphine 0.05 to 0.1 mg/kg IV or hydromorphone 5 to 10 μg/kg IV, may also be initiated in the PACU if needed. It is important to recognize that these agents have a longer time to peak effect, and unintended respiratory depression may occur after transfer to floor or home if the patient is prematurely discharged. Patient-controlled analgesia (PCA) and nurse-controlled analgesia (NCA) have been shown to provide superior pain control as opposed to physician-ordered boluses and are associated with higher patient satisfaction ratings.

Codeine should not be used in children because of individual variability of metabolism, which can result in over- or under-dosing. Meperidine should also be administered with caution because of the epileptic potential of its metabolite, normeperidine.

Regional Anesthesia

Neuraxial and regional anesthesia is generally performed intraoperatively under general anesthesia in the pediatric population. In the PACU, attention must be directed at determining whether the block or catheter is functional. Evidence of success of the regional technique includes decreased intraoperative anesthetic requirement, confirmation of catheter placement via ultrasound or radiographic contrast administration, determination of motor blockade, or, in older, verbal children, identification of sensation level.

Adjuncts, such as opioids or clonidine, may be added to local anesthetics and may increase duration of pain relief. Systemic analgesia, either PO or IV, should be initiated in the PACU, *prior* to resolution of the block, to reduce any possible gap in pain control.

POSTOPERATIVE NAUSEA AND VOMITING

In children, the risk of postoperative nausea and vomiting (PONV) is related to age. Neonates and infants are unlikely to be affected by PONV. The incidence increases during childhood and reaches its peak in adolescence. PONV is more likely to occur after tonsillectomy, strabismus repair, hernia repair, orchiopexy, and middle ear procedures. The type of anesthetic (lower risk with a propofol-based anesthetic vs. higher risk with use of nitrous oxide) may also contribute to the incidence of PONV. Symptoms in children may be difficult to differentiate because of their inability to communicate and may include crying, retching, vomiting, and complaining of upset stomach.

Prophylaxis against PONV with multimodal therapy is recommended in high-risk patients. 5-HT$_3$ antagonists, such as ondansetron 0.05 to 0.1 mg/kg

IV, are the first-line treatment for both prophylaxis and rescue therapy in children. Intraoperative dexamethasone 0.1 to 0.5 mg/kg IV has also been shown to be effective in reducing PONV but has little effect as rescue treatment. Other rescue therapies in the PACU include metoclopramide 0.1 to 0.15 mg/kg IV, promethazine 0.25 to 0.5 mg/kg (in children >2 years), and prochlorperazine 0.1 to 0.15 mg/kg IV; however, recognition that these drugs are associated with dystonic reactions diminishes their utility. Scopolamine has not been approved for use in children; however, case reports of early intraoperative use of scopolamine 10 to 20 μg/kg IM/IV/SC have demonstrated a reduced incidence of PONV.

Other techniques that should be considered for minimizing risk of PONV include reducing administration of opioids and using nonopioid adjunctive medications such as ketorolac and acetaminophen. In addition, adequate hydration should be assured.

TEMPERATURE

Hypothermia is defined as temperature <96.8°F (36°C) and is associated with altered metabolism of medications, prolonged emergence from anesthesia, and delayed return of cognitive function in both children and adults. It may also contribute to physical discomfort, bleeding, infections, delayed wound healing, and cardiovascular instability. Neonates and infants are at high risk for hypothermia because of their larger skin surface-to-volume ratio (via radiation and convection) and higher MV per kilogram (via evaporation).

Forced-air warming blankets, which work by convection, are currently the most effective techniques in maintaining normal body temperature in children. Radiant heaters may also be used; however, overly aggressive rewarming can result in burn injury or hyperthermia if devices are not used properly or carefully. Prewarmed blankets and sheets will reduce conductive heat loss. Warming PACU rooms prior to the child's arrival will prevent heat loss by radiation.

Postoperative hyperthermia is defined as temperature >101°F (38.3°C) and is less common in the pediatric patient. Hyperthermia in the PACU is most frequently iatrogenic in nature secondary to aggressive warming techniques; however, it may also be a sign of an emerging underlying disease process, such as infection, viscera perforation, respiratory complication, thyroid storm, neuroleptic malignant syndrome, or malignant hyperthermia and thus warrants immediate investigation and treatment of the developing process.

COMMON PEDIATRIC PROCEDURES

Tonsillectomy and Adenoidectomy

These procedures are frequently performed as therapy for children with obstructive sleep apnea. Although the surgery itself may relieve mechanical obstruction, these children may still have a "central" apnea component and can be prone to respiratory pauses. Vigilant respiratory monitoring in the PACU should be performed. Patients may be hypersensitive to opioids *after* tonsillectomy and adenoidectomy (T&A); thus, these medications should be used with extreme caution. PONV may be prevalent, and dexamethasone 0.2 to 0.7 mg/kg IV has been demonstrated to be both an effective antiemetic and analgesic for these patients. Additional PACU concerns include acute postoperative bleeding and swelling, which may require emergent reintubation and surgical consult. Tracheal reintubation should be performed with a smaller ET tube than the one used intraoperatively.

Myringotomy and Tympanostomy

This is the most common surgery performed in pediatric patients between 1 and 3 years of age. The procedure includes making a small incision in the tympanic membrane and placing a drainage tube into the incision, typically to treat middle ear infections. The actual procedure is brief, and recovery is usually uneventful. Pain may manifest as irritability or grabbing or hitting of the ears or the head. Intranasal fentanyl, ketorolac IM, and/or topical anesthetic ear drops are typically adequate for analgesia. PONV may also be present and should be treated with the medications described previously.

Circumcision

This is another very common pediatric surgery, typically with minimal complications. Pain, anxiety, and, rarely, bleeding may be seen in the PACU. Younger children may be especially inconsolable, and determining whether the cause is pain, anxiety, or altered sensation (a penile block is frequently performed intraoperatively) may be challenging. Frequently, a bolus of fentanyl 0.5 to 1 μg/kg IV is sufficient to provide both analgesia and anxiolysis for the child.

Endoscopy

Upper (esophageal) or lower (colonoscopy) endoscopy procedures should not result in extreme pain in the recovery room; however, visceral stretching owing to insufflation of air during the procedure or sore throat from passing the endoscope may manifest as discomfort. Pain out of proportion to what is expected or pain associated with a tense abdomen and peritoneal signs suggests the possibility of viscera perforation. Likewise, a temperature >101.5°F (38.6°C) may indicate perforation. Aspiration may be observed after endoscopy because many of these procedures are performed for reflux disease. A persistent oxygen requirement may suggest this diagnosis.

APNEA OF PREMATURITY

Preterm infants (<36 weeks' gestation) are at risk for apnea and subsequent bradycardia after both sedation and general anesthesia. This risk decreases with increasing postconceptual age (PCA), which is defined as the sum of gestational age (GA) and postnatal age (PNA). Spinal anesthesia, solely with local anesthetic, decreases the risk of pulmonary and cardiovascular complications, but does not fully eliminate the risk of postoperative apnea.

Preterm infants who are younger than 55 weeks' PCA, anemic (hematocrit <30%), with major cardiorespiratory or neurologic disorders, and with current, ongoing apnea should be admitted for monitoring. An apnea-free period of 12 hours should be demonstrated prior to consideration for discharge. Preterm infants who are 55 weeks' PCA or older, not anemic, and without ongoing apnea should be observed for an extended period of time and may be discharged later if stable.

Full-term infants who are 50 weeks' PCA or older may be discharged if stable. Full-term neonates younger than 30 days, full-term infants with a history of apnea and bradycardia, or those with a family history of sudden infant death syndrome (SIDS) should be observed for an extended period of time and may require hospitalization for overnight monitoring.

DISCHARGE CRITERIA

Recovery from anesthesia in the PACU can be divided into two stages. Phase I includes confirmation of a stable, patent airway with return of airway reflexes, return of baseline motor function, stabilization of vital signs and oxygen saturation, and adequate pain control. Phase II includes presence of adequate hydration and fluid status, minimal emesis, appropriate ambulation and mental status, and continued stable vital signs.

Various criteria are used to determine readiness for discharge, whether it is to a pediatric floor for monitoring or to the patient's home. The modified

Aldrete score is the most common system used in the PACU, with the addition of postoperative pain and nausea assessment (Table 30.6).

To be considered eligible for general discharge from the PACU, the child should be awake, alert, and at his or her original level of consciousness (Table 30.7).

The blood pressure and HR should be within 20% of the preoperative values. The patient should not require additional airway support, and oxygen saturation should be >92% on 3 L/minute nasal cannula or at the patient's baseline. These hemodynamic and respiratory parameters should remain stable for at least 30 minutes for inpatients and 60 minutes for outpatients. Temperature should be between 97.0°F and 100.8°F. Pain control should be optimal. Nausea and vomiting should be controlled. The surgical site should be appropriate without signs of abnormal bleeding. Lab values, electrocardiograms, and chest radiographs should be reviewed and abnormalities addressed.

Of note, tolerating oral intake is not required for discharge. Similarly, voiding postoperatively is also not a requirement for discharge. An appropriate recovery time (generally 1 to 2 hours) should be decided by the PACU anesthesiologist and may be influenced by the child's medical history and procedure.

The decision to discharge a patient should be based on the clinical judgment of the anesthesiologist staffing the PACU. Children should be discharged home under the care of a competent adult caregiver. Either the surgical or anesthesia team should answer all questions asked by the caregiver. Both written and verbal instructions should be distributed and should include

TABLE 30.6	Modified Aldrete Scoring System		
	0	**1**	**2**
Activity	Four extremities	Two extremities	No extremities
Respiration	Able to breathe deeply and cough freely	Dyspnea, shallow or limited breathing	Apnea
Circulation	Blood pressure within 20 mm Hg of preop level	Blood pressure within 20–50 mm Hg of preop level	Blood pressure >50 mm Hg of preop level
Consciousness	Fully awake	Arousable on calling	Unresponsive
Oxygen saturation	Saturation >90% when breathing room air	Needs oxygen to maintain saturation >90%	Saturation <90% with oxygen

TABLE 30.7	Level of Consciousness Criteria
0	Reflexes absent, no response to verbal commands
1	Reflexes present, no response to verbal commands
2	Eyes open to verbal command or in response to name
3	Lightly asleep, eyes open intermittently
4	Fully awake, eyes open, conversing

postprocedural side effects and activity limitations, dietary restrictions, and anticipated postanesthesia side effects. Discharge instructions should include a 24-hour emergency phone number.

Suggested Readings

American Society of Peri Anesthesia Nurses. *2012–2014 Perianesthesia Nursing Standards, Practice Recommendations, and Interpretive Statements.* Cherry Hill, NJ: ASPAN; 2012.

Basker S, Singh G, Jacob R. Clonidine in paediatrics—a review. *Indian J Anaesth* 2009;53(5):270–280.

Behrman RE, Kliegman RM, Jenson HB. *Nelson Textbook of Pediatrics.* 17th ed. Philadelphia, PA: WB Saunders; 2004.

Cote CJ, Lerman J, Anderson B. *A Practice of Anesthesia for Infants and Children.* 5th ed. Philadelphia, PA: Saunders; 2013.

EMT National Training. EMT Basic Airway Management Module 2.1. Downloaded March 11, 2015 from http://www.ceu-emt.com/airway-ceu.php. Accessed March 26, 2017.

Hampson-Evans D, Morgan P, Farrar M. Pediatric laryngospasm. *Pediatr Anesth* 2008;18:303–307.

Horimoto Y, Tomie H, Hanzawa K, et al. Scopolamine patch reduces postoperative emesis in paediatric patients following strabismus surgery. *Can J Anaesth* 1991;38(4 Pt 1):441–444.

Kattwinkel J, Perlman JM, Aziz K, et al. Special report—neonatal resuscitation: 2010 American Heart Association guidelines for cardiopulmonary resuscitation and emergency cardiovascular care. *Circulation* 2010;122:S909–S919.

Kleinman ME, Chameides L, Schexnayder SM, et al. Pediatric advanced life support: 2010 American Heart Association guidelines for cardiopulmonary resuscitation and emergency cardiovascular care. *Circulation* 2010;122:S876–S908.

Maloney E, Meakin GH. Acute stridor in children. *Contin Educ Anaesth Crit Care Pain* 2007;7(6):183–186.

Merkel SI, Voepel-Lewis T, Shayevitz JR, et al. The FLACC: a behavioral scale for scoring postoperative pain in young children. *Pediatr Nurs* 1997;23:293–297.

Miller RD, Eriksson LI, Fleisher LA, et al. *Miller's Anesthesia.* 7th ed. Philadelphia, PA: Churchill Livingstone Elsevier; 2010.

Schnabel A, Reichl S, Poepping DM, et al. Efficacy and safety of intraoperative dexmedetomidine for acute postoperative pain in children: a meta-analysis of randomized controlled trials. *Pediatr Anesth* 2013;23(2):170–179.

Sikich N, Lerman J. Development and psychometric evaluation of the pediatric anesthesia emergence delirium scale. *Anesthesiology* 2004;100:1138–1145.

Vlajkovic GP, Sindjelic RP. Emergence delirium in children: many questions, few answers. *Anesth Analg* 2007;104:84–91.

Wong DL, Hockenberry-Eaton M, Wilson D, et al. *Wong's Essentials of Pediatric Nursing.* 6th ed. St. Louis, MO: Mosby Inc.; 2001.

Woods BD, Sladen RN. Perioperative considerations for the patient with asthma and bronchospasm. *Br J Anaesth* 2009;103(suppl 1):i57–i65.

31

The Morbidly Obese Patient

Yasuko Nagasaka and Jean Kwo

I. INTRODUCTION

Excess body weight is associated with an increased risk of death, because an elevated body mass index (BMI) increases the risk for type 2 diabetes mellitus (T2DM), cardiovascular disease, pulmonary disease, metabolic syndrome, and obstructive sleep apnea (OSA). Patients with high BMIs challenge clinicians during the postoperative period secondary to acute complications or exacerbations of chronic comorbidities and often present with complex clinical pictures. In this chapter, we will summarize the pathophysiology of obesity, postoperative management and monitoring, and pharmacologic approaches of the morbidly obese patients. Our goal is to provide a better understanding of why obese patients may deteriorate postoperatively, with a hope to further improve patient care.

II. DEFINITION

Obesity is a medical condition in which excess body weight causes increased health risks and reduced longevity. The diagnosis of obesity is based on BMI because it correlates with the amount of body fat.

$$\text{BMI} = \frac{\text{Body weight (kg)}}{(\text{Height (m)})^2}$$

The World Health Organization classifies BMI as:

Normal: 18.5 to 24.9
Overweight: 25 to 29.9
Obese: >30

Obesity is further categorized into Class I (BMI 30 to 34.9), Class II (BMI 35 to 39.9), and Class III (BMI >40). The distribution of fat is also important in the risk of developing comorbid diseases. Central or abdominal obesity, as reflected by the ratio of the circumference of the waist to that of the hips (waist–hip ratio), is associated with increased insulin resistance, dyslipidemia, and risk of atherosclerotic heart disease. Relative to healthy weight women, overweight women have been shown to be 3 to 6 times more likely to have mobility disability.

III. PATHOPHYSIOLOGY

Obesity causes systemic oxidative stress and inflammatory changes resulting in increased levels of inflammatory markers, such as tumor necrosis factor alpha and interleukin 6, which result in changes that affect multiple body systems.

A. Cardiac

1. **Coronary artery disease (CAD):** Obese individuals have a higher prevalence of CAD than nonobese individuals. The prevalence of high total cholesterol (defined as ≥240 mg/dL) is higher with increased BMI. In a meta-analysis of 19,388 bariatric surgery patients, 7% had a history of CAD.

2. **Cardiomyopathy** can develop due to increased total blood volume, resulting in left ventricular chamber dilation. Fatty infiltration of the myocardium can develop resulting in a pattern of restrictive cardiomyopathy. Approximately 31% of individuals with extreme obesity develop obesity-related cardiomyopathy.

3. **Heart failure:** An increase in blood volume leads to an increase in stroke volume, resulting in left ventricular overload, dilation and left ventricular hypertrophy, and finally culminating in heart failure.

4. **Pulmonary hypertension and biventricular dysfunction:** Prolonged exposure to cardiotoxic factors such as insulin resistance, steatosis, neurohumoral overactivation, and nocturnal hypoxia and hypercarbia associated with OSA can eventually conclude in the development of pulmonary hypertension and biventricular dysfunction.

5. **Arrhythmias:** There is an association between obesity and atrial fibrillation (AF). Patients with a BMI >40 have a 2.3-fold increased risk of postoperative AF compared to a 1.2-fold increased risk in those with a BMI between 25 and 30.

6. **Hypertension:** A recent cohort study with a median follow-up period of 46 years disclosed that those who were overweight or obese in early adulthood or middle age were at higher risk of developing hypertension later in life.

7. **Metabolic syndrome** is a group of conditions that increase the risk of cardiovascular disease and T2DM. A recent definition includes elevated waist circumference (value determined by individual populations) plus any two of the following: elevated triglycerides ($\geq$150 mg/dL), reduced high-density lipoprotein C ($\leq$40 mg/dL in males, $\leq$50 mg/dL in females), hypertension (systolic $\geq$130 and/or diastolic $\geq$85 mm Hg), and elevated fasting glucose ($\geq$100 mg/dL).

B. **Respiratory**

Increased BMI adversely impacts respiratory function with significant impairment observed once BMI exceeds 45. Coexisting polycythemia may suggest long-standing hypoxemia.

1. **Obstructive sleep apnea (OSA):** OSA affects approximately 94% of patients presenting for weight loss surgery and is often undiagnosed. OSA increases perioperative morbidity and mortality and is significantly associated with a composite endpoint of death, venous thromboembolism, reintervention, or failure to be discharged by 30 days after surgery. Treating patients with continuous positive airway pressure (CPAP) or bilevel positive airway pressure for several weeks to months preoperatively combined with postoperative pulse oximetry monitoring has been shown to reduce postoperative complications. The American Society of Anesthesiologists recommends perioperative initiation of CPAP if OSA is severe, and continuation of CPAP or noninvasive positive pressure ventilation in the perioperative period unless contraindicated.

2. **Anatomic airway changes:** Ever-increasing weight is associated with the deposition of adipose tissue around pharyngeal structures and a reduction in airway caliber. This results in impaired of pharyngeal dilator activity and an increased risk of airway collapse. These changes can lead to difficulty with laryngoscopy and intubation.

3. **Obesity hypoventilation syndrome** (defined as BMI >30 kg/m^2, chronic alveolar hypoventilation, and sleep-disordered breathing) and overlap syndrome (coexisting OSA and chronic obstructive pulmonary disease without pathologic link) are often seen in the morbidly obese. These patients are at higher risk of developing pulmonary hypertension.

4. **Asthma:** Obese individuals (BMI >30) are nearly twice as likely to develop asthma as individuals with a BMI <25. Weight loss is associated with improved asthma control.

C. **Hepatobiliary/Gastrointestinal**

1. **Liver disease:** In bariatric patients, the prevalence of nonalcoholic fatty liver disease (NAFLD) and nonalcoholic steatohepatitis (NASH) has been estimated to be as high as 91% and 37%, respectively. Risk factors for metabolic syndrome are concurrent risk factors for NAFLD and NASH.

2. **Gastroesophageal reflux disease (GERD):** Obese individuals are at higher risk of GERD due to mechanical and hormonal changes. However, in otherwise healthy obese patients, gastric emptying appears normal.

3. **Gallstones:** Obesity is a risk factor for the formation of cholesterol gallstones and exposes patients to an increased risk of gallstone-related complications and need for cholecystectomy. Female gender and rapid weight loss are major risk factors for postoperative cholelithiasis.

D. **Renal**

Obesity is associated with an increased risk of developing Stage 3 chronic kidney disease when studied in a cohort with over 20 years of follow-up.

E. **Central Nervous System**

1. **Stroke:** Obesity is associated with stroke and has a significantly higher prevalence in patients with younger age as compared to nonobese patients.

2. **Psychosocial aspects and depression:** Individuals with obesity have elevated psychologic risk factors for developing psychologic strains and thus, this patient population exhibits a higher prevalence of depression.

F. **Hematology**

1. **The blood volume** of obese patients is increased and can be estimated by the following equation:

$$\text{Indexed blood volume} = \frac{70}{\sqrt{\text{patient's BMI}/22}}$$

2. **Hypercoagulability:** Obesity is associated with an overproduction of procoagulant agents and increased thrombin generation resulting in hypercoagulability.

3. **Venous thromboembolism (VTE):** The obesity-related state of chronic inflammation and impaired fibrinolysis place patients with elevated BMIs at an increased risk for postoperative thromboembolic events. The rate of VTE in patients undergoing bariatric surgery is 2%. Risk factors for postoperative VTE include increased age, high BMI, male gender, and history of prior VTE. Patients undergoing surgery should receive chemoprophylaxis with either low-dose unfractionated heparin or low-molecular weight heparin in addition to mechanical prophylaxis with elastic stockings or intermittent pneumatic compression. Because most VTE occurs after discharge, continuing chemoprophylaxis after hospital discharge should be considered in high-risk patients (e.g., those with history of deep venous thrombosis).

G. **Endocrine**

1. **Type 2 diabetes mellitus:** Obesity promotes insulin resistance and the development of T2DM. Adults with a BMI ≥40 are 7 times more

likely to have diabetes compared to normal weight individuals. Patients with poorly controlled diabetes are more prone to developing wound infections, acute renal failure, and postoperative wound dehiscence.

2. **Thyroid:** Obesity has been strongly associated with thyroid cancer, perhaps via the increase of insulin or insulin-like growth factor 1 that results from insulin resistance.

H. Cancer

Obesity has been linked to 20% of all cancer deaths in women and 14% in men. Increased BMI is associated with a higher risk of both common and less common cancers. In men, significant positive associations with obesity were noted with rectal and prostate cancers. In women, positive associations were found with endometrial, gastrointestinal, and postmenopausal breast cancers. Underlying pathophysiologic mechanisms of cancer susceptibility in patients with elevated BMIs are related to genetic factors, insulin/IGF-I signaling axis, chronic low-grade inflammation, adipokine secretion, and gut microbiota.

I. Other Conditions

1. **Polycystic ovarian syndrome** is characterized by obesity, insulin resistance, cardiometabolic features, ovarian cysts, hirsutism, and infertility. Weight gain exacerbates reproductive and metabolic risks.

2. **Pediatric obesity syndromes:** The most recent data from the National Health and Nutrition Examination Survey report a 5.5% decrease in the prevalence of obesity among 2- to 5-year-olds between 2003 to 2004 and 2011 to 2012. Children with obesity are at risk for adult conditions such as T2DM, hypertension, and dyslipidemia. Certain congenital conditions are associated with morbid obesity. These include Prader–Willi syndrome, Alstrom syndrome, Cohen syndrome, Albright hereditary osteodystrophy (pseudohypoparathyroidism), Carpenter syndrome, MOMO syndrome, and Rubinstein–Taybi syndrome.

IV. PERIOPERATIVE RISK ASSESSMENT

A. Cardiac Risk Assessment

Cardiac risk assessment requires an analysis of the patient's personal risk factors and functional status in conjunction with the planned procedure. The American College of Cardiologist and the American Heart Association guidelines do not recommend cardiac testing if the risk of a major adverse cardiac event (MACE) is <1%. If the MACE risk is ≥1%, functional status should guide whether further cardiac testing is necessary.

Surgical risk scoring indices: There are several validated tools to help assess perioperative cardiac risk, including the following:

1. **American College of Surgeons National Surgical Quality Improvement Program Risk Calculator** can be accessed at http://www.surgicalrisk calculator.com

2. **The Revised Cardiac Risk Index** (Table 31.1) uses six categories to risk-stratify patients for adverse cardiac events after noncardiac surgery.

B. Diabetes Risk

Poorly controlled diabetes is associated with increased perioperative complications such as wound infections, surgical anastomotic breakdown, and acute renal failure. In patients undergoing bariatric surgery, a glycohemoglobin (Hgb A1c) value of <6.5% was associated with a 10% less complication rate when compared to Hgb A1c value of >8%.

Revised Cardiac Risk Index

One point for each factor:
1. High-risk surgery (intraperitoneal, intrathoracic, and suprainguinal vascular procedures)
2. Ischemic heart disease
3. History of congestive heart failure
4. History of cerebrovascular disease
5. Insulin therapy for diabetes mellitus
6. Preoperative serum creatinine >2.0 mg/dL

Number of Factors	Rates of Major Cardiac Complications (%)
0	0.5
1	0.9–1.3
2	3.6–6.6
≥3	9.1–11

Adapted from Lee TH, Marcantonio ER, Mangione CM, et al. Derivation and prospective validation of a simple index for prediction of cardiac risk of major noncardiac surgery. *Circulation* 1999;100: 1043–1049.

STOP-Bang Questionnaire

Snoring: Do you snore loudly (loud enough to be heard through closed doors)?
Tired: Do you often feel tired, fatigued, or sleepy during daytime?
Observed: Has anyone observed you stop breathing during your sleep?
Blood **P**ressure: Do you have or are you being treated for high blood pressure?
BMI: BMI more than 35 kg/m^2?
Age: Age over 50 years old?
Neck circumference: Neck circumference greater than 40 cm?
Gender: Male?

High risk of OSA	Yes to three or more questions
Low risk of OSA	Yes to less than three questions

BMI, body mass index; OSA, obstructive sleep apnea.
Adapted from Chung F, Yegneswaran B, Liao P, et al. STOP questionnaire: a tool to screen patients for obstructive sleep apnea. *Anesthesiology* 2008;108:812–821.

C. Liver Disease Risk

Predictors of liver disease include elevated liver enzymes, increased BMI, male gender, and history of T2DM. A triglyceride level >150 mg/dL is associated with a 3.4-fold greater risk of developing NASH. Conversely, an elevated level of high-density lipoprotein C is associated with a decreased likelihood of NASH.

D. OSA-Related Risk

Patients with OSA have an increased risk of postoperative cardiopulmonary complications. The STOP-Bang questionnaire (Table 31.2) is a screening tool for OSA developed specifically for use in surgical patients. In obese patients, a score of 0 to 3 indicates a low risk of OSA; a score of 4 and 5, an intermediate risk of OSA; and a score of 6 to 8, a high risk of OSA. The degree of postoperative monitoring required for patients with OSA should be based on clinical predictors, surgical risk, and risks associated with sedation (Fig. 31.1).

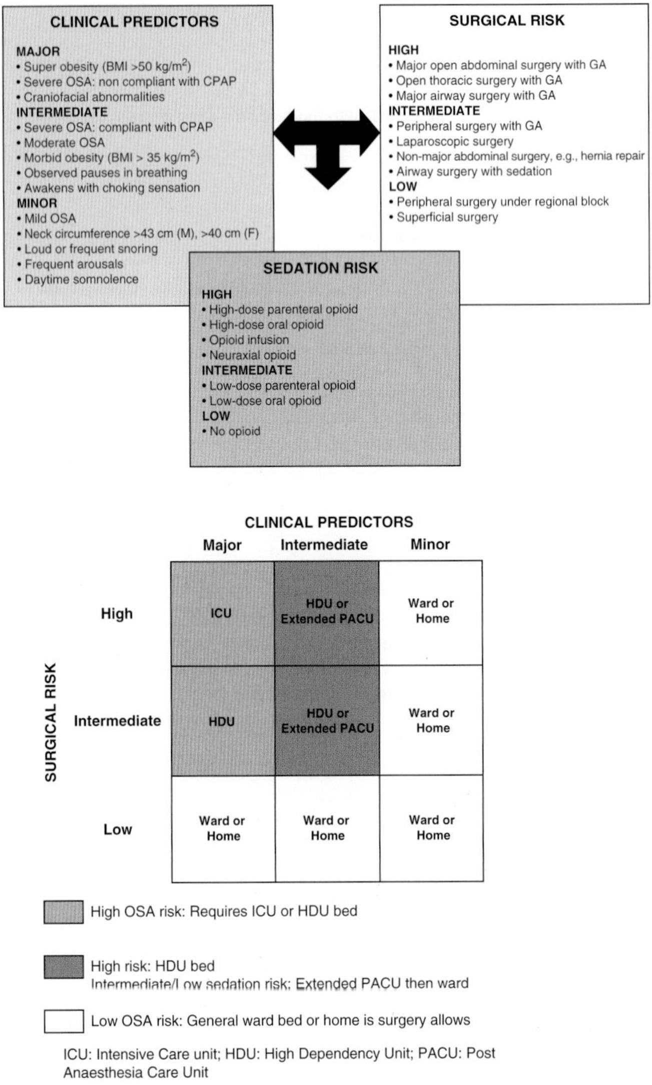

CLINICAL PREDICTORS

MAJOR
- Super obesity (BMI >50 kg/m²)
- Severe OSA: non compliant with CPAP
- Craniofacial abnormalities

INTERMEDIATE
- Severe OSA: compliant with CPAP
- Moderate OSA
- Morbid obesity (BMI > 35 kg/m²)
- Observed pauses in breathing
- Awakens with choking sensation

MINOR
- Mild OSA
- Neck circumference >43 cm (M), >40 cm (F)
- Loud or frequent snoring
- Frequent arousals
- Daytime somnolence

SURGICAL RISK

HIGH
- Major open abdominal surgery with GA
- Open thoracic surgery with GA
- Major airway surgery with GA

INTERMEDIATE
- Peripheral surgery with GA
- Laparoscopic surgery
- Non-major abdominal surgery, e.g., hernia repair
- Airway surgery with sedation

LOW
- Peripheral surgery under regional block
- Superficial surgery

SEDATION RISK

HIGH
- High-dose parenteral opioid
- High-dose oral opioid
- Opioid infusion
- Neuraxial opioid

INTERMEDIATE
- Low-dose parenteral opioid
- Low-dose oral opioid

LOW
- No opioid

CLINICAL PREDICTORS

SURGICAL RISK	Major	Intermediate	Minor
High	ICU	HDU or Extended PACU	Ward or Home
Intermediate	HDU	HDU or Extended PACU	Ward or Home
Low	Ward or Home	Ward or Home	Ward or Home

High OSA risk: Requires ICU or HDU bed

High risk: HDU bed
Intermediate/Low sedation risk: Extended PACU then ward

Low OSA risk: General ward bed or home is surgery allows

ICU: Intensive Care unit; HDU: High Dependency Unit; PACU: Post Anaesthesia Care Unit

FIGURE 31.1 Perioperative bed resource allocation for patients with obstructive sleep apnea (OSA). (Redrawn after Weinberg L, Tay S, Lai CF, et al. Perioperative risk stratification for a patient with severe obstructive sleep apnoea undergoing laparoscopic banding surgery. *BMJ Case Rep* 2013, with permission.)

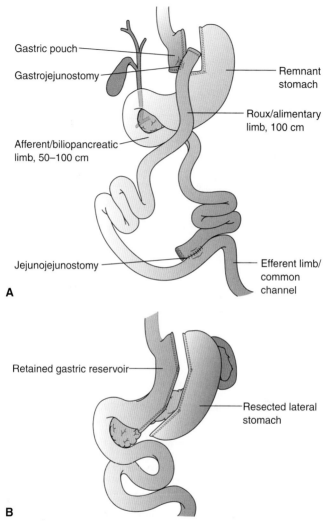

FIGURE 31.2 Types of bariatric surgery. **A:** Roux-en-Y gastric bypass: It involves the creation of a small pouch from the body of the stomach and the formation of a direct, Y-shaped connection to the duodenum. These modifications bypass portions of the stomach and small intestine, thereby restricting food intake and limiting absorption. **B:** Vertical sleeve gastrectomy: It consists of removal of 80% to 90% of stomach to create a gastric sleeve. This slows food absorption and restricts the amount of food that can be consumed. **C:** Adjustable gastric banding: This involves the placement of an adjustable band around the upper body of the stomach to create a small pouch. The band tension can be adjusted through the instillation or removal of fluid via an implanted subcutaneous port. The procedure restricts food intake and slows digestion. (From O'Rourke RW. Management of obesity. In: Mulholland MW, Lillemoe KD, Doherty GM, et al, eds. *Greenfield's Surgery: Scientific Principles and Practice.* 6th ed. Philadelphia, PA: Wolters Kluwer; 2017:742–744.)

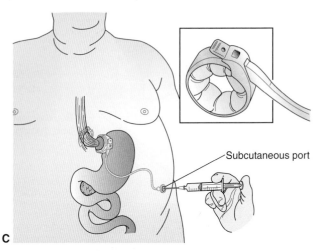

C

FIGURE 31.2 *(continued)*

E. **Surgical Procedure Risk**

Although obese patients are at an increased risk for perioperative complications, surgery in and of itself is an independent risk factor. For example, the open Roux-en-Y gastric bypass procedure is associated with an increased rate of adverse outcomes as compared to the laparoscopic Roux-en-Y gastric bypass procedure. Thus, it is pivotal to have an understanding of what has been done in the operating room and what to expect. The three most common bariatric surgeries are summarized in Figure 31.2.

V. **POSTOPERATIVE MANAGEMENT AND MONITORING**

Postoperative complications occur with greater frequency in the obese patient. Table 31.3 provides a summary of major complications that clinicians often encounter during the early postoperative period and their management. Although there is an increased risk of complications, mild obesity may confer a survival benefit. This benefit has been coined the term the "obesity paradox" and has been demonstrated in sepsis, patients undergoing coronary intervention, and heart failure.

VI. **POSTOPERATIVE DRUG ADMINISTRATION STRATEGY**

The physiologic changes produced by obesity affect the distribution, binding, and elimination of drugs. These can be further altered in the postoperative period due to changes in protein binding. Therefore, each drug warrants cautious titration according to their pharmacologic properties as well as the patient's conditions. Table 31.4 summarizes recommended dosing regimens for some frequently used perioperative medications.

VII. **CONCLUSION**

Patients with elevated BMIs carry increased risks for postoperative complications. A thorough preoperative assessment, early planning for the placement of postoperative patients, and monitoring may facilitate timely recognition of complications to improve patient care, and reduce morbidity and mortality.

TABLE
31.3

Etiology, Monitoring, and Management of Postoperative Complications in Morbidly Obese Patients

Complication	Etiology	Monitoring/Diagnosis	Management
Hypoxemia	Atelectasis	SpO_2, RR, TV, MV, CXR, ABG as needed	Elevate head of the bed to 30 degrees, incentive spirometry, early ambulation, CPAP/BiPAP as needed
	Aspiration		Elevate head of the bed to 30 degrees, H_2 blocker if patient is intubated
	Pneumonia		Antibiotics, airway clearance, early ambulation, incentive spirometry
	Asthma		Bronchodilators (inhaled or systemic), ipratropium (inhaled), steroids (inhaled and systemic), magnesium, intubation if severe
	Airway obstruction		Open airway: jaw thrust, chin lift, oral/nasal airway
			Reverse: residual neuromuscular blockade, opioid-induced respiratory depression
			Ventilation-assisted devices: CPAP/BIPAP, mechanical ventilation
	Pneumothorax		Conservative therapy: watch with serial chest x-rays
			Invasive therapy: chest tube insertion, surgical intervention
	Pulmonary embolism (PE)	Above + low end-tidal CO_2 with high $PaCO_2$, PE-CT, TTE/TEE, pulmonary angiography, V/Q scan	Medical management: anticoagulation, thrombolysis
			Invasive management: surgical intervention, interventional thrombectomy

(continued)

TABLE 31.3	Etiology, Monitoring, and Management of Postoperative Complications in Morbidly Obese Patients (continued)		
Complication	Etiology	Monitoring/Diagnosis	Management
Hypotension	Acute coronary syndrome[a]	Continuous EKG monitoring, ABP, TTE/TEE, troponin, 12-lead EKG	Aspirin, nitroglycerin, percutaneous coronary intervention, anticoagulation, surgical intervention if necessary
	Arrhythmias	Continuous EKG, 12-lead EKG, check electrolytes, TTE/TEE, electrophysiology exam	Correct hypokalemia and hypomagnesemia, antiarrhythmic pharmacotherapies, treat underlying causes (e.g., uncontrolled infection)
	PE	See above	See above
	Sepsis	Culture potential sites of infection, radiographic studies to detect source of infection including x-rays and CT/MRI, TEE versus TTE for endocarditis	Antibiotics to treat the intravascular organisms and perfused areas, source control (drainage of abscess)
	Bleeding	Abdominal US, aspiration of fluid, x-ray/CT/MRI, check coagulation status, serial CBCs	Source control, correct coagulopathy, red blood cell transfusion, hemodynamic management
	Abdominal compartment syndrome	Measure bladder pressure	Consider surgical decompression
	GI tract leak	Serial abdominal exams, abdominal US/CT	Medical (drainage) versus surgical management
	Hypothermia	Find cause, check thyroid function (TSH), antipsychotics may cause hypothermia	Treat underlying cause and warm patient
	Metabolic	Hypokalemia, hyperkalemia, acidosis, hypocalcemia (especially after transfusion)	Treat underlying cause and correct electrolyte disturbance
Hypertension	Essential	Titrate antihypertensive agents, resume home antihypertensive medications	
	Pain	Determine origin of pain, rule out other factors (secondary pain and anxiety)	Titrate pain medications to patient's needs
	Stroke/intracerebral hemorrhage	Serial neurologic exams, CT/MRI, TTE/TEE to look for PFO	Consult neurologist, consider thrombolysis for acute ischemic stroke, treat hyper/hypoglycemia, do not overtreat hypertension
	Alcohol withdrawal	CIWA questionnaire, monitor BP/HR	Scheduled benzodiazepines and cardiovascular medications

Tachycardia	Bleeding		See above
	Arrhythmias		See above
	Sepsis		See above
	Abdominal compartment syndrome		See above
	Hyperthermia	Consider serotonin syndrome, malignant hyperthermia, or infection	Treat underlying cause
	Endocrine (hyperthyroid, diabetes exacerbation)	Check TSH, blood glucose	Treat underlying cause
	Alcohol withdrawal		See above
Bradycardia	Arrhythmias		See above
	Acute coronary syndrome		See above
	Sepsis		See above
Altered mental status	Hypoglycemia, electrolyte disturbances	Check blood glucose/electrolytes	Treat underlying cause
	Acidosis	Check blood glucose, anion gap, lactate, base deficit	Treat underlying cause
	Toxins (excess medications vs. withdrawal from alcohol, benzodiazepine or opioids)	Medical history, physical exam (e.g., pinpoint pupils)	Naloxone for opioid overdose, flumazenil for benzodiazepine overdose
	Liver failure	Check LFTs, ammonia level	Supportive care, lactulose for encephalopathy

(continued)

TABLE
31.3

Etiology, Monitoring, and Management of Postoperative Complications in Morbidly Obese Patients (*continued*)

Complication	Etiology	Monitoring/Diagnosis	Management
Oliguria	Prerenal	Check urine electrolytes, calculate fractional excretion of sodium, check urinalysis and urine sediment, renal ultrasound	Adequate hydration
	Renal (acute on chronic renal failure, acute tubular necrosis, drug induced)		Dose medications renally, control sepsis, support renal perfusion, avoid nephrotoxic drugs
	Postrenal		Remove obstruction
Acidosis	Diabetic ketoacidosis	Measure blood sugar, ketones	Insulin infusion to treat hyperglycemia, follow electrolytes (especially potassium), correct hypovolemia
	Hyperosmolar, hyperglycemic state		Insulin infusion to treat hyperglycemia, treat underlying causes, correct hypovolemia, follow electrolytes (especially potassium)
	Pressure-induced rhabdomyolysis	Measure creatine phosphokinase levels (CPK), assess for compartment syndrome	Hydration if CPK >10,000; fasciotomy for compartment syndrome

SpO$_2$, oxygen saturation; RR, respiratory rate; TV, tidal volume; MV, minute volume; CXR, chest radiograph; ABG, arterial blood gas; CPAP, continuous positive airway pressure; BiPAP, bilevel positive airway pressure; PE-CT, CT scan with pulmonary embolism protocol; TTE, transthoracic echocardiogram; TEE, transesophageal echocardiogram; EKG, electrocardiogram; MRI, magnetic resonance imaging; CBC, complete blood count; GI, gastrointestinal; US, ultrasound; PFO, patent foramen ovale; CIWA, Clinical Institute Withdrawal Assessment for Alcohol; BP/HR, blood pressure/heart rate; LFT, liver function tests.

TABLE 31.4	Medication Dosing Guidelines for Morbidly Obese Patients		

Medication		Loading Dose	Maintenance Dose
Analgesics/ opioids	Fentanyl	ABW	$0.8 \times$ IBW
	Morphine	IBW	IBW
	Remifentanil	IBW	IBW
	Sufentanil	ABW	Reduced
Sedatives/ hypnotics	Benzodiazepines	ABW	IBW
	Propofol	ABW	IBW + titration versus ABW
	Thiopental	ABW	IBW
	Ketamine	ABW	IBW
	Etomidate	ABW	—
Neuromuscular blockers	Succinylcholine	ABW	—
	Rocuronium	ABW	ABW versus reduced infusion rate
	Vecuronium	IBW	IBW
	Cisatracurium	Prolonged effect when given 0.2 mg/kg in obese women	—
Antiarrhythmics	Amiodarone	IBW	IBW
β-Blockers	Metoprolol	IBW	IBW
	Esmolol	IBW	IBW
	Propranolol	IBW	IBW
	Labetalol	IBW	IBW
Calcium channel blockers	Diltiazem (intravenous)	ABW	Titrate to HR/BP goal
	Verapamil	ABW	IBW
Catecholamines	Dobutamine	—	IBW + 0.4 (ABW − IBW)
Other cardiac medications	Adenosine	IBW	IBW
	Digoxin	IBW	IBW
Anticoagulants	Heparin	IBW + 0.4 × (ABW − IBW)	Adjust according to PTT
	Enoxaparin	TBW if <144 kg	Consider using bid dosing, monitor anti-Xa levels 4 hours after dose
Anticonvulsants	Carbamazepine		IBW
	Phenytoin	IBW + 1.33 (ABW − IBW)	IBW
	Valproic acid		IBW

(*continued*)

TABLE 31.4	Medication Dosing Guidelines for Morbidly Obese Patients (*continued*)		
Medication		**Loading Dose**	**Maintenance Dose**
Antibiotics	β-Lactams		IBW + 0.3 (ABW − IBW)
	Aminoglycosides		IBW + 0.4 (ABW − IBW)
	Vancomycin		ABW, adjust dosage to trough levels
	Fluoroquinolones		IBW + 0.45 (ABW − IBW)
Antifungals	Amphotericin		ABW
	Fluconazole		6 mg/kg/d
Corticosteroids	Methylprednisolone- lone	IBW	IBW
GI drugs	H₂ blockers		Standard dosing

ABW, actual body weight; IBW, ideal body weight; IBW for men = 49.9 kg + 0.89 kg/cm above 152.4 cm height; IBW for women = 45.4 kg + 0.89 kg/cm above 152.4 cm height.
Adapted with modifications from Watson N, Bittner E. Medication dosing guidelines for morbidly obese patients in the ICU. In: Ortiz V, Wiener-Kronish J, eds. *Perioperative Anesthetic Care for the Obese Patient*. Boca Raton, FL: CRC Press; 2009, with permission.

Suggested Readings

Bamgbade OA, Rutter TW, Nafiu OO, et al. Postoperative complications in obese and nonobese patients. *World J Surg* 2007;31:556–560.

Chung F, Yang Y, Liao P. Predictive performance of the STOP-Bang score for identifying obstructive sleep apnea in obese patients. *Obes Surg* 2013;23:2050–2057.

Flum DR, Belle SH, King WC, et al. Perioperative safety in the longitudinal assessment of bariatric surgery. *N Engl J Med* 2009;361:445–454.

McCullough PA, Gallagher MJ, Dejong AT, et al. Cardiorespiratory fitness and short-term complications after bariatric surgery. *Chest* 2006;130:517–525.

Ortiz V, Wiener-Kronish J, eds. *Perioperative Anesthetic Care for the Obese Patient*. Boca Raton, FL: CRC Press (Informa Healthcare USA Inc.); 2009.

Perna M, Romagnuolo J, Morgan K, et al. Preoperative hemoglobin A1c and postoperative glucose control in outcomes after gastric bypass for obesity. *Surg Obes Relat Dis* 2012;8:685–690.

Quidley AM, Bland CM, Bookstaver PB, et al. Perioperative management of bariatric surgery patients. *Am J Health Syst Pharm* 2014;71:1253–1264.

Weinberg L, Tay S, Lai CF, et al. Perioperative risk stratification for a patient with severe obstructive sleep apnoea undergoing laparoscopic banding surgery. *BMJ Case Rep* 2013. doi:10.1136/bcr-2012-008336.

Weingarten TN, Flores AS, McKenzie JA, et al. Obstructive sleep apnea and perioperative complications in bariatric patients. *Br J Anaesth* 2011;106:131–139.

The Geriatric Patient

Elie P. Ramly and Haytham M. A. Kaafarani

INTRODUCTION

Older patients constitute a substantial proportion of the current surgical population, with more than half of all operations in the United States being performed on patients aged 65 or above.[1] With decreased physiologic reserves and preexisting comorbidities, the geriatric patient warrants special consideration, meticulous monitoring, and careful care. This holds especially true following invasive surgical procedures that innately possess increased risks for intraoperative or postoperative complications.

POSTOPERATIVE COMPLICATIONS IN THE GERIATRIC SURGICAL PATIENT

When caring for elderly patients in the postoperative period, it is important to keep in mind that complications in the elderly often have atypical presentations. For example, delirium may be the first presenting sign of infection.[2] Elderly patients may also easily slip into physiologic decompensation once a complication occurs, because of their low overall reserve. Hence, utmost care must be taken to: (1) prevent intraoperative surgical or anesthesia complications, (2) monitor for early signs of distress or decline, (3) avoid errors, adverse events, or harm during the immediate and short-term postoperative period, and (4) mitigate the sequelae of any complication when it occurs.

Respiratory Complications

Postoperative pulmonary complications include atelectasis, bronchospasm, aspiration, pneumonia, pulmonary embolism (PE), pleural effusion, and exacerbation of chronic lung disease.[3] Inherent anatomic, physiologic, and immunologic age-related changes place the elderly at an increased risk for pulmonary complications.

Respiratory Failure

Elderly patients are at increased risk for respiratory failure requiring mechanical ventilation.[4] In patients who develop hypoxemia after abdominal surgery, positive pressure ventilation can be used to increase mean airway pressure, recruit collapsed alveoli, increase minute ventilation, and maintain airway patency.[5] If patients fail to improve with noninvasive measures, endotracheal intubation is warranted. Early tracheostomy should be considered particularly in the elderly patient, because it may decrease the overall time needed for mechanical ventilation.[6]

Aspiration Pneumonia

Elderly patients are at a particularly high risk for aspiration pneumonia because of age-related physiologic changes, such as weakened respiratory muscles, cough and swallowing reflexes, mucociliary clearance mechanisms, and immune function. Not uncommonly, elderly patients will also have poor oral hygiene, gastroesophageal reflux disease, or neurologic disease, which may exacerbate the process.[5] Routine postoperative use of nasogastric tubes may increase the risk for aspiration, and is therefore reserved for patients requiring enteral nutrition or bowel decompression.[7,8]

Pulmonary Embolism
Older patients are also at a higher risk for perioperative PE, because of prevalent comorbidities, preoperative functional dependence, and further reduced mobility postoperatively. When assessing a geriatric patient suspected of having a PE, caution and thoughtful judgment should be exercised upon the use of contrast-enhanced computed tomography scanning or pulmonary angiography, because of the high prevalence of kidney dysfunction and an especially elevated risk of contrast-induced acute kidney injury in the elderly. When attempting to screen for PE using D-dimer levels, the physician should only rely on *age-adjusted D-dimer screening cutoffs*, because D-dimer levels are commonly elevated in the elderly.[9,10] Age does not affect the use of pharmacologic and/or mechanical deep vein thrombosis prophylaxis when indicated, or anticoagulation and thrombolytic treatment, as indicated, in the event of a PE. Vena cava filters are an alternative option when anticoagulation is contraindicated such as in the patient with a recent cranial hemorrhage and a concomitant deep vein thrombosis.[11]

Cardiac Complications
Myocardial Infarction
Myocardial ischemia and myocardial infarction are the most commonly encountered postoperative cardiovascular complications in the elderly. Elderly patients with myocardial ischemia or infarction are more likely to develop heart failure as well as other noncardiac morbidity, such as renal failure, and have an overall higher postoperative mortality risk because of these events.[12] Monitoring of this patient population should be most intense during the first 3 to 5 days after surgery, when most myocardial infarctions will occur.

Myocardial ischemic events are silent in over 80% of elderly patients, and incisional pain, residual anesthetic effects, and postoperative analgesia may mask symptoms.[12] Tachycardia, hypotension, dyspnea, respiratory failure, syncope, confusion, nausea, and excessive hyperglycemia in diabetics are all alert signals during the postoperative period, and should prompt a comprehensive evaluation that includes electrocardiography and measurements of cardiac enzymes such as CK, CK-MB isoenzyme, and troponin T and I levels. In appropriately selected high-risk patients, there may be a role for prophylactic β-blocker therapy in attenuating the impact of myocardial infarction and associated in-hospital mortality.[13] Currently, the American College of Cardiology and the American Heart Association recommend perioperative β-blockers for patients who were already receiving β-blockers or to patients with particularly high perioperative cardiac risk a priori that are undergoing major vascular surgery.[14–16]

Congestive Heart Failure
Congestive heart failure is present preoperatively in 10% of patients over 65 years of age, and is a major risk factor for subsequent postoperative cardiopulmonary complications.[17] Elective surgery should be deferred, when possible, in the setting of decompensated severe heart failure (New York Heart Association class IV symptoms) until the patient is medically optimized.[5] Postoperative heart failure, manifesting as pulmonary edema, usually occurs by the third postoperative day, and should prompt an immediate assessment for possible myocardial ischemia. Treatment includes

angiotensin-converting enzyme inhibitors and diuretics, with special monitoring for hypotension and electrolyte disturbances. β-Blockers can be considered with caution in patients with associated myocardial ischemia, whereas digoxin is considered in patients with associated atrial fibrillation in the setting of heart failure.[12,18]

Arrhythmias

Postoperative atrial arrhythmias are seen in 6% of elderly patients undergoing noncardiac surgery,[19] particularly in patients undergoing thoracic lung or esophageal surgery and are commonly associated with electrolyte disturbances, MI, congestive heart failure, hemodynamic instability, postoperative acute respiratory or heart failure. Rapid diagnosis and treatment is necessary, because the elderly rely on the atrial contribution for adequate ventricular filling and cardiac output. Management of atrial fibrillation consists of heart rhythm and/or rate control and prevention of thromboembolism. The authors' preferred medication for rhythm control is amiodarone, a class III antiarrhythmic agent. Rate control can also be achieved with intravenous β-blockers or calcium channel blockers, and risk stratification using the Congestive Heart Failure-Hypertension-Age >75-Diabetes-Stroke (CHADS2) or CHADS2-VASC score should be used to decide on the risks versus benefits of therapeutic anticoagulation with heparin or vitamin K antagonists in the immediate perioperative phase.[12,19,20]

Nervous System Complications
Delirium

Delirium, stroke, and peripheral injuries are important postoperative complications in the elderly. Delirium is the most common neurologic complication in this group of patients, with an incidence ranging between 15% and 53%, depending on the type of the surgical procedure performed.[21] Impaired mobility, high ASA classification, undertreatment of postoperative pain, and administration of medications that alter sensorium such as benzodiazepines, tramadol, or meperidine are among many known risk factors, whereas the type of anesthesia or analgesia technique does not seem to have a significant effect.[22] Structured clinical protocols focused on delirium risk factor modification have been shown to have a strong preventative role.[23,24] Prophylactic administration of low-dose haloperidol (1.5 mg/day) may not definitively reduce the incidence of postoperative delirium, but has been suggested to decrease the severity and duration of the delirium episodes in elderly hip patients undergoing hip surgery.[24] Postoperative delirium is often one of the early signs for other postoperative complications in evolution.

Gastrointestinal Complications
Dysphagia

Age-related neurodegeneration affecting the enteric nervous system contributes to dysphagia, gastrointestinal reflux, and constipation in the elderly.[25,26] Previous neurologic conditions and prolonged intubation can also result in a slow recovery of swallowing function, which puts elderly patients at an increased risk for aspiration. Preoperative nutritional habits and the presence of dentures should be taken into consideration when initiating postoperative diet, in order to ensure simultaneously a safe and adequate nutritional intake. Assessment of the nutritional and swallowing status of the patient should be performed when needed, and accordingly, formulation and maintenance of a nutritional plan should be established, with continuous reassessment for nausea, vomiting, difficulty chewing/swallowing or other signs of food aspiration or intolerance, and implementation of aspiration precautions.[27]

Postoperative Ileus
Elderly patients are especially prone to the development of postoperative ileus. Minimally invasive surgery and regional anesthesia (thoracic epidural blockade) are two methods that potentially decrease the incidence of postoperative ileus. The management of postoperative ileus includes optimization of the underlying medical conditions, and correction of electrolyte or acid–base abnormalities. Discontinuation or reduction in the dose of opioid analgesics, when possible, should be attempted. The use of nonsteroidal anti-inflammatory drugs may have an alleviating role, by reducing the opioid requirement for analgesia, and reducing inflammation, but its use should be weighed against the risk of acute kidney injury, platelet dysfunction, and gastritis. Cisapride, erythromycin, or metoclopramide are kinetic agents that may be used as part of a multimodal strategy to improve food tolerance.[28]

Urinary Tract and Renal Complications
Urinary Tract Infections
Identifiable common preexisting conditions such as benign prostate hypertrophy, urinary incontinence, or decreased mobility in elderly patients frequently require prolonged bladder catheterization, which increases the risk of urinary tract infections (UTIs). Special attention to medications that may cause urinary retention, and avoidance or early discontinuation of urinary catheters are always recommended in order to decrease the risk of UTIs.

Wound Complications
Wound Healing and Surgical Site Infections
Malnutrition, diabetes mellitus, prior treatment with steroids, chemotherapy, and radiotherapy are all common conditions in the elderly that affect wound healing. Elderly patients with surgical site infections (SSIs) are at increased risk for longer hospital stays, readmissions, and mortality. Therefore, prevention of SSIs and their associated morbidity requires a continuous effort of vigilance throughout the pre-, intra-, and postoperative phases, including prophylactic administration of antibiotics within 60 minutes from the surgical incision, maintenance of normothermia intraoperatively, the avoidance of shaving the surgical site, and perioperative euglycemia. Postoperatively, patients should be examined carefully and routinely by uncovering the incision site and monitoring for erythema and/or purulent drainage from the wound or organ space. Systemic signs of infection may be subtle or atypical in the older patient, and patients may rapidly fall into physiologic decompensation. Close monitoring, adequate drainage, and consideration of antibiotics usage as appropriate for the pathogens expected from the operative procedure are recommended.[12]

Pressure Ulcers
Approximately 10% of hospitalized patients develop pressure ulcers. Elderly patients are at an increased risk for those wounds, especially in the setting of peripheral neuropathy, paraplegia or tetraplegia, immobility, and/or critical illness. Age-related loss in fat and muscle mass accentuates bony prominences, creating sites for pressure ulcers to occur, specifically, the presacral area, heels, and occipital scalp. Incontinence can lead to maceration and facilitate shear back or perineal injuries, which can initiate pressure ulcers. Once a pressure ulcer develops, treatment is difficult and recurrence rates are high. Frequent patient repositioning off the bony prominences, as well as early recognition and treatment of stage I ulcers constitute the mainstay of treatment.[29] In advanced stages of a sacral decubitus, surgical debridement and complex skin, soft tissue or muscle flaps might be required.

CONCLUSION

Care of the elderly postoperative surgical patients is particularly challenging because their comorbidities predispose them to a wide range of cardiac, pulmonary, neurologic, gastrointestinal, and dermatologic complications. Primary prevention of these perioperative complications is crucial, but so is their early recognition and the immediate initiation of measures to mitigate their effects and rescue the patients when they occur.

References

1. Yang R, Wolfson M, Lewis MC. Unique aspects of the elderly surgical population: an anesthesiologist's perspective. *Geriatr Orthop Surg Rehabil* 2011;2(2):56–64.
2. Fong TG, Tulebaev SR, Inouye SK. Delirium in elderly adults: diagnosis, prevention and treatment. *Nat Rev Neurol* 2009;5(4):210–220.
3. Smetana GW. Preoperative pulmonary evaluation. *N Engl J Med* 1999;340(12): 937–944.
4. Sevransky JE, Haponik EF. Respiratory failure in elderly patients. *Clin Geriatr Med* 2003;19(1):205–224.
5. Ramly E, Kaafarani HMA, Velmahos GC. The effect of aging on pulmonary function: implications for monitoring and support of the surgical and trauma patient. *Surg Clin North Am* 2015;95(1):53–69.
6. Terragni PP, Antonelli M, Fumagalli R, et al. Early vs late tracheotomy for prevention of pneumonia in mechanically ventilated adult ICU patients: a randomized controlled trial. *JAMA* 2010;303(15):1483–1489.
7. Cheatham ML, Chapman WC, Key SP, et al. A meta-analysis of selective versus routine nasogastric decompression after elective laparotomy. *Ann Surg* 1995;221(5):469–476; discussion 476–478.
8. Nelson R, Tse B, Edwards S. Systematic review of prophylactic nasogastric decompression after abdominal operations. *Br J Surg* 2005;92(6):673–680.
9. Schouten HJ, Geersing GJ, Koek HL, et al. Diagnostic accuracy of conventional or age adjusted D-dimer cut-off values in older patients with suspected venous thromboembolism: systematic review and meta-analysis. *BMJ* 2013;346:f2492.
10. Righini M, Van Es J, Den Exter PL, et al. Age-adjusted D-dimer cutoff levels to rule out pulmonary embolism: the ADJUST-PE study. *JAMA* 2014;311(11):1117–1124.
11. Berman AR. Pulmonary embolism in the elderly. *Clin Geriatr Med* 2001;17(1):107–130.
12. Lagoo-Deenadayalan SA, Newell MA, Pofahl WE. Common perioperative complications in older patients. In: Rosenthal RA, Zenilman ME, Katlic MR, eds. *Principles and Practice of Geriatric Surgery.* 2nd ed. New York, NY: Springer; 2011:361–376.
13. Lindenauer PK, Pekow P, Wang K, et al. Perioperative betablocker therapy and mortality after major noncardiac surgery. *N Engl J Med* 2005;353:349–361.
14. Fleischmann KE, Beckman JA, Christopher EB, et al. 2009 ACCF/AHA focused update on perioperative beta blockade. *J Am Coll Cardiol* 2009;54(22):2102–2128.
15. POISE Study Group, Devereaux PJ, Yang H, Yusuf S, et al. Effects of extended-release metoprolol succinate in patients undergoing non-cardiac surgery (POISE trial): a randomised controlled trial. *Lancet* 2008;371(9627):1839–1847.
16. Kaafarani HM, Atluri PV, Thornby J, et al. beta-Blockade in noncardiac surgery: outcome at all levels of cardiac risk. *Arch Surg* 2008;143(10):940–944.
17. Loran DB, Hyde BR, Zwischenberger JB. Perioperative management of special populations: the geriatric patient. *Surg Clin North Am* 2005;85:1259–1266.
18. Gilmore JC. Heart failure and treatment: part II. Perianesthesia management. *J Perianesth Nurs* 2003;18:242–246.
19. Amar D, Zhang H, Leung DHY, et al. Older age is the strongest predictor of postoperative atrial fibrillation. *Anesthesiology* 2002;96:352–356.
20. Gage BF, Waterman AD, Shannon W, et al. Validation of clinical classification schemes for predicting stroke: results from the National Registry of Atrial Fibrillation. *JAMA* 2001;285:2864–2870.
21. Inouye SK. Delirium in older persons. *N Engl J Med* 2006;354(11):1157–1165.
22. Zhang H, Lu Y, Liu M, et al. Strategies for prevention of postoperative delirium: a systematic review and meta-analysis of randomized trials. *Crit Care* 2013;17(2):R47.
23. Sieber FE, Barnett SR. Preventing postoperative complications in the elderly. *Anesthesiol Clin* 2011;29(1):83–97.

24. Bourne RS, Tahir TA, Borthwick M, et al. Drug treatment of delirium: past, present and future. *J Psychosom Res* 2008;65(3):273–282.

25. Ahmed T, Haboubi N. Assessment and management of nutrition in older people and its importance to health. *Clin Interv Aging* 2010;5:207–216.

26. Saffrey MJ. Ageing of the enteric nervous system. *Mech Ageing Dev* 2004;125(12):899–906.

27. Nohra E, Bochicchio GV. Management of the gastrointestinal tract and nutrition in the geriatric surgical patient. *Surg Clin North Am* 2015;95(1):85–101.

28. Holte K, Kehlet H. Postoperative ileus: a preventable event. *Br J Surg* 2000;87(11):1480–1493.

29. Greenhalgh DG. Management of the skin and soft tissue in the geriatric surgical patient. *Surg Clin North Am* 2015;95(1):103–114.

Suggested Readings

Glance LG, Osler TM, Neuman MD. Redesigning surgical decision making for high-risk patients. *N Engl J Med* 2014;370(15):1379–1381.

Griffiths R, Beech F, Brown A, et al. Peri-operative care of the elderly 2014: Association of Anaesthetists of Great Britain and Ireland. *Anaesthesia* 2014;69(Suppl 1):81–98.

Kwok AC, Semel ME, Lipsitz SR, et al. The intensity and variation of surgical care at the end of life: a retrospective cohort study. *Lancet* 2011;378(9800):1408–1413.

Scandrett KG, Zuckerbraun BS, Peitzman AB. Operative risk stratification in the older adult. *Surg Clin North Am* 2015;95(1):149–172.

Sheetz KH, Krell RW, Englesbe MJ, et al. The importance of the first complication: understanding failure to rescue after emergent surgery in the elderly. *J Am Coll Surg* 2014;219(3):365–370.

The Pregnant Patient

Naveen F. Sangji and Haytham M. A.
Kaafarani

I. INTRODUCTION

Pregnant women may present with obstetric and nonobstetric conditions (e.g., trauma, appendicitis, cholecystitis, bowel obstruction) whose definitive care cannot be postponed until the postpartum phase. The incidence of nonobstetric operations needed to treat such diseases during pregnancy is estimated at 0.15% to 0.75%. In the last few decades, surgery and surgical care of the pregnant patient have been proven to be feasible and safe, as long as the care team is aware of the special considerations needed in her care. Postoperative care of the pregnant patient presents particular challenges, not only in relationship to the presence of a vulnerable fetus that may get harmed by any of the radiologic tests performed, medications administered, or instruments used in patient care, but also intimately related to the physiologic and anatomic changes encountered in a pregnant woman that puts her, in addition to the fetus, at a different and higher risk profile compared to the nonpregnant woman. The American College of Obstetrics and Gynecologists (ACOG) recommends preoperative obstetrics consultation for any pregnant women undergoing surgery.

In this chapter, we will discuss some of the general strategies needed to take care of the pregnant postoperative patient, with particular emphasis on tips to ensure the safety of both the mother and the fetus. Specifically, we will: (1) briefly delineate the stages of fetal development and explore the maternal anatomic and physiologic changes of pregnancy, (2) suggest systematic physiologic monitoring of the patient and her fetus postoperatively, (3) develop a basic understanding of pain control, medication administration, and transfusion practices in pregnancy, and (4) discuss the safety of different radiologic modalities in pregnancy.

A. Fetal Development

In the first trimester (up to 12 weeks) of pregnancy, the major fetal organs have formed and the uterus is palpable at the level of the symphysis pubis. During the second trimester (13 to 28 weeks), the fetus undergoes growth, and lung maturity is the primary determinant of survival in the case of preterm labor. Growth continues during the third trimester (29-40 weeks). The gestational age of the fetus should be calculated preoperatively. As a general rule, whenever possible, surgery should be performed during the second trimester, when the risk of preterm labor and spontaneous abortion is less likely.

B. Maternal Physiology: The Anatomic and Physiologic Changes of Pregnancy

Pregnancy induces major physiologic changes to the cardiovascular, pulmonary, and hematologic systems, which include, among many, an increase in the cardiac output (CO), a decrease in the functional residual capacity (FRC), dilutional anemia, and hypercoagulability.

A brief summary of the major physiologic and anatomic changes during pregnancy follows, which should be taken into consideration to guide the postoperative care of the pregnant patient. The major physiologic and laboratory changes noted during pregnancy are summarized in Tables 33.1 and 33.2, respectively.

TABLE 33.1 Selected Changes in Clinical Parameters During Pregnancy

Clinical Parameter	Nonpregnant Woman	Pregnant Woman	Direction of Change
Heart rate (beats/min)	60–75	75–95	Increased
Systolic blood pressure (mm Hg)/diastolic blood pressure (mm Hg)	100–140/60–90	100–140/50–80	Unchanged/decreased
Cardiac output (L/min)*	4.6–6.8	5.5–9.8†	Increased
Lung tidal volume (mL/min)	450	650	Increased

*Supine position lowers cardiac output by 25% to 30%.
†Second trimester values.
Adopted from Tamirisa, Borahay, Kilic. *Care in Special Situations: The Pregnant Surgical Patient.* Scientific American Surgery; Decker Intellectual Properties Inc., 2015.

TABLE 33.2 Normal Laboratory Values During Pregnancy

Laboratory Value	Normal Range in Nonpregnant Women	Normal Range During Pregnancy	Direction of Change
Alkaline phosphatase (unit/L)	33–96	17–229	Increased
ALT (unit/L)	7–41	2–33	Unchanged/decreased
AST (unit/L)	12–38	3–32	Unchanged/decreased
Amylase (unit/L)	20–96	15–83	Unchanged/decreased
Bilirubin (total) (mg/dL)	0.3–1.3	0.1–1.1	Unchanged/decreased
BUN (mg/dL)	7–20	3–13	Decreased
Creatinine (mg/dL)	0.5–0.9	0.4–0.9	Unchanged
HCO_3 (mmol/L)	22–30	20–24	Decreased
Hematocrit (g/dL)	35.4–44.4	30–39*	Decreased
Hemoglobin (g/dL)	12–15.8	9.7–14.8*	Decreased
Lipase (unit/L)	3–43	21–112	Increased
Sodium	136–146	129–148	
Prothrombin time (s)	12.7–15.4	9.5–13.3*	Decreased
Partial thromboplastin time (s)	26.3–39.4	22.9–38.1*	Decreased
PaO_2 (mm Hg)	93	101–106	Increased
$PaCO_2$ (mm Hg)	37	26–30	Decreased
WBC ($\times 10^3/\mu L$)†	3.5–9.1	5.6–16.9	Increased

*Second trimester values.
†Neutrophils also increase.
Adopted from Tamirisa, Borahay, Kilic. *The Pregnant Surgical Patient.* Scientific American Surgery; 2015.

1. **Cardiovascular system**
    a. In order to meet the perfusion needs of the fetus and the enlarged uterus, the pregnant woman increases her stroke volume and heart rate (HR); this leads to the CO increasing by up to 50% during pregnancy. Maternal HR increases starting during the first trimester and peaks during the third trimester to 15 to 20 beats/minute higher than normal. Systemic vascular resistance will initially decrease, secondary to the vasodilatory effect of progesterone until 20 weeks, and then increases slowly to term. CO therefore increases starting in the sixth week and peaks during the third trimester. Systolic blood pressure remains constant throughout the duration of pregnancy; however, the diastolic blood pressure decreases.
    b. Anatomically, the gravid uterus displaces the diaphragm upward, which displaces the heart upward and the left ventricle laterally. Heart compliance increases and the ventricles dilate to maintain ejection fraction.
    c. The uterus receives 25% of the maternal CO during pregnancy. After the second trimester, the gravid uterus compresses the inferior vena cava when supine, and therefore pregnant patients should be placed in the left lateral decubitus position when in a hospital bed. Beginning as early as 8 weeks, supine position can lower the CO by 25% to 30%. Blood pressure readings in pregnant patients should be taken at a 30-degree tilt rather than supine for accurate measurements.
    d. In cases of refractory hypotension despite left lateral decubitus position and fluid resuscitation, vasopressor administration can be utilized in critically ill pregnant patients.
2. **Respiratory system**
    a. Due to an enlarged neck circumference and relative pharyngeal and laryngeal edema, a pregnant woman may require the use of a smaller endotracheal tube for intubation compared to a nonpregnant patient of similar height and weight.
    b. In pregnancy, the diaphragm is elevated because of the increasing size of the fetus, which results in a decrease in the FRC. In pregnancy, the chest wall expands, but compliance decreases, with resultant decreases in the total lung capacity, the residual volume, and expiratory reserve volume.
    c. Pregnancy increases inspiratory capacity by increasing tidal volume (first trimester) while preserving respiratory rate; this, in turn, leads to increased minute ventilation (30% to 50% more than normal values). Subsequently, a physiologic respiratory alkalosis occurs (Table 33.1). This is a common cause of dyspnea during pregnancy. However, less common causes such as pulmonary embolism and cardiac etiologies mist also be worked up and excluded when a pregnant woman presents with worsening dyspnea.
    d. A pregnant patient needing ventilation postoperatively should have the minute ventilation adjusted to a lower than usual target $PaCO_2$ of 30 to 32, with a corresponding pH of 7.40 to 7.47.
    e. Due to decreased FRC, apnea in a pregnant patient can lead to rapid hypoxemia and oxygen desaturation. Pregnant patients should be preoxygenated with 100% oxygen by face mask for 3 to 5 minutes prior to intubation.
3. **Hematologic system**
    a. Plasma volume increases by up to 15% during the first trimester because of fluid retention and systemic vasodilation. Red blood

cell mass increases as well, but not in proportion to the increase in plasma volume, and therefore, there is a resulting dilutional anemia that ensues during pregnancy in the second trimester.

    b. Leukocytosis with neutrophilia is a normal physiologic change seen during the second trimester through 1 month postpartum.

    c. Pregnancy induces a prothrombotic state, which can persist until 6 weeks postpartum. The risk of venous thromboembolism (VTE) is four- to fivefold higher among pregnant or postpartum women. The risk is highest in the postpartum period. Inherited thrombophilia, prior VTE, and acute illness will further increase this risk.

    d. Gestational thrombocytopenia can be seen; however, severe thrombocytopenia should be worked up for a more serious underlying disorder.

4. Gastrointestinal system

    a. The enlarged uterus displaces intraabdominal organs, particularly the stomach and small bowel.

    b. Increased progesterone circulation causes delayed gastric emptying and decreased lower esophageal sphincter tone, which causes reflux symptoms in 80% of pregnant patients. Aspiration risk increases with endotracheal intubation, which is important to consider if postoperative reintubation is required.

II. POSTOPERATIVE CARE

A. Maternal and Fetal Monitoring

1. Maternal monitoring

Following nonobstetric surgical procedures in pregnant patients, the rate of premature labor has been estimated at 3.5%, fetal loss at 2.5%, and prematurity rate at 8.2%. Studies have failed to reveal a benefit from the use of perioperative prophylactic tocolytic agents. Patients should be monitored for contractions; however, specific guidelines are lacking with regard to the duration of monitoring in the postoperative setting.

2. Fetal monitoring

As previously stated, the gestational age of the fetus should be determined preoperatively.

    a. For a previable fetus (less than 24 weeks): document fetal heart rate (FHR) before and after the procedure.

    b. For a viable fetus (greater than 24 weeks): FHR and contraction monitoring should be undertaken before and after surgery.

    c. Tocolytic therapy can be used in the setting of preterm contractions postoperatively under the guidance of an obstetrician and should be discussed preoperatively.

B. Pain Control/Anesthesia

According to the ACOG guidelines, opioids are safe for use during pregnancy for the management of labor pain. However, there are limited studies on opioid use during pregnancy and fetal outcomes, and therefore, the risks associated with opioid use during pregnancy are not fully understood. Most prescription opioids are classified as category C for use during pregnancy, indicating evidence of harm in animal studies and the absence of human studies. Oxycodone is one exception, classified as category B, indicating no harm in animal studies but absence of human studies. Nevertheless, although in general, studies on opioid use during pregnancy have been inconclusive for outcomes such as fetal growth parameters and preterm labor, there is some evidence to suggest that oxycodone use could contribute to preterm labor.

First trimester opioid use by pregnant patients has been shown to have higher rates of birth defects such as cardiac anomalies, gastroschisis, and spina bifida. Nonsteroidal anti-inflammatory medications should be avoided in the first trimester because of the risk of fetal malformations. Moreover, NSAID use should be averted in the third trimester to prevent premature closure of the ductus arteriosus and because of the risk of bleeding. Acetaminophen is considered safe for use throughout pregnancy

C. **Transfusions**

Transfusions in pregnant patients carry the risk of maternal immune reactions. Maternal antibody formation or alloimmunization with transplacental passage of these antibodies into the fetal circulation can lead to hemolytic disease in the fetus or neonate, depending on the degree of antigenicity and the amount and type of antibodies. Any blood products needed should be matched for maternal Rh compatibility.

D. **Venous Thromboembolism**

Pregnant patients have a moderate to high risk of VTE during nonlabor-related hospitalization, which persists up until 4 weeks following discharge from the hospital. Distinctive guidelines for thromboprophylaxis for hospitalized pregnant patients in the absence of prior VTE or preexisting thrombophilias are lacking, and therefore, the risks and benefits of chemical thromboprophylaxis should be tailored to each individual patient. Pregnant patients, like all patients, should be encouraged to return to normal activity and ambulation as soon as possible postoperatively.

1. When thromboprophylaxis is deemed appropriate, low-molecular-weight heparin (LMWH) and unfractionated heparin are both safe for use in pregnancy. ACOG guidelines recommend the use of LMWH over unfractionated heparin during pregnancy.
2. Warfarin (Coumadin) is teratogenic and should not be used during pregnancy.
3. Oral direct thrombin inhibitors and factor Xa inhibitors lack safety and efficacy data and should therefore be avoided during pregnancy.
4. Bilateral sequential compression devices are recommended as VTE prophylaxis before surgery and until discharge from the hospital.

E. **Antibiotic Administration**

Prophylactic antibiotic guidelines for the pregnant patient are similar to those for nonpregnant patients. However, antibiotics that should be avoided in pregnancy include gentamicin, tetracyclines, and fluoroquinolones given risk of ototoxicity, bone growth inhibition, and arthropathy, respectively, to the fetus. Cephalosporins and penicillins are generally considered safe (Table 33.3).

F. **Imaging/Radiation**

Radiation can cause carcinogenesis and germ cell mutations, and has serious teratogenic effects on the fetus. On the other hand, delays in diagnosis of life-threatening diseases or injuries can also cause damage to both the mother and the fetus. Therefore, the pros and cons of imaging should always be considered and discussed thoroughly with the mother and all generalists/specialists taking care of the patient.

The impact of ionizing radiation exposure depends on the gestational age of the fetus as well as the radiation dose. Fetal loss has been observed with exposures greater than 1 Gy (equivalent to 100 rad). Central nervous system effects are greatest during 8 to 15 weeks gestational age at doses in the 60 to 310 mGy range (6 to 31 rad). Fetal loss or anomalies have not been reported below 50 mGy (5 rad). Carcinogenesis risk to the fetus is unclear, but is generally considered to be small. A 10 to 20 mGy (1 to 2 rad) exposure may increase the risk of leukemia by a factor of 1.5 to 2.0. For some commonly used tests, the typical radiation exposure

TABLE 33.3	Antibiotic Safety During Pregnancy
Antibiotic	**Safety Category*: Side Effects During Pregnancy**
Azithromycin	B: Limited data; animal studies suggest low risk
Cephalosporins	B: Safe
Clindamycin	B: Safe
Doxycycline	D: Contraindicated; bone growth inhibition
Ertapenem	B: No human data; probably safe
Erythromycin	B: Compatible (excludes estolate salt)
Fluoroquinolones	C: Avoid; irreversible arthropathy
Gentamicin	D: Avoid; 8th nerve toxicity
Metronidazole	B: Likely low risk; avoid during breast-feeding
Nitrofurantoin	B: Risk in third trimester
Penicillins	B: Safe
Trimethoprim	C: Contraindicated at term; ototoxicity
Vancomycin	B: Safe

*Safety classes—B: Animal studies demonstrate no risk to fetus, C: Animal studies demonstrate adverse effects on fetus, D: Evidence of fetal risk but potential benefits may warrant use of the drug despite risks. Adopted from Tamirisa, Borahay, Kilic. *The Pregnant Surgical Patient.* Scientific American Surgery; 2015.

TABLE 33.4	Radiation Doses of Imaging
Imaging Modality	**Radiation Dose (mrad)***
Chest x-ray	0.02–0.07
Abdominal x-ray	100
Hip x-ray	7–20
Computed tomography scan:	
Head or chest	<1 rad
Abdomen/lumbar spine	3.5 rad
Pelvis	250

*1 rad is equivalent to 10 mGy.
Adopted from Tamirisa, Borahay, Kilic. *The Pregnant Surgical Patient.* Scientific American Surgery; 2015, and ACOG Committee Opinion No. 656: Guidelines for diagnostic imaging during pregnancy and lactation. *Obstet Gynecol* 2016;127(2):e75–e80.

is outlined in Table 33.4. It is worth noting that the levels of radiation exposure known to cause fetal harm are not typically used in current diagnostic imaging. For patients needing high-dose or repeated imaging, a radiation physicist consultation is recommended to determine the fetal exposure to radiation.

Magnetic resonance imaging and ultrasonography do not include ionizing radiation and are considered safer in pregnancy. Radioactive iodine administration is contraindicated during pregnancy. Oral contrast administration for computed tomography has no known side effects to the fetus. Iodinated contrast administered intravenously can cross the placenta, but has also not shown to cause any teratogenic effects; however, its use is recommended only when absolutely necessary.

III. SUMMARY AND RECOMMENDATIONS

Despite the significant need for guidance in the perioperative management of the pregnant patient, few evidence-based recommendations currently exist. Monitoring and treatment approaches can be extrapolated from current guidelines for pregnant women in labor. For pregnant patients diagnosed with a surgical problem, treatment should not be delayed. Preoperative obstetric consultation should be requested and fetal age documented. The risks and benefits of various postoperative therapies should always be discussed with all providers and with the patient to determine the best approach to her care.

Suggested Readings

Abdul Sultan A, West J, Tata LJ, et al. Risk of first venous thromboembolism in pregnant women in hospital: population based cohort study from England. *BMJ* 2013;347:f6099.

American College of Obstetricians and Gynecologists: ACOG Practice Bulletin No. 75: Management of alloimmunization during pregnancy. *Obstet Gynecol* 2006;108(2):457–464.

American College of Obstetricians and Gynecologists: ACOG Practice Bulletin No. 100: Critical care in pregnancy. *Obstet Gynecol* 2009;113(2 Pt 1):443–450.

American College of Obstetricians and Gynecologists: ACOG Practice Bulletin No. 138: Inherited thrombophilias in pregnancy. *Obstet Gynecol* 2013;122(3):706–717.

Bates SM, Greer IA, Pabinger I, et al. Venous thromboembolism, thrombophilia, antithrombotic therapy, and pregnancy: American College of Chest Physicians Evidence-Based Clinical Practice Guidelines (8th Edition). *Chest* 2008;133(6 Suppl):844s–886s.

Broussard CS, Rasmussen SA, Reefhuis J, et al. Maternal treatment with opioid analgesics and risk for birth defects. *Am J Obstet Gynecol* 2011;204(4):314.e1–314.e11.

Cheek TG, Baird E. Anesthesia for nonobstetric surgery: maternal and fetal considerations. *Clin Obstet Gynecol* 2009;52(4):535–545.

Cohen-Kerem R, Railton C, Oren D, et al. Pregnancy outcome following non-obstetric surgical intervention. *Am J Surg* 2005;190(3):467–473.

Committee Opinion No. 656: Guidelines for diagnostic imaging during pregnancy and lactation. *Obstet Gynecol* 2016;127(2):e75–e80.

Horowitz KM, Ingardia CJ, Borgida AF. Anemia in pregnancy. *Clin Lab Med* 2013;33(2):281–291.

James A. Practice Bulletin No. 123: Thromboembolism in pregnancy. *Obstet Gynecol* 2011;118(3):718–729.

Kallen B, Reis M. Ongoing pharmacological management of chronic pain in pregnancy. *Drugs* 2016;76(9):915–924.

Kort B, Katz VL, Watson WJ. The effect of nonobstetric operation during pregnancy. *Surg Gynecol Obstet* 1993;177(4):371–376.

Mazze RI, Kallen B. Reproductive outcome after anesthesia and operation during pregnancy: a registry study of 5405 cases. *Am J Obstet Gynecol* 1989;161(5):1178–1185.

Ni Mhuireachtaigh R, O'Gorman DA. Anesthesia in pregnant patients for nonobstetric surgery. *J Clin Anesth* 2006;18(1):60–66.

San-Frutos L, Engels V, Zapardiel I, et al. Hemodynamic changes during pregnancy and postpartum: a prospective study using thoracic electrical bioimpedance. *J Matern Fetal Neonatal Med* 2011;24(11):1333–1340.

Tan EK, Tan EL. Alterations in physiology and anatomy during pregnancy. *Best Pract Res Clin Obstet Gynaecol* 2013;27(6):791–802.

Visser BC, Glasgow RE, Mulvihill KK, et al. Safety and timing of nonobstetric abdominal surgery in pregnancy. *Dig Surg* 2001;18(5):409–417.

Yazdy MM, Desai RJ, Brogly SB. Prescription opioids in pregnancy and birth outcomes: a review of the literature. *J Pediatr Genet* 2015;4(2):56–70.

Postoperative Care of Patients with a History of Substance Use

Connie Wang, Sheri Berg, and Carlos Fernandez-Robles

Substance abuse remains a major problem in the United States, and physicians can often encounter postsurgical patients who have addiction issues. Treating a patient with either acute intoxication or chronic use/abuse in the postoperative period can be quite challenging. Often, pain control can be hard to manage and could be misconstrued with drug-seeking behavior. Withdrawal symptoms should be monitored for and appropriately treated.

I. ALCOHOL

Alcohol is one of the most commonly abused substances in the United States. Up to 28% of surgical patients can have alcohol dependency.

A. Pharmacology

Alcohol is a term frequently used to refer to the substance ethanol. By binding to the γ-aminobutyric acid (GABA)$_A$ receptor, ethanol affects the central nervous system (CNS) by increasing the inhibitory effects of the GABA neurotransmitter. Ethanol also inhibits N-methyl-D-asparate receptors and can lead to an upregulation of glutamate to maintain the CNS homeostasis. It is thought that both the decrease in both brain GABA levels and GABA-receptor sensitivity and the activation of glutamate systems have been implicated in the development of dependence, craving, and withdrawal.

B. Effects of Drug

Both acute intoxication and chronic alcohol use carry significant risks in the postoperative period. Patients who are acutely intoxicated in the postoperative setting can have increased sedation, impaired judgment, combativeness, and confusion. These patients are at increased risk for aspiration and can be at risk of injuring oneself or others. Chronic alcohol use can lead to liver disease, coagulapathies, immune deficiency, cardiomyopathy, increased risk for delirium, and electrolyte and glucose disturbances. Thus, they are at higher risk for postoperative bleeding, surgical wound infections, and electrolyte abnormalities, and they can be more susceptible to anesthetic side effects given impaired ability to metabolize these medications. Chronic alcoholics are also at increased risk for developing postoperative delirium.

C. Withdrawal Symptoms

Alcohol withdrawal onset occurs between 6 and 12 hours after ingestion of the last drink. Early symptoms include tremors, diaphoresis, nausea/vomiting, hypertension, tachycardia, hyperthermia, and tachypnea, but as the syndrome progress more serious complications can occur including visual and tactile disturbances, diffuse, tonic–clonic seizures, and fluctuating level of consciousness paired with severe autonomic symptoms known as delirium tremens (DT). Alcohol withdrawal symptoms can last up to 7 days and carry a 10% risk of mortality. It is important to consider that some agents commonly used for anesthesia such as propofol and methohexital can increase GABA-mediated inhibitory tone in the CNS and postpone the onset of alcohol withdrawal.

D. Treatment

For sedated and combated patients who are acutely intoxicated, it is important to ensure that proper restraints and airway management equipment are available if needed. Treatment of alcohol withdrawal can be carried out with a combination of medications used to target the different symptoms associated with the syndrome. Benzodiazepines stimulate GABA receptors and are the gold standard agents in the management of alcohol withdrawal and prevention of complicated forms of it, with a reduction in the incidence of seizures, DT, and the associated risk of mortality. Recent clinical trials have found anticonvulsants such as carbamazepine and valproic acid, and barbiturates to also be efficacious in the treatment of alcohol withdrawal.

E. Potential Difficulties in Care Postoperatively

For chronic abusers of alcohol, alcohol withdrawal can be a life-threatening complication. The most dangerous complication of alcohol withdrawal is DT which can occur 2 to 4 days without alcohol. Seizures occurring during alcohol withdrawal are best treated with benzodiazepines. Agitation and hallucinations occurring during alcohol withdrawal should be treated with neuroleptics. Clonidine and β-blockers can serve as sympatholytics for controlling the autonomic manifestations of withdrawal. If clonidine and neuroleptics are used in conjunction, care must be taken to monitor QTc prolongation. Securement of the airway may be necessary when administering a large amount of sedatives to control symptoms.

II. HEROIN

Since 2007, the number of people who have started to use heroin has steadily risen. Part of the reason may be that heroin is more readily available and is cheaper than prescription opioids.

A. Pharmacology

Heroin is a drug of abuse that is a derivative of morphine. Users most often abuse the drug by injection, but it can also be administered by smoking, suppository (anal or vaginal insertion), insufflation (snorting), and ingestion (swallowing). Heroin, like all opioids, activate μ-, κ-, and δ-receptors. The μ-receptor is responsible for the reward and analgesic properties of opioids as well as the respiratory depression and constipation effects. Chronic use of opioids leads to up regulation of cyclic adenosine monophosphate along with gene transcription changes which may cause cellular tolerance.

B. Effects of Drug

Use of heroin can cause feelings of euphoria, sedation, and respiratory depression. People who use heroin on a long-term basis are at increased risk of addiction and infections from injection. The most dangerous complication of heroin use is overdose, which can lead to death.

C. Withdrawal Symptoms

Heroin withdrawal may present in the postoperative setting 6 to 24 hours after the last use of the substance. Symptoms may include nausea, dysphoria, anxiety, insomnia, rhinorrhea, gastrointestinal upset such as vomiting and diarrhea, and restlessness.

D. Treatment

Heroin withdrawal is not life-threatening, although it is unpleasant. Acute detoxification with long-acting agent methadone reduces symptoms dramatically. α_2-Agonists such as clonidine can also be used in suppressing autonomic symptoms, but should be used in conjunction with other drugs that can alleviate other withdrawal symptoms. However, acute detoxification is rarely a sustainable solution, and people often relapse after completing it. Opioid replacement therapy has proven to be a more efficacious strategy reducing harm associated with heroin use; it consists of substituting heroin with noneuphoric agents such as methadone or buprenorphine. Psychosocial interventions need to be enacted and maintained to prevent relapse in the future.

E. **Potential Difficulties in Care Postoperatively**

Patients who are chronic users can be quite tolerant to opioids and typically need more medication to achieve the euphoric effects of opioid analgesics. Acute pain in the postoperative setting could be hard to treat. Quantification and conversion of a patient's daily heroin use to opioid equivalents should be carried out. These patients should receive their baseline requirement in opioids minding that cross-tolerance between opioid agents is incomplete, hence adjustments are often needed to avoid accidental overdoses. Additionally, a short-acting opioids agents should be added for the treatment of acute pain postoperatively. Multimodal analgesics should also be added in order to achieve better pain control. Whenever possible, regional anesthesia should be implemented. A proper transition should occur between the acute postoperative pain management period and the discharge period. Appropriate follow-up after discharge should be coordinated.

III. **RECOVERING/ABSTINENT HEROIN USERS**

There may often be a fear to expose patients who are recovering or abstinent users to opioids in the postoperative setting. However, it is important to remember that increased pain without proper treatment could promote relapse after discharge from the hospital. Therefore, the appropriate course of action for these patients is treatment with short-acting opioid analgesics along with multimodal analgesics. After the acute pain management period, a taper plan for the opioids should be given and proper outpatient follow-up should be arranged to help prevent relapse.

IV. **METHADONE**

A. **Pharmacology**

Methadone is a long-acting μ-receptor agonist and N-methyl-D-aspartate antagonist that is used to treat patients with chronic pain or opiate abuse. Methadone has a half-life of 15 to 60 hours and its analgesic action can last between 6 and 8 hours.

B. **Effects of Drug**

Methadone's effects are similar to those of other opioids. Other effects that methadone have include dizziness, vomiting, and sleep problems. Methadone can prolong QTc and cause heart arrhythmias. If used in conjunction with other QTc prolonging medications, frequent electrocardiography should be done to monitor for prolonged QT.

C. **Withdrawal Symptoms**

Methadone withdrawal presents similarly to withdrawal from other opioids. It usually begins 24 hours after the patient's last dose. Common symptoms include chills, sweating, cravings, diarrhea, tachycardia, anxiety, irritability, insomnia, nausea, and vomiting.

D. **Treatment**

If a patient is withdrawing from methadone, he or she should be given the usual home dose of methadone. If the health care provider wants to ultimately have the patient come off of methadone, a strict taper schedule should be implemented. Psychosocial follow-up should be provided.

E. **Potential Difficulties in Care Postoperatively**

Patients on methadone may have a resistance to the euphoric effects of intravenous narcotics. Cross-tolerance with methadone does not occur; thus, these patients may need higher doses of pain medication than would be required of patients who are not on methadone. When indicated, opioid analgesics should be given for pain in the postoperative setting in addition to the usual dose of maintenance methadone therapy. For patients on methadone maintenance therapy, the usual dosage of methadone should be continued after confirmation with the patient's prescriber. If patients are not yet taking medications by mouth after surgery, parenteral methadone can be administered after the appropriate dose conversion.

V. BUPRENORPHINE

A. Pharmacology

Buprenorphine is a μ-receptor partial agonist and a κ-receptor antagonist that is used for the treatment of chronic pain or opiate abuse. Buprenorphine has a strong affinity for the μ-receptor and will displace full μ-agonists. This can make treating postoperative pain with other narcotics difficult in the postoperative period.

B. Effects of Drug

Buprenorphine's side effects are similar to those of opioids. They include drowsiness, dry mouth, nausea, vomiting, headache, and itching. Buprenorphine is unique in that it shows a ceiling effect for respiratory depression.

C. Withdrawal Symptoms

Withdrawal symptoms can occur from 48 hours after the last dose and can last up to 10 days. Symptoms of withdrawal include nausea, vomiting, drowsiness, cravings, irritability, and insomnia. Depression and cravings can occur up to several months.

D. Treatment

The usual dose of buprenorphine should be given if the patient experiences withdrawal in the postoperative setting. If the patient needs detoxification, the health care provider should provide a taper schedule for the buprenorphine and arrange proper outpatient psychosocial follow-up.

E. Potential Difficulties in Care Postoperatively

Patients on buprenorphine can be especially difficult to treat from a pain management perspective. If the patient has stopped buprenorphine therapy for 3 days or more prior to surgery, pain can be managed with opioid analgesia and should be readily provided in the postoperative setting for acute pain. If the patient has continued buprenorphine therapy, adequate pain control may require higher than normal doses and shorter than normal administration intervals of short-acting opioid agonists. Adjunct analgesic agents should also be given for opioid sparing effects. Another strategy for managing pain in the postoperative setting for patients on buprenorphine therapy includes converting the patient's usual buprenorphine dose to methadone equivalents. The methadone would prevent withdrawal, and additional opioid analgesics can be given to treat acute postsurgical pain in the postoperative setting. Methadone has a weaker affinity for the μ-receptor than does buprenophine, making any additional opioid agonist analgesics more effective. When acute postoperative pain resolves for the patient, opioid analgesics can be tapered off and buprenorphine maintenance therapy can be resumed by the appropriate inpatient service or the patient's outpatient provider. A patient should be in mild opioid withdrawal before restarting buprenorphine, because restarting buprenorphine itself can lead to opioid withdrawal if taken in the presence of opiates.

VI. COCAINE

Cocaine is the second most frequently used illegal drug. It is a stimulant that can be smoked, snorted, or injected.

A. Pharmacology

Initially cocaine affects the CNS through inhibiting monoamine uptake. Most importantly, it affects the dopamine transporter protein by inhibiting its reuptake function, causing dopamine accumulation in the synaptic cleft. Because dopamine is part of the reward circuit in the brain, buildup of this neurotransmitter causes the feelings of cocaine's high. Chronic cocaine use can lead to downregulation of dopamine receptors and depletion of synaptic dopamine. When alcohol is taken in conjunction with cocaine, cocaethylene, an active metabolite with a longer half-life and stronger cardiotoxic effects, is produced by liver sterases.

B. Side Effects

Acute cocaine intoxication leads to euphoria, hypersensitivity, irritability, anorexia, rapid speech and thought processes, and extreme energy. Cocaine-induced psychosis is characterized by paranoia, visual and auditory, and tactile hallucinations. Autonomic symptoms such as tachycardia, diaphoresis, dilated pupils, hyperreflexia, tremors, hyperthermia, and restlessness can occur. Overdosing on cocaine can lead to death, especially if the substance has been mixed with other drugs of abuse such as alcohol or heroin. Causes of death due to overdose may include heart arrhythmias, cocaine-induced vasospastic events (strokes and myocardial infarcts), and seizures.

C. Withdrawal Symptoms

Patients who are long-term users of cocaine will experience withdrawal with cessation of the drug. Withdrawal symptoms include depression, irritability, insomnia or hypersomnia, fatigue, and increased appetite.

D. Treatment

The selection of medications to treat cocaine-induced hypertension and tachycardia postoperatively include agents such as phentolamine, an α-antagonist, or nitroprusside to induce vasodilation. β-Blockers such as esmolol (a selective β_1 receptor blocker) can be used to counter the stimulation of the sympathetic nervous system. Labetalol, which has both α_1 and nonselective β_1 and β_2 antagonism, has been used successfully in the treatment hypertension of patients with acute cocaine intoxication. However, there is still a risk of unopposed α-adrenergic stimulation, because the β-blocking effects of labetalol are more potent than the α-blocking effects. Cocaine-induced psychosis can lead to agitation and combativeness, in these cases high doses of benzodiazepines are recommended, and neuroleptics, typically used in other forms of psychosis, should be avoided because of the risk of potentially fatal hyperthermia. Intravenous benzodiazepines should be used to control convulsions. For signs of cocaine withdrawal, treatment is usually supportive, because symptoms are often quite minor. For more severe forms of withdrawal, drugs that enhance CNS catecholamine transmission such as amantadine may have some beneficial effects.

E. Potential Difficulties in Care Postoperatively

Patients who are addicted to cocaine have not been shown to have a cross-tolerance to opioids, but it is important to keep in mind that people who use cocaine are at higher risk of exposure to other substances of abuse such as heroin.

VII. CANNABIS

Cannabis is the most used psychoactive recreational drug. Medical cannabinoids has been increasingly legalized in a growing number of states to reduce nausea and vomiting, increase appetite, and treat chronic pain.

A. Pharmacology

Tetrahydrocannabinol (THC) is the main psychoactive component of cannabis and affects the endocannabinoid system. The endocannabinoid system is located in the central and peripheral nervous systems and contains neuromodulatory lipids and receptors. The body naturally produces cannabinoids and they interact with endocannabinoid system to regulate different body functions and importantly, how a person feels and reacts. THC attaches to cannabinoid receptors throughout the body and interferes with communication between neurons. It can affect memory and reaction time. It also affects the reward circuit of the brain and creates a feeling of being high.

B. **Side Effects**

Acute intoxication can lead to euphoria, increased awareness of sensation, distortion of perception of time and space, dry mouth, erythematous conjunctiva, and impaired short-term memory and motor skills and at higher doses can cause paranoia, hallucinations, ataxia, and in more severe cases dissociation. Chronic users can be at risk of pulmonary issues.

C. **Withdrawal**

Patients who use cannabis regularly are at risk of withdrawal symptoms such as depressed mood, craving, irritability, boredom, anxiety, hyporexia, and sleep disturbances.

D. **Treatment**

For heavy users of cannabis, withdrawal can begin the first 24 hours after the last dose and symptoms peak around 48 to 72 hours. Symptoms can last for several weeks and should lessen over time. Withdrawal is usually milder than other substances such as alcohol or benzodiazepines. Treatment is usually supportive.

E. **Potential Difficulties in Care Postoperatively**

For acute pain control, these patients can receive the usual doses of opioids because there does not seem to be a cross-tolerance. There also does not appear to be an increased risk of opioid dependency if opiates are used in the setting of acute pain.

VIII. **AMPHETAMINES/METHAMPHETAMINES**

Psychostimulants are drugs that enhance alertness and wakefulness. It can be used as a prescription medication to treat narcolepsy disorder and attention-deficit hyperactivity disorder or illegally as a street drug.

A. **Pharmacology**

Amphetamines exist as two enantiomers: levoamphetamine and dextroamphetamine. Methamphetamine is also a potent stimulant of the CNS and exists as two enantiomers: dextrorotary and levorotary. Amphetamines/methamphetamines can be taken orally, smoked, snorted, or injected. These agents exert their action by increasing the synaptic dopamine via the release of it into the synaptic space. Additionally, methamphetamine also blocks the dopamine reuptake transporter. Its effects are more potent and longer lasting than those of cocaine.

B. **Side Effects**

Short-term effects of stimulants include increased alertness/energy, tachycardia, hypertension, hyperthermia, seizures, and arrhythmias. When stimulants are used with alcohol, their effects may mask the depressant effects of alcohol and increase the risk of alcohol overdose. Chronic use can lead to depression, brain dysfunction, weight loss, and psychosis. Other distinctive features of chronic use include dental problems, muscle cramps, constipation, nasal perforation, and excoriated skin lesions.

C. **Withdrawal**

Symptoms of withdrawal from stimulants can occur 24 to 72 hours after the last dose which include tiredness, sleep problems, and depression and occur a few hours to several days after last using the substance.

Symptoms should subside by 18 days, but depression and cravings may continue for several weeks or months.

D. Treatment

If a patient experiences withdrawal in the postoperative setting, the health care provider should monitor for suicide ideation and depression. Sometimes, antidepressants may be used to help with depression. Haloperidol or low-dose second-generation antipsychotics can be used in the acute management of amphetamine-induced psychosis. Benzodiazepines can be used to treat agitation and insomnia.

E. Potential Difficulties in Care Postoperatively

Pain medication should be given for pain control for patients who take psychostimulants in the postoperative setting. Patients have not been shown to have a cross-tolerance to opioids, but may be at risk of addiction to other substances such as heroin.

IX. BARBITURATES

Barbiturates are depressants of the CNS and have been replaced mainly by benzodiazepines. They have been used for treatment of anxiety, for general anesthesia, for treatment of headaches, and for its anticonvulsant properties. Barbiturates have a strong addictive potential and there is a significant risk for overdose.

A. Pharmacology

Barbiturates are agonists of $GABA_A$ receptors and inhibit the CNS by increasing the duration of chloride ion channel opening at the $GABA_A$ receptor. Additionally, these agents block the α-amino-3-hydroxy-5-methyl-4-isoxazolepropionic acid receptor, a non-NDMA glutamate receptor with excitatory properties. Because it causes a direct opening of the chloride channel, it has increased toxicity compared to benzodiazepines, which only increase the frequency of chloride channel opening.

B. Side Effects

The effects of barbiturates are sedative and acute intoxication presents similarly to that of alcohol, but an overdose can be marked by drowsiness, shallow breathing, sluggishness, and reduced reflexes. Although tolerance can develop, there is no concomitant increase in the lethal dose, thus barbiturate overdose should always be considered potentially life-threatening. Long-term users can have symptoms such as memory loss, irritability, and decreased functioning. If barbiturates are combined with alcohol, there is an even further risk of respiratory depression.

C. Withdrawal

Patients taking barbiturates can develop a tolerance. With all GABAergic medications, withdrawal can be fatal. The symptoms of barbiturate withdrawal include tremors, seizures, sweating, nausea, hallucinations, psychosis, hyperthermia, and circulatory failure. If not properly treated, barbiturates are one of the few substances that can result in death with withdrawal.

D. Treatment

Careful history regarding use and average daily dose should be obtained when possible, and equivalent doses should be continued. If a patient experiences withdrawal from barbiturates in the postoperative settings, benzodiazepines or barbiturates can be substituted. A taper process can then occur in the subsequent days after surgery.

E. Potential Difficulties in Care Postoperatively

For chronic users of barbiturates, severe agitation, hallucinations, and seizures may occur. Seizures can be treated with benzodiazepines or barbiturates. Neuroleptics can be helpful as an adjunct in treating agitation and hallucinations. Clonidine and β-blockers are used for controlling the autonomic manifestations of withdrawal.

X. BENZODIAZEPINES

Benzodiazepines can be used to treat a variety of conditions, most commonly of which include anxiety disorders, certain sleep disorders, and convulsive disorders. Benzodiazepines use can lead to a strong physiologic and psychologic dependence. Different benzodiazepines have different potencies and half-lives.

1. High-potency benzodiazepines, short half-life: alprazolam, lorazepam, triazolam.
2. High-potency long half-life: clonazepam.
3. Low-potency, short half-life: oxazepam, temazepam.
4. Low-potency, long half-life: chlordiazepoxide, clorazepate, diazepam, flurazepam.

A. Pharmacology

Benzodiazepines work by binding to the GABA$_A$ receptor and acts as a positive allosteric modulator increasing the conduction of chloride ions that flow across the neuronal cell membranes. Benzodiazepines, barbiturates, and ethanol all have similar effects on a common receptor type and have cross-tolerance. Benzodiazepines can thus be used in alcohol withdrawal and alcohol detoxification.

B. Side Effects

Benzodiazepines can cause drowsiness, decreased alertness, dizziness, and impaired attention and concentration. Toxicity can lead to confusion, nystagmus stupor, coma respiratory depression, and cardiorespiratory arrest.

C. Withdrawal

For short-acting benzodiazepines, withdrawal usually starts within 6 to 8 hours after the last dose. For long-acting benzodiazepines, withdrawal starts around 24 to 48 hours after the last dose. Symptoms of benzodiazepine withdrawal are similar to those described for other GABA active agents and include tachycardia, hypertension, tremors, diaphoresis, insomnia, and seizures. DT could also occur. The time frame of withdrawal corresponds to the half-life of the benzodiazepine that the patient has been using. Withdrawal symptoms such as anxiety, depression, and insomnia can be protracted for months.

D. Treatment

In the postoperative period, it is imperative to monitor for withdrawal symptoms in patients who regularly take benzodiazepines. One can prevent withdrawal by keeping the patient on his or her home dose or an equivalent dose with a substitute agent. Sudden cessation or a dramatically reduction of the baseline dose of the drug can be dangerous. If acute withdrawal does occur, benzodiazepines can be substituted to the patient to counter the hyperexcitation symptoms of the CNS. If the health care provider hopes the patient to come off of the drug, a gradual taper can be carried out in the days subsequent to surgery. Benzodiazepine toxicity can be equally dangerous; treatment consists in providing adequate supportive measures, and in severe cases respiratory support. Reversal agent, flumanezil, is not routinely recommended given risk of inducing seizures and cardiac arrhythmias.

E. Potential Difficulties in Care Postoperatively

Severe agitation, hallucinations, and seizures may occur in chronic users of benzodiazepines. Seizures are best treated by administering either benzodiazepines or barbiturates. Neuroleptics can be helpful as an adjunct in treating agitation and hallucinations. Clonidine and β-blockers be used for controlling the autonomic manifestations of withdrawal.

XI. OPIOIDS

An opioid is a drug with morphine-like effects used to relieve pain. Opioids can be natural, semi-synthetic, or fully synthetic. Natural opiates include morphine and codeine. Semi-synthetic opioids are made from natural opiates or morphine esters and include hydromorphone, hydrocodone, oxycodone, and oxymorphone. Fully synthetic opioids include fentanyl, methadone, and tramadol. People who take opioids can develop tolerance, dependence, and abuse.

A. Pharmacology

Opioids bind to μ-, δ-, and κ-receptors in the CNS. However, it is the activation of μ-receptors that leads to analgesia, euphoria, and dependence.

B. Side Effects

The effects of opioids include pain relief, slowed breathing, nausea, vomiting, pruritus, euphoria, constipation, and sedation/cognitive impairments. Accidental overdose or use with other depressant drugs can lead to dangerous bradycardia and respiratory depression leading to death.

C. Withdrawal

When the substance is discontinued or the dose drastically decreased, symptoms of withdrawal can occur. For short-acting opioids, withdrawal symptoms can occur as early as 6 to 12 hours after the last dose. Whereas for long-acting opioids, withdrawal can occur around 24 to 48 hours. Symptoms to monitor for include cravings, diarrhea, insomnia, restlessness, vomiting, and muscle and bone pain. Sudden withdrawal symptoms can also occur if opioid antagonists (e.g., naloxone) are given in a patient who is chronically taking opioids.

D. Treatment

If the patient is in acute withdrawal, opioid agonists can be given. Methadone and buprenorphine can also be used to relieve withdrawal symptoms and help with detoxication in the long run. Clonidine can be given to reduce anxiety and agitation caused by opioid withdrawal. Antiemetics can be given to control nausea and vomiting, whereas muscle relaxants can help with muscle aches.

E. Potential Difficulties in Care Postoperatively

Treatment of postoperative pain in patients who have been using opioids for greater than 2 weeks may be harder due to tolerance. Use of adjuvant medications and regional techniques such as neuraxial or nerve blocks will result in opioid sparing in the postoperative setting. For management of acute pain in the postoperative setting, the baseline dose of opioids should be given. Additional short-acting opioids should be given to treat additional pain. Only a relatively small amount of opioid is needed to prevent withdrawal ($<$50% of preoperative dose). However, it is important to note that depending on the surgery, pain could be either alleviated or exacerbated. Sometimes, opioid doses can be decreased after surgery.

Suggested Readings

Alford D, Compton P, Samet J. Acute pain management for patients receiving maintenance methadone or buprenorphine therapy. *Ann Intern Med* 2006;144(2): 127–134.

Kork F, Neumann T, Spies C. Perioperative management of patients with alcohol, tobacco and drug dependency. *Curr Opin Anaesthesiol* 2010;23(3):384–390.

Moran S, Isa J, Steinemann S. Perioperative management in the patient with substance abuse. *Surg Clin North Am* 2015;95(2):417–428.

Prince V. Pain management in patients with substance-use disorders. In: *Chronic Illnesses I, II, and III—PSAP-VII, Book 5*. Lenexa, KS: American College of Clinical Pharmacology; 2011.

Pulley DD. Preoperative evaluation of the patient with substance use disorder and perioperative considerations. *Anesthesiol Clin* 2016;34(1):201–211.

Voigt L. Anesthetic management of the cocaine abuse patient. *AANA J* 1995;63(5): 438–443.

Ethico-Legal Issues and PACU Administration

SECTION IV

Ethico-Legal Issues and PACU Administration

Legal and Ethical Issues in the PACU

Caroline B. G. Hunter and Sheri Berg

I. INTRODUCTION

The postanesthesia care unit (PACU) is a complex and dynamic environment that provides both medical and ethical challenges to the anesthesiologist. Ethical challenges often arise in the setting of providing medical care and specific treatments in the postoperative period, while respecting patient autonomy. This chapter explores the complexities of the perioperative period, medical decision-making and obtaining informed consent in the PACU, special postanesthetic patient populations, and caring for the "do not resuscitate" (DNR)/"do not intubate" (DNI) patient in the perioperative period.

II. PERIOPERATIVE PERIOD

The **perioperative period** is defined in several ways:
- A. The **physical definition** includes time and location of care in the hospital or ambulatory care facility, including preoperative evaluation of the patient in the preoperative clinic or holding area, administration of anesthesia in the operating or procedure room, and postoperative care until the patient is discharged from the PACU.
- B. The **physiologic definition** includes the interval of altered physiology that begins with the onset of surgical illness and ends with the return to baseline that was present prior to surgical illness.
- C. It is important to note that the patient's perioperative physiology may resolve while the patient physically remains in the PACU.
   1. Institutional guidelines vary regarding patient care in the physical location of the PACU after a patient meets PACU criteria for discharge but has not physically left the PACU.
      a. Health care providers need to be aware of the specific guidelines in their institution.
         1. Unfortunately, these do not always exist and this is often a "gray" area.
         2. The providing clinician must always communicate with the patient and/or health care proxy if patient physiology changes.
   2. The resolution of the patient's perioperative physiology should be well defined and well documented, particularly if the patient is still physically in the PACU location.

III. DECISION-MAKING AND OBTAINING INFORMED CONSENT

- A. Patient **autonomy** is a highly valued, guiding ethical principle in the practice of medicine in the United States. Adult patients with decision-making capacity may choose to accept or refuse medical therapies.
- B. Decision-making **capacity** is determined by a medical doctor and is based on the elements of communication, understanding, reasoning, and values.
- C. Autonomy can be very difficult to incorporate into medical decision-making in the PACU because of patients' dynamic physiologic states.

329

1. During the postoperative period, the neurologic state of the patient may be altered secondary to lingering effects of anesthetic medications, and therefore patients may be unable to communicate, understand, or reason as effectively as they normally would. It should also be noted that many patients often do not recall making decisions while in the PACU.

2. Postoperative care units are often seen as an "area of coercion," and therefore medical decisions made under such pretenses can be misinterpreted by the patient or the provider.

3. Postoperative patients are sometimes medically unstable as they enter the PACU and may require emergent medical or surgical treatments. In this circumstance, an advance directive should be employed, given one does exist.

D. An **advance directive**, or living will, is a legal document specifying the types of the treatment that the patient wishes to receive or reject should future need arise and often includes a designated surrogate.

1. The surrogate (health care proxy or power of attorney for health care) has the legal charge to execute the patient's wishes should he/she become unable to do so.

   a. The surrogate offers substituted judgment for the patient, providing decisions that the patient would make if capable.

   b. If the patient has not designated a surrogate before becoming unable to make medical decisions, the next of kin may become the de facto surrogate in some states.

   c. In some circumstances where no family is living or available, a trusted friend may act as the patient's surrogate.

   d. A court-appointed legal guardian may be necessary in rare instances in which no family member or friend is able to make decisions in the best interest of the patient.

2. In emergency situations, physicians may need to act in the best interest of the patient until the patient's wishes, either directly from the patient or from an advance directive, can be elucidated.

E. **Informed consent** should be considered in the PACU for invasive procedures, testing of patients' blood for blood-borne pathogens, and surgical reexploration. When a patient provides informed consent for anesthesia, the consent includes care extending through the perioperative period and including the PACU.

1. Consent for **invasive procedures** should be obtained in the absence of an emergency from the patient or from the patient's surrogate. This includes new placement or replacement of invasive lines or epidural catheters.

2. Consent for **testing of patient blood** for blood-borne pathogens (including HIV) should be obtained in the event of an intraoperative needle-stick injury.

   a. Institutions have protocols in place regarding this process and they often involve some form of consent from the patient, either verbal or written.

   b. Although timeliness is important, this does not qualify as an emergency, and one may have to wait a period of time for anesthetic effects to abate in order for the patient to be capable to provide informed consent.

3. **Surgical reexploration** may be required in the postoperative period in the event of bleeding, hemodynamic instability, or suboptimal intraoperative results.

   a. In an emergency, consent is not required in order to act in the best interest of the patient.

      b. When the circumstance is not an emergency, consent should be obtained from the patient or surrogate.

      c. Any time informed consent is reobtained, the risk/benefit profile of the intervention should be discussed with the patient, taking into account that the clinical situation may have changed.

  F. Conflict can sometimes occur in the setting of medical decision-making.

    1. Conflict resolution best occurs via ongoing discussion with the individuals involved. The physician must recognize and respect cultural differences that influence a patient's decision.

    2. The institutional ethics committee best addresses irresolvable conflict among family members, health care team members, or between the family and medical care team.

      a. When the ethics committee is requested to consult on a case, the question to be answered or the nature of the conflict should be clearly stated. The patient's condition and prognosis should be documented.

      b. Members of the ethics committee may help organize and/or attend a family meeting to facilitate decision-making.

  G. There are **legal implications** of decision-making in the PACU.

    1. Physicians who engage in an honest, open communication with patients and their families about ethical issues rarely find themselves facing such issues in a court of law.

    2. Legal precedent is clear that patient autonomy is primary in decision-making.

      a. Under this tenet, patients may refuse life-sustaining or other therapies if they are capable to do so.

      b. Similarly, care once rendered may be withdrawn.

      c. However, as previously stated, the postoperative and perioperative period are often open to interpretation and vary between institution and even practitioners.

      d. It is necessary to speak with patient or their health care proxy and surgical team prior to surgical procedures.

        1. This allows for open communication and realistic expectations across all parties.

    3. Physicians also have legal rights and they are not bound to provide care that they deem futile.

      a. However, determination of futility may be problematic and may cause conflict with patient or family.

      b. In this case, it is advisable for the physician to pursue every avenue of conflict resolution, including removing him/herself from the patient's care, before exercising this dictum against patient or family wishes.

IV. SPECIAL PATIENT POPULATIONS

  A. The **pediatric patient** deserves special consideration where ethical issues are concerned.

    1. Legally, such decisions are deferred to the parents.

    2. Ethically, the patient may participate in these decisions to provide assent, depending on his/her developmental level and decision-making capacity. If the child is too immature to participate in decision-making, parents are relied upon to make decisions in the best interest of the child, incorporating family values as well as weighing the benefit versus risk of the planned therapy.

  B. Jehovah's Witnesses generally do not accept transfusions of blood products based on religious beliefs.

    1. Each Jehovah's Witness must be assessed individually.

   a. Some will accept blood subfractions, products made from recombinant DNA, autotransfused blood, salvaged autologous blood, or albumin.
   b. Careful documentation of preoperative discussions is paramount to appropriate postanesthetic care.
   c. In the PACU, the wishes of the Jehovah's Witness patient regarding blood transfusion should be reconfirmed once he/she is capable of decision-making.
   2. Special considerations may apply if the patient is a minor, does not have capacity to make his/her own medical decisions, has responsibilities for dependents, and in certain emergency situations where the patient's wishes are not known.
   3. Law and judicial practices vary from state to state, and health care providers should be familiar with their particular state's statutes or seek advice from hospital legal counsel.
   4. Legal precedent generally supports patient autonomy regarding the acceptance of transfusion.

V. THE DNR/DNI PATIENT
A. **DNR orders** should not be automatically suspended when a patient enters the operating room. Rather, the institution's written policy regarding this situation should be followed.
   1. The American Society of Anesthesiologists recognizes patients' right to self-determination and recommends that preexisting advance directives be discussed with the patient (or surrogate) and other involved parties (e.g., surgeon and primary physician) before initiating anesthetic care.
   2. Specific aspects of the anesthetic that might be considered "resuscitation" in another setting (e.g., endotracheal intubation) may be necessary to provide successful anesthesia intraoperatively.
   3. All communications regarding DNR orders should be documented in a chart and used to guide anesthetic care.
      a. Precise communication with the patient and primary surgical team is imperative in order to appropriately optimize patient care.
B. **Resuscitation courses of action** may be defined in three categories:
   1. A full resuscitation status is implemented for the anesthetic and perioperative period, suspending the "DNR" status completely.
   2. A limited, procedure-directed resuscitation is implemented for the anesthetic and perioperative period.
      a. For example, a patient may accept an endotracheal tube, which may be necessary for the surgical procedure, but may reject chest compressions in the event of cardiac arrest.
   3. A limited, goal-directed resuscitation based on patient values is followed for the perioperative period.
      a. For example, the patient may allow resuscitation for events that are deemed to be reversible and known complications of the anesthetic (e.g., hypotension), but may not allow resuscitation for events that, in the judgment of the anesthesiologist, are likely irreversible (e.g., pulseless electrical activity in the setting of large venous air embolism).
      b. Similarly, a patient may define a priori based on his/her values, circumstances that would result in an unacceptable quality of life, and may request limitation of life-sustaining therapies in those circumstances.
C. Anesthesiologists often find it difficult to enact limited resuscitation goals because it puts them in a position to either feel unprepared to manage a situation or to make judgments about the consequences of

their actions. Patient autonomy should guide decisions and the anesthesiologist should not try to coerce the patient into any one resuscitative plan.

D. These patients should ideally be seen preoperatively in a multidisciplinary discussion between the patient and/or surrogate, primary care physician, surgeon, anesthesiologist, and PACU physician.

E. The patient's wishes should be well documented so that the PACU team understands them when PACU care begins.

  1. The duration of the perioperative period should be defined and well documented in the patient record. As described previously, the perioperative period may be defined in different ways, based on either temporal or physiologic measures.

  2. Ongoing discussions should occur with the patient and/or surrogate regarding patient goals, particularly in the event that the perioperative period becomes prolonged or the patient's clinical situation changes.

Suggested Readings

American Society of Anesthesiologists. Ethical guidelines for the anesthesia care of patients with do-not-resuscitate orders or other directives that limit treatment. Available at: http://www.asahq.org/~/media/Sites/ASAHQ/Files/Public/Resources/standards-guidelines/ethical-guidelines-for-the-anesthesia-care-of-patients.pdf. Approved October 17, 2001. Last affirmed October 22, 2008.

Ewanchuk M, Brindley PG. Ethics review: perioperative do-not-resuscitate orders—doing 'nothing' when 'something' can be done. *Crit Care* 2006;10:219.

Jenkins K, Baker AB. Consent and anaesthetic risk. *Anaesthesia* 2003;58:962–984.

Kelly T, Berg S. Ethical and end-of-life issues. In: Pino R, ed. *Clinical Anesthesia Procedures of the Massachusetts General Hospital*. 9th ed. Philadelphia, PA: Lippincott Williams & Wilkins; 2016.

Roy RC, Calicott RW. Anesthesia practice models, perioperative risk, and the future of anesthesiology. *ASA Newsl* 2007;71(10):14–17.

Truog RD, Waisel DB, Burns JP. DNR in the OR: a goal-directed approach. *Anesthesiology* 1999;90:289–295.

Waisel DB. Unrecognized barriers to perioperative limitations on potentially life-sustaining medical treatment. *J Clin Anesth* 2014;26:171–173.

PACU Admission and Discharge Criteria

Yuriy Bronshteyn and William Schoenfeld

I. INTRODUCTION

A postanesthesia care unit (PACU) is a specialized intensive care ward that serves the brief, yet intense medical needs of patients after a surgical procedure. Such requirements arise from the dual physiologic insult of surgery and anesthesia on the human body. There are occasional needs to deliver emergent cardiovascular and respiratory support postoperatively to patients, and PACUs are equipped to provide the same level of intensive care that a surgical intensive care unit is capable of. Further, because of continual traffic between the operating suite and the PACU, the two are usually located near one another within a hospital.

II. HISTORY

As early as 1801, some British hospitals had areas dedicated to the care of patients recovering from operations and also those who were severely ill. Soon after the discovery of the anesthetic properties of ether, which opened the door to a considerable growth in surgery, Florence Nightingale suggested in 1863 that postoperative patients in the U.S. be cared for in a specialized ward. Apparently, however, such units did not become commonplace in the hospitals of the developed world until the first half of the 20th century. These units did not receive "intensive care unit" status until the later decades of the 20th century.

III. VULNERABILITIES OF THE POST-OP PATIENT

The trauma of an operation and the residual effects of anesthetic drugs alter human physiology in predictable ways. Surgery typically begets bleeding and inflammation. Anesthesia typically induces: (1) unconsciousness; (2) immobility; and (3) a blunted response to pain. Emergence from these anesthetic effects is a time of instability, characterized by upper airway obstruction, delirium, pain, nausea/vomiting, hypothermia, and autonomic lability.

In multiple studies over the past few decades, the two most common life-threatening postoperative complications affecting patients have been respiratory insufficiency and cardiovascular instability. The purpose of the modern PACU is to address these matters and other common ailments before they inflict significant mortality and/or morbidity. Further, modern PACU discharge criteria emphasize respiratory and cardiac stability as a prerequisite to PACU discharge (see PACU Discharge Criteria in this chapter).

Several retrospective, single-center studies have examined the prevalence and types of postoperative complications in the recovery room. The first study published in the era of pulse oximetry examined 18,000 anesthetics and found that the three most common post-op complications were: (1) nausea/vomiting (42% of complications); (2) need for upper airway support (29%); and (3) hypotension (13%). Fourteen years later, another study of over a thousand patients found a similar 23% overall rate of post-op complications. However, the distribution of complications differed a bit. The three most common types were: (1) need for upper airway support

(40% of complications); (2) nausea/vomiting (31%); and tachycardia (13%). Most recently, a study of over a thousand patients in Qatar found a much lower overall rate of post-op complications in the PACU (4%). Of these complications, the three most common were: (1) desaturation (40% of complications); (2) hypo- or hyperthermia (25%); and (3) postoperative nausea and vomiting (PONV; 15%). The discrepancies in complication prevalence and distribution can be attributed, at least in part, to marked heterogeneity between the studies related to, among other things: (1) case mix (e.g., rate of ENT and gynecologic surgeries known to be high risk for PONV); (2) provider level of expertise; and (3) data collection (i.e., lack of universal criteria for defining various complications).

The analysis of national adverse event databases is probably more relevant. In 1989, Zeitlin published a review of the recovery room cases found in the American Society of Anesthesiologists (ASA) closed claims database. Such cases represented 7% of the over 1,100 incidents in the database. Most of these occurred in the era before pulse oximeters became widely used. Not surprisingly, respiratory incidents comprised the majority of the cases (49 of the 84), whereas cardiovascular incidents represented a minority (9 of 84). In 2002, Kluger et al published a similar analysis of the Anaesthetic Incident Monitoring Study (AIMS) database in Australia. Of the over 8,000 total cases, 5% occurred in the recovery room. The three most common cases were: (1) respiratory/airway issues (43%); (2) cardiovascular problems (24%); and (3) drug errors (11%).

A. Respiratory

Respiratory insufficiency in the PACU is usually partially secondary to residual anesthetic effects. All of the medications given intraoperatively to enable tolerance of airway manipulation and surgical stimulation can undermine normal respiratory function postoperatively. Opioids and hypnotics depress respiratory drive, airway reflexes, and airway patency. Central nervous system depressants also put patients at risk of laryngospasm. Residual neuromuscular blockade contributes to upper airway obstruction and hypoventilation. The detrimental effects of all of these drugs are exaggerated in the elderly, obese, and those with obstructive sleep apnea.

B. Cardiovascular

Common cardiovascular problems in the PACU include hypotension, hypertension, or tachycardia.

Surgery results in bleeding, nonhematologic volume losses (e.g., evaporative and interstitial), and inflammation. Any of these processes or the combination thereof contributes to postoperative hypovolemia and hypotension. Residual anesthetics such as opioids and hypnotics can also lower arteriolar and venous tone, resulting in decreased preload and afterload.

When postoperative pain control is inadequate, nociceptive signaling from the surgical site can trigger sympathetically mediated tachycardia and hypertension. Although hypotension is more immediately life threatening, tachycardia and hypertension are associated with increased risk of ICU admission and mortality. The mechanism of mortality may be related to the metabolic burden placed on the heart in this transient hyperdynamic state. For instance, it is known that most perioperative myocardial infarctions occur 24 to 48 hours postoperatively and likely arise from supply–demand mismatch rather than plaque rupture events.

IV. PACU STANDARDS AND GUIDELINES

The ASA publishes and regularly updates practice standards that define the minimum expectations of care in the postanesthetic period. The standards are, at times, vague (e.g., standard #1 below) and can certainly be exceeded at a clinician's discretion. From the standpoint of these standards, "anesthesia" refers to any combination of general, regional, and monitored anesthesia care. The ASA's five minimum expectations for postanesthetic care are summarized below (Anesthesiologists Approved by the House of Delegates on Oct 12, 1998 and last ammended on Oct 21, 2009):

A. A patient who receives anesthesia should receive appropriate post-anesthesia care.

B. During transport to the PACU, a patient should be accompanied and constantly evaluated and supported by a member of the anesthesia team knowledgeable about the patient's condition.

C. Upon arrival in the PACU, the anesthesia team member should reevaluate the patient and provide a verbal report to the accepting PACU nurse.

D. The patient should be evaluated continually while in the PACU.

E. A physician should be responsible for discharge of the patient from the PACU.

In contrast to standards, guidelines provide "suggestions" rather than "requirements" for care. The Practice Guidelines for Postanesthetic Care are developed by the ASA Taskforce on Postanesthetic Care. They integrate current scientific literature and the opinion of groups of experts, including, separately, the (1) members of the ASA Taskforce (a group of anesthesiologists and epidemiologists); (2) PACU consultants; and (3) ASA members at large.

The guidelines encourage vigilance in the PACU for the common postoperative complications and appropriate treatment when such complications arise. Specifically, the guidelines recommend regular monitoring for and support of the following:

1. Respiratory function
   a. Airway patency, respiratory rate, and oxygen saturation
2. Cardiovascular function
   a. Pulse, blood pressure, and/or electrocardiographic monitoring
   b. Euvolemia judged by hemodynamics and the balance of fluid intake and output (including the output of urine and surgical drains)
3. Neurologic function
   a. Mental status and neuromuscular function
4. Miscellaneous
   a. Normothermia, pain control, shivering control, and nausea/vomiting prevention/treatment

V. PACU ADMISSION CRITERIA

In accordance with the ASA Standards, at our institution, any patient who receives a general or regional anesthetic is transported to the PACU. Patients receiving conscious sedation can either be brought to the PACU or delivered to stage 2 recovery (see Phases of Postanesthetic Recovery in this chapter) at the discretion of the anesthesiologist.

A. Phases of Postanesthetic Recovery

Postanesthetic recovery for ambulatory surgery patients is often divided into three phases: early, intermediate, and late.

1. Phase I (Early): from the discontinuation of the anesthetic until the return of protective airway reflexes and baseline cardiovascular and respiratory function (i.e., when patient meets PACU discharge criteria described below). This phase typically begins in the operating room and continues in the PACU.

2. Phase 2 (Intermediate): starts when the patient meets PACU discharge criteria. This phase occurs in a step-down unit or ambulatory surgery unit (ASU) and ends when the patient is ready to be safely discharged home. Notably, all ambulatory surgery patients

discharged home should be accompanied by an adult, per ASA Guidelines.

3. Phase 3 (Late): continues at home until the patient returns to their preoperative psychomotor state. For ambulatory surgery patients, this often takes 1 to 3 days.

For hospitalized inpatients, phases 2 and 3 both occur on an inpatient ward. Because of the speed with which newer anesthetics are eliminated by the body, patients can sometimes bypass phase 1 and proceed straight from the operating room to phase 2, thus liberating PACU personnel and efficiently decreasing resource utilization. This practice is sometimes called "fast-tracking." Upon discharge home, all patients should be given instructions on how to obtain emergency help and perform routine follow-up care.

VI. DISCHARGE CRITERIA

Distinct discharge criteria exist for the PACU (phase 1), the ASU (phase 2), and fast-track patients (i.e., those that skip phase 1 and pass directly to phase 2).

A. Criteria for Discharge from Phase 1 (PACU) to Phase 2 (ASU)

The main goal of the PACU (phase 1 recovery) is to monitor and treat the postoperative patient until they are no longer at risk for respiratory insufficiency or cardiovascular instability. To that end, in 1970 Aldrete adapted the Apgar scoring system (used for neonatal assessment) for the assessment of all patients postoperatively. He replaced the testing of neonatal reflexes with assessment of consciousness, but otherwise maintained the same 5-category system, with a maximum of 2 points per category: (1) activity; (2) respiration; (3) circulation; (4) consciousness; and (5) color (pink vs. pale vs. cyanotic). With the widespread adoption of pulse oximetry, Aldrete changed the last category from the subjective "color" to the objective oxygen saturation. The current system is shown in Table 36.1. For ambulatory surgery patients, an Aldrete score of 9 is generally considered a prerequisite for discharge from the PACU to phase 2 recovery. For inpatients undergoing surgery, an Aldrete score of 8 is considered to be sufficient to qualify them for transition to phase 2, recognizing that medical assessment will continue on the floor, albeit at a greater patient-to-nurse ratio than in the PACU. Ultimately, a physician is responsible for a patient's discharge from the PACU.

B. "Fast-track" Criteria for Discharge from the OR to Phase 2 Recovery (ASU)

To screen ambulatory surgery patients for "fast-track" eligibility (i.e., to bypass phase 1), White proposed and validated a revised version of the modified Aldrete score that also includes pain and nausea scores (see Table 36.2). Patients achieving a score of 12 (with no less than a single point in each category) are deemed eligible for transfer directly from the OR to the ASU. A hemodynamically stable patient with normal respiratory function and good pain and nausea control is unlikely to burden the resource-scarce phase 3 recovery area.

C. Criteria for Discharge from Phase 2 Recovery (ASU) to Home (Phase 3)

To safely discharge a patient home postoperatively from day surgery, one ought to feel comfortable that the patient's postoperative needs can be met in a home environment. Though there are multiple scoring systems available, the most widely used is the Post Anesthesia Discharge Score (PADS) developed by Chung. The original iteration of the system emphasized (1) vital sign stability, (2) ability to ambulate, (3) pain and nausea control, (4) control of surgical bleeding, and (5) ability to void and tolerate oral intake. However, subsequent studies showed that imposing the last criterion on all patients causes more harm than benefit. Forcing patients to trial oral intake before discharge resulted in significantly

TABLE 36.1 Modified Aldrete Scoring System for PACU Discharge	
Category	**Points**
Activity	
Moves all 4 extremities	2
Moves 2 extremities	1
Unable to move	0
Respiration	
Able to cough and deep breathe	2
Dyspneic or hypoventilating	1
Apneic	0
Circulation	
BP within 20% of presedation level	2
BP within 50% of presedation level	1
BP $>$ 50% of presedation level	0
Consciousness	
Fully awake and alert	2
Arousable to voice only	1
Unarousable/unresponsive	0
Oxygen saturation	
O_2 sat $>$92% on room air	2
Requires supplemental O_2 to keep O_2 sat $>$92%	1
O_2 sat $<$92% with supplemental O_2	0

Adapted from Aldrete JA. The post-anesthesia recovery score revisited. *J Clin Anesth* 1995;7(1):89–91.

TABLE 36.2 White Fast-Tracking Additions to the Modified Aldrete Score	
Category	**Points**
Pain	
None or mild discomfort	2
Moderate to severe requiring IV analgesia	1
Refractory severe pain	0
Nausea	
None or mild nausea	2
Transient vomiting or retching	1
Refractory moderate/severe nausea and vomiting	0

Adapted from White PF, Song D. New criteria for fast-tracking after outpatient anesthesia: a comparison with the modified Aldrete's scoring system. *Anesth Analg* 1999;88(5):1069–1072.

more nausea and vomiting (especially in patients receiving opioids) than allowing patients to wait to trial orals when their appetite returns at home. Furthermore, forcing patients to stay in the hospital until they void only benefits patients at high risk of urinary retention (i.e., older age, male sex, pelvic surgery, neuraxial anesthesia, duration of surgery $>$60 minutes, intraoperative fluids $>$750 mL). Patients at low risk of retention are highly likely to void adequately at home in due time, so keeping them in the hospital until they void only delays their discharge by hours. Awad proposed that: (1) patients at low risk of retention be instructed to return to the hospital if they are unable to void within 6 to

Category	Points
Modified PADS Criteria for Discharge from Phase 2 Recovery to Home	
Vital signs	
Within 20% of preoperative values	2
20%–40% of preoperative values	1
>40% of preoperative values	0
Activity level	
Steady gait without dizziness/back to baseline	2
Requires assistance	1
Unable to ambulate/assess	0
Nausea and vomiting	
Mild/none—no treatment needed	2
Moderate—treatment effective	1
Severe—refractory to treatment	0
Pain	
VAS 0–2 (mild or no pain)	2
VAS 4–6 (moderate pain)	1
VAS 7–10 (severe pain)	0
Surgical bleeding	
Minimal—does not require dressing change	2
Moderate—bleeding stopped with 2 dressing changes	1
Severe—continues to bleed despite 3 dressing changes	0

Modified from Awad IT, Chung F. Factors affecting recovery and discharge following ambulatory surgery. *Can J Anaesth* 2006;53(9):858–872.

8 hours and (2) patients at high risk of retention should be required to both void and demonstrate a postvoid residual <300 mL measured by ultrasound; a postvoid residual >600 mL should prompt catheterization prior to discharge home (Awad and Chung, 2006). The latest ASA Practice Guidelines now advise against holding up a patient's discharge for a voiding trail or oral tolerance except for selected patients.

The modified PADS criteria (see Table 36.3) thus exclude trials of voiding and oral intake and separate pain and nausea control into segregated categories (to maintain a total of 5 categories and thus a maximum score of 10).

VII. DISCHARGE CRITERIA FOR REGIONAL AND NEURAXIAL ANESTHESIA

Patients receiving regional and neuraxial anesthesia can be screened for phase 1 and 2 discharge eligibility using the same criteria described for patients receiving general anesthesia. Additional steps should also be taken specific to the anesthetic. In patients who received a neuraxial anesthetic that is expected to be receding, it is important to test for and document regression of the block in motor and sensory modalities. Block regression can be detected using these ascending signs: return of perineal sensation (S4–5), ability to plantar-flex the foot (S1–2), and proprioception of the big toe (L5).

Patients being discharged home after single-shot nerve blocks should be given explicit verbal and written instructions of how to avoid accidental injury (including thermal and mechanical). Patients being discharged home with continuous peripheral nerve catheters should, in addition to the aforementioned counseling, be advised about the potential for toxicity from catheter migration (including intravascular, epidural, intrathecal, etc., as relevant). Such patients should also be given clear instructions on how to reach a member of the anesthesia team 24 hours a day while the catheter is infusing medications.

Suggested Readings

Aldrete JA. The post-anesthesia recovery score revisited. *J Clin Anesth* 1995;7(1):89–91.

Allen A, Badgwell JM. The post anesthesia care unit: unique contribution, unique risk. *J Perianesth Nurs* 1996;11(4):248–258.

American Society of Anesthesiologists. Standards for Postanesthesia Care. (Approved by the ASA House of Delegates on October 27, 2004, and last amended on October 15, 2014.) http://www.asahq.org/coveo/~/media/sites/asahq/files/public/resources/standards-guidelines/standards-for-postanesthesia-care.pdf. Accessed June 3, 2017.

Apfelbaum JL, Silverstein JH, Chung FF, et al. Practice guidelines for postanesthetic care: an updated report by the American Society of Anesthesiologists Task Force on Postanesthetic Care. *Anesthesiology* 2013;118(2):291–307.

Awad IT, Chung F. Factors affecting recovery and discharge following ambulatory surgery. *Can J Anaesth* 2006;53(9):858–872.

Butterworth J, Mackey DC, Wasnick F, eds. Postanesthesia care. In: *Morgan and Mikhail's Clinical Anesthesiology*. 5th ed. New York, NY: McGraw-Hill; 2013.

Chinnappa V, Chung F. What criteria should be used for discharge after outpatient surgery? In: Fleisher LA, ed. *Evidence-Based Practice of Anesthesiology*. Philadelphia, PA: Saunders; 2009:305–313.

Chung F, Chan VW, Ong D. A post-anesthetic discharge scoring system for home readiness after ambulatory surgery. *J Clin Anesth* 1995;7(6):500–506.

Faraj JH, Vegesna AR, Mudali IN, et al. Survey and management of anaesthesia related complications in PACU. *Qatar Med J* 2013;2012(2):64–70.

Hines R, Barash PG, Watrous G, et al. Complications occurring in the postanesthesia care unit: a survey. *Anesth Analg* 1992;74(4):503–509.

Kluger MT, Bullock MF. Recovery room incidents: a review of 419 reports from the Anaesthetic Incident Monitoring Study (AIMS). *Anaesthesia* 2002;57(11):1060–1066.

Landesberg G. The pathophysiology of perioperative myocardial infarction: facts and perspectives. *J Cardiothorac Vasc Anesth* 2003;17(1):90–100.

Nicholau D. The postanesthesia care unit. In: Miller RD, ed. *Miller's Anesthesia*. Vol 2. Philadelphia, PA: Churchill Livingstone; 2010.

Nightingale F. *Notes on Hospitals*. London, UK: Roberts & Green; 1863.

Pinsker MC. Anesthesia: a pragmatic construct. *Anesth Analg* 1986;65(7):819–820.

Rose DK, Cohen MM, Wigglesworth DF, et al. Critical respiratory events in the postanesthesia care unit. Patient, surgical, and anesthetic factors. *Anesthesiology* 1994;81(2):410–418.

Tarrac SE. A description of intraoperative and postanesthesia complication rates. *J Perianesth Nurs* 2006;21(2):88–96.

White PF, Song D. New criteria for fast-tracking after outpatient anesthesia: a comparison with the modified Aldrete's scoring system. *Anesth Analg* 1999;88(5):1069–1072.

Yip PC, Hannam JA, Cameron AJ, et al. Incidence of residual neuromuscular blockade in a post-anaesthetic care unit. *Anaesth Intensive Care* 2010;38(1):91–95.

Zeitlin GL. Recovery room mishaps in the ASA Closed Claims Study. *ASA Newsl* 1989;53(7):28–30.

Quality Assurance, Organization,
Policies, and Management in the
Postanesthesia Care Units (PACUs)

Edward George

I. POSTANESTHESIA CARE UNITS QUALITY ASSURANCE

A. Introduction

Postanesthesia care units (PACUs) often vary in the scope and the nature of practice as a function of the services provided in a given institution. The spectrum of operational requirements ranges from ambulatory surgical centers, where a PACU can serve as an admission, recovery, and discharge facility, to the largest of medical centers with multiple PACU, often providing services to a unique subset of patients, to include an integrated function to the surgical intensive care units. Moreover, in the setting of extreme operational demands, such as seen with natural disasters or mass casualty/emergency response situations, the PACU may be required to expand the scope of practice to serve in capacities ranging from general care units to ICU.

Regardless of the nature of services provided by the PACU, it is vital that all units maintain an active program in quality assurance and patient safety. Although the design, implementation, and maintenance of such programs are driven by the practice within the institution or medical group, the requirement for a comprehensive system is critical to every facility. Although individual PACUs are organized to serve the unique need(s) of a specific practice site, there are commonalities of program structure and function that are present in all programs.

B. Definition

In the domain of health care, quality assurance and patient safety activities and programs are designed to assure or improve the quality of care in either a defined medical setting or a program. This concept encompasses the assessment and/or evaluation of the quality of care, identification of problems or shortcomings in the delivery of care, designing activities to correct/overcome these deficiencies, and monitoring processes to ensure effectiveness of corrective steps.

Health care facilities commonly maintain a department or functionality in quality assurance and patient safety. Most often, major services, such as medicine, surgery, and neurology, will also organize a quality assurance/patient safety process that will provide an ongoing system of surveillance and oversight germane to the quality and safety challenges of a given department/specialty. These local activities are often subordinate to institutional quality programs and depend upon a coordinated process at higher levels of management to ensure that events with potential interdepartmental implications are appropriately managed in a timely manner.

PACUs present a unique challenge with regard to the organization of quality and safety programs, in that the PACU represents the operational domain of several departments within a hospital, all functioning in a close and coordinated fashion. Typically, the departments of anesthesia and nursing maintain key leadership roles in the operation of the

PACU and collaborate closely with the department of surgery, as well as other subspecialties (interventional radiology, gastroenterology, etc.).

As such, any program designed to oversee unit functionality must be represented by experienced personnel from all disciplines. As previously suggested, this may also be further complicated by the unique role many PACUs play in providing clinical services to specialties outside of the typical surgical domains, such as the endoscopic services of the department of medicine and the interventional services of the department of radiology. Institutions may approach such challenges of coordination by developing a robust reporting system to organizational functions from departments that may function as a component of an integrated service, or a middle-level functionality that serves as a perioperative oversight service described as a perioperative quality assurance committee.

Regardless of the structure and organization of the quality assurance programs, it is critical to maintain a clear and discrete process for reporting and evaluation of events related to quality assurance. Furthermore, it is essential that the system be designed to facilitate any subsequent analysis in a manner that serves institutional quality assurance and patient safety requirements, as well as providing the opportunity to contribute to departmental and institutional quality improvement processes.

C. Operational Significance

Industry has utilized quality assurance and quality control programs for decades. However, the manner in which quality assurance has been embraced by the health care industry has its roots in the safety programs that have emerged from the world of aviation with a clear pioneer of the process resident in the military aviation community beginning around the World War II era.

The adoption of checklists and policies to engage and empower personnel at every level of clinical care, now seen as commonplace in the practice of medicine, evolved directly from the experiences of army and navy aviation programs. With roots in the years preceding World War II, these processes have been refined over decades in both the military and civilian communities and have been recognized as providing the fundamentals of quality and safety programs in professions ranging from manufacturing to law enforcement to medicine.

Capitalizing on the ability to learn from experience gained, not only in clinical care but also in industrial applications, has resulted in the development of a systems-based approach to analysis, employing the fundamental concepts of root cause analysis. Coupled with the philosophy that quality assurance and patient safety are institutional priorities, these programs have provided the ability to bring the vital elements of direct patient care to an integrated process engaging institutional expertise and resources.

In addition, adopting a philosophy where the culture of blame is replaced by an approach driven by evaluation of data in a manner that can separate performance versus system's based challenges offers the ability to optimize processes of assessment without attaching any stigma related to individual execution. This practice results in a more complete evaluation in that personnel are more comfortable offering details associated with an event, without fear of retribution, as well as positioning the process in a manner that can better offer assistance to individuals involved in what may often be emotionally challenging events. Programs such as peer support and peer counseling have grown from the evolution of quality assurance and patient safety programs over the past decade or more, and now provide a vital service to caregivers involved in quality-related events.

D. Structure/Development of a Quality Assurance Program

Although the requirements for a formal quality assurance program reflect the nature of practice in a given institution, basic program elements fall into a set of common components as follows:

- Concept of operations
- Structure
- Reporting system
- Data acquisition/analytic function
- Review process
- Determination/findings
- Dissemination
- Review

1. Concept of operations

The concept of operations is ordinarily a reflection of institutional values that are stipulated by departmental leadership and, although variable, generally address the spirit of a comprehensive program to improve care and evaluate and improve shortcomings in practice at the individual and departmental levels. Interests in the integration of quality improvement functions are often specified as an element of operational concepts, as are relationships within a department. It is important to appreciate that operational concepts are often dynamic, adjusting to address changing practice(s).

2. Structure

The organization of a quality assurance activity may range from a dedicated administrative activity, staffed by permanent personnel, to a function within a clinical care unit, with personnel assigned to the process by additional/ancillary duties. Regardless of the structure, it is imperative that personnel possess appropriate clinical insight and are provided with adequate time and resources to effectively manage the program.

3. Reporting system

The design and implementation of a reporting system is integral to the success of any quality assurance program. Systems range from the most simple and straightforward, using a simple form and transfer to a database, to computerized systems, integrating key elements of clinical care over the spectrum of perioperative services, with automated elements directly providing information to institutional leadership. Regardless of the degree of sophistication, the reporting system must be simple to use, comprehensive in scope, and accessible to all, yet appropriately protecting patient confidentiality and offering anonymity to personnel. Although typically engaged by staff involved in direct patient care, the ability to accept input from leadership, as well as to integrate reports from elements such as patient advocacy offices, offers the best chance to ensure all issues are evaluated in the most comprehensive fashion.

4. Data acquisition/analytic function

In the setting of a reported event, or that of an occurrence that is directed to the quality assurance functionaries, the ability to obtain accurate information comprehensively is vital to any successful quality assurance activity. Information is often obtained from multiple sources. In addition to the event notice, critical information may often involve perioperative records (perioperative evaluation, intraoperative records, etc.) as well as interviews with involved individuals, often including the patient. Personnel involved in the analysis must possess appropriate clinical experience, as well as the ability to consult with individuals with expertise germane to the event being evaluated.

5. **Review process**

A systematic process must be utilized in the evaluation of all safety-related issues. Institutions will maintain a quality assurance/safety office often providing format and guidance to subordinate departments regarding specific requirements for process review and reporting. Individuals at the unit level assigned to a quality/safety function must have relevant clinical experience and must be provided with the opportunity for education/training in quality and safety areas. The review process can be straightforward, examining any deviation from a standard of care, or may require in-depth and interdepartmental analysis and collaboration. Unit leadership must maintain an oversight function through all phases of the process.

6. **Determination/findings**

At the completion of the analytic phase(s), the quality and safety personnel must determine whether an issue is, in fact, of concern, as well as the root cause factors that contributed to the compromise. This component will require a formal report to leadership, often set in a standardized format specifying the event, individuals involved, findings of fact, and recommendations for follow-up.

7. **Dissemination**

Leadership personnel, at the unit, departmental, or institutional levels, are responsible for the dissemination of the results of analysis. Because those elements of a quality or safety issue may involve issues of confidentiality, it is vital that those involved in quality and safety processes not only maintain detailed records but also ensure that the patient, as well as the clinician's personal information, remains protected. This anonymity of sorts both safeguards sensitive information and provides a sense of reassurance on the part of all involved individuals that are concerned about retribution associated with reporting of incidents.

8. **Review**

All programs addressing quality and safety issues must be reviewed by clinical leadership with unit/clinical responsibilities, as well as by departmental and institutional elements responsible for pertinent quality and safety programs. This process provides the ability to review findings, as well as the process used in all steps of the analysis.

Many clinical units schedule a regular review session, with appropriate attention to confidentiality, for staff personnel and leadership to present key cases for discussion. This can afford opportunities for improvement in reporting, analysis, and, perhaps most importantly, implementing necessary change(s) to ensure that avoidable events do not reoccur.

II. PACU ORGANIZATION, MANAGEMENT, AND POLICIES

A. Introduction

Recovery of patients after procedures requiring anesthesia or sedation is most commonly performed in a PACU or recovery room. As specialized areas designed for the observation, treatment, and discharge of postoperative patients, a PACU's role(s) and function can be as varied as the scope of practice within the individual institution. An ambulatory care/day surgery clinic may maintain a PACU staffed by perioperative nurses, with medical oversight provided by an anesthesiologist who may also be involved in supervising cases in the operating room; whereas a large-scale academic hospital, such as a Level I trauma center, may have multiple, geographically distinct PACUs. These units, supporting various functions, often with subspecialty segregation, can provide intermediate critical care requirements, with medical oversight provided by dedicated anesthesiologists and/or surgical intensivists.

Optimally located near the operating room, thereby minimizing transport time for the patient, and affording rapid access to anesthesiologists and surgeons, the PACU is staffed by specially trained nurses and nurse practitioners proficient in the care of patients in the immediate postoperative period. Under the supervision of an anesthesiologist, the PACU provides care to a broad crosssection of postprocedural patients, with the majority being subsequently transferred in a timely manner from the PACU to a general care floor of the hospital, or, as in the case of an ambulatory care facility, discharged home. A broad diversity characterizes patients admitted to the PACU as well as the surgical procedures. Many patients are healthy and have an uneventful hospital course, whereas some experience a more complex perioperative course influenced by their preexisting medical history and/or a complicated intraoperative course.

Patients are admitted into the PACU at the conclusion of procedures requiring anesthesia or sedation. Patients are most often admitted after surgical procedures in the operating room. However, interventions under anesthesia may also take place outside of the main operating rooms in other departments such as radiology, cardiology, or gastro-enterology. In such cases, care can be provided in areas removed from the hospital's main recovery areas and may require coordination with the PACU. Personnel trained and experienced in the recovery of these patients should be present to oversee the recovery phase and must be able to obtain immediate help in the event of an urgent or acute change in a patient's condition.

Given the wide range of patients undergoing recovery in the PACU, the potential issues are also quite varied. Being able to anticipate common issues in advance may facilitate the initiation of appropriate action(s) in a timely manner and may help avoid the complications associated with more urgent interventions.

Healthy patients may undergo procedures as either inpatients or outpatients, depending on the severity of the surgical intervention. Some complex surgical procedures, even in an otherwise healthy subject, may require prolonged postoperative care in the hospital. In such cases, the planned length of the hospital stay is influenced by the period required for functional recovery, as well as possible postoperative complications. An uncomplicated recovery in the PACU is generally anticipated for most patients. However, patients often present to the PACU with comorbid conditions that may influence their postoperative course, both in the PACU and during their subsequent hospital stay. While patients with multiple medical conditions are routinely discharged home on the same day of surgery, comorbidities are often a major factor in the decision to admit a patient to the hospital after surgery.

Regardless of the nature and complexity of patients admitted to the PACU, it is important to remember that the goal of any PACU is to facilitate the recovery of a postprocedural patient to the point that permits this patient to continue on the anticipated clinical course, be it discharge from the hospital or transfer to a general care unit in the institution. This evolution may be as simplified as observing a patient during recovery from a simple procedure. Or it may involve elements of resuscitation; analgesia and additional means of support to ensure all patients' needs are anticipated before leaving the PACU. Although the majority of patients passing through a PACU present few clinical challenges to an experienced staff, a small percentage can require extended monitoring and may require aggressive treatment. That the evolution of current day ICU present in all hospitals came from the experience gained in PACU and recovery rooms of only a few decades ago is testimony to the variability of demands seen in today's PACUs.

B. Organization

The PACU is typically staffed by anesthesiologists, specially trained recovery room nursing staff, and support personnel. In addition to providing the ability to appropriately monitor patients and provide routine postoperative care, the PACU also affords the capability to provide mechanical ventilation and invasive monitoring, as well as the emergency equipment and skilled personnel able to conduct emergency resuscitation and provide advanced/critical care in anticipation of short-term (24 to 36 hours) requirements, or in preparation for transfer to an ICU.

The staff assigned to the PACU must have a thorough understanding of the surgeries performed and be familiar with potential complications associated with both the anesthetic provided and the surgical procedure, as well as with the patient's pertinent past medical and surgical history. The American Society of Anesthesiology (ASA) standards for postanesthesia care specifically identify principles of care intended to encourage quality patient care (Table 37.1). Standards for PACU operations were established in 1988 by the American Society of Anesthesiologists' House of Delegates and amended in 2014. Standards include guidelines for admission, patient transport and the transfer of care from the operating room team to the PACU team patient care in the PACU, as well as discharge guidelines and procedures.

TABLE 37.1	Standards for Postanesthesia Care

Committee of Origin: Standards and Practice Parameters
(Approved by the ASA House of Delegates on October 27, 2004, and last amended on October 15, 2014)

These standards apply to postanesthesia care in all locations. These standards may be exceeded based on the judgment of the responsible anesthesiologist. They are intended to encourage quality patient care, but cannot guarantee any specific patient outcome. They are subject to revision from time to time as warranted by the evolution of technology and practice.

Standard I

All patients who have received general anesthesia, regional anesthesia or monitored anesthesia care shall receive appropriate postanesthesia management.[a]

1. A postanesthesia care unit (PACU) or an area which provides equivalent postanesthesia care (e.g., a surgical intensive care unit) shall be available to receive patients after anesthesia care. All patients who receive anesthesia care shall be admitted to the PACU or its equivalent *except* by specific order of the anesthesiologist responsible for the patient's care.

2. The medical aspects of care in the PACU (or equivalent area) shall be governed by policies and procedures, which have been reviewed and approved by the department of anesthesiology.

3. The design, equipment, and staffing of the PACU shall meet requirements of the facility's accrediting and licensing bodies.

TABLE
37.1 Standards for Postanesthesia Care (*continued*)

Standard II

A patient transported to the PACU shall be accompanied by a member of the anesthesia care team who is knowledgeable about the patient's condition. The patient shall be continually evaluated and treated during transport with monitoring and support appropriate to the patient's condition.

Standard III

Upon arrival in the PACU, the patient shall be reevaluated and a verbal report provided to the responsible PACU nurse by the member of the anesthesia care team who accompanies the patient.

1. The patient's status on arrival in the PACU shall be documented. From Committee on Standards and Practice Parameters 409-1.3 (PA). Subject: Standards for Post anesthesia Care (Clean) Page 2. Date: March 2, 2014. Information concerning the preoperative condition and the surgical/anesthetic course shall be transmitted to the PACU nurse.

2. The member of the anesthesia care team shall remain in the PACU until the PACU nurse accepts responsibility for the nursing care of the patient.

Standard IV

The patient's condition shall be evaluated continually in the PACU.

1. The patient shall be observed and monitored by methods appropriate to the patient's medical condition. Particular attention should be given to monitoring oxygenation, ventilation, circulation, level of consciousness, and temperature. During recovery from all anesthetics, a quantitative method of assessing oxygenation such as pulse oximetry shall be employed in the initial phase of recovery.[b] This is not intended for application during the recovery of the obstetric patient in whom regional anesthesia was used for labor and vaginal delivery.

2. An accurate written report of the PACU period shall be maintained. Use of an appropriate PACU scoring system is encouraged for each patient on admission, at appropriate intervals prior to discharge, and at the time of discharge.

3. General medical supervision and coordination of patient care in the PACU should be the responsibility of an anesthesiologist.

4. There shall be a policy to assure the availability in the facility of a physician capable of managing complications and providing cardiopulmonary resuscitation for patients in the PACU.

Standard V

A physician is responsible for the discharge of the patient from the PACU.

1. When discharge criteria are used, they must be approved by the department of anesthesiology and the medical staff. They may vary depending upon whether the patient is discharged to a hospital room, to the ICU, to a short stay unit or home.

2. In the absence of the physician responsible for the discharge, the PACU nurse shall determine that the patient meets the discharge criteria. The name of the physician accepting responsibility for discharge shall be noted on the record.

[a]Refer to Perianesthesia Nursing Standards, Practice Recommendations and Interpretive Statements, published by ASPAN, for issues of nursing care.
[b]Under extenuating circumstances, the responsible anesthesiologist may waive the requirements; it is recommended that when this is done, it should be so stated (including the reasons) in a note in the patient's medical record.

Specialized nurses, certified by the American Society of Peri-Anesthesia Nurses (ASPAN), are essential to provide care for postoperative patients. Nursing standards for recovery established by ASPAN are similar to those developed by the ASA for physicians. These standards are designed to optimize the care of postoperative patients. The similarity between the ASA and ASPAN standards for patient care represents a significant convergence for physicians and nurses in providing optimum care to the patient in the immediate postoperative period.

Standard monitors capable of displaying vital signs are used for all patients arriving in the PACU. An oxygen supply and a method for providing suction are also required. Adequate supplies used for patient care (dressings, respiratory equipment, drains, etc.) as well as intravenous fluids and medications must be available. A method for providing emergency positive pressure ventilation (i.e., self-inflating bag-valve-mask or "Ambu bag") must be present at each bed station. Importantly, emergency equipment and personnel trained in emergency resuscitation must be immediately available. Also, the ability to provide invasive monitoring and support at the level of an ICU's capability must be considered for every PACU.

C. Management

The management of a PACU is related to the nature of clinical practice being supported. Smaller facilities uniquely providing ambulatory care surgeries may choose to incorporate PACU management with operating room management, with appropriate involvement of anesthesiologists in policy and clinical oversight. Institutions with a more diversified practice will commonly utilize a dedicated management team, consisting of anesthesiologists and perioperative nurses to provide direct leadership to the multiple phases of PACU operations. In addition to direct patient care, these requirements can include training, continuing education (such as basic life support [BLS] and advanced cardiovascular life support [ACLS]), personnel, and data management, as well as logistic support. In the setting of multiple PACUs, coordination of support can mandate several tiers of management, coordinated by PACU leadership's integration to the institution's perioperative management team.

Regardless of the scope of practice supported by a PACU, there must be a clear delineation of responsibilities, with regard to both clinical care provided and overall operational management. Given that the care of a postoperative patient may entail multiple disciplines, the need for clear and concise communication through phases of care is vital and must be conducted in a collaborative manner. Although care in the PACU is most often directed by an anesthesiologist, the surgeon (or other proceduralists) must be kept abreast of a patient's condition and be available to offer guidance regarding the patient's care germane to the procedure performed and the anticipated clinical course. In this manner, patients are afforded the most comprehensive care without the potential compromise caused by all specialties involved in the patient's overall management individually guiding care in a manner that may influence other elements of the postoperative evolution without fully appreciating decisions made by other groups collaborating in the care of the patient in the PACU.

D. Operations

As described in the preceding sections, PACU scope of practice can vary as a function of clinical activities in a given institution. Despite this variability in practice, there is a commonality of clinical scenario that all clinicians providing care in that setting must be able to effectively manage in a timely manner. Most often arising as routine sequelae to the surgical procedure and anesthetics, clinical issues encountered in the PACU include hypoxia, hypotension, tachycardia, pain, and postoperative nausea/vomiting. Even the simplest clinical challenges, such as hypertension, can in fact be the harbinger of serious postoperative complications. These variable interpretations of seemingly routine parameters underscore the absolute need for all clinicians providing care in the PACU to be completely cognizant of the procedure performed, the clinical issues germane to the patient, and the potential challenges/complications associated with given procedures.

Institutional policies will drive various aspects of PACU operations. Regardless of the scope of practice in the PACU, there must be clearly delineated roles, responsibilities, and guidelines for all PACUs. A clear plan for communication with clinicians involved in the care of the patient, as well as with the leadership engaged in managing the operating rooms and the direction/assignment of patient disposition after recovery, is vital to the efficient functioning of all components of patient care.

E. Policies and Procedures

Although the routine recovery of the postoperative patient and the overall operations of a PACU may seem straightforward, the diversity of any patient population, as well as of the institutions providing care, requires that clear and concise plans and policies are in place to optimize efficiency. With more specialized care, the need for such guidelines may be more complex; however, there are commonalities in care that link all providers, regardless of institutional focus. Several basic requirements, although certainly not be viewed as limiting, are offered for consideration as operational standards are framed by individuals responsible for the management of a PACU, because these facilities are often called upon to demonstrate the widest capability of patient care functions and are often considered an institution's buffer during periods of increased operational tempo.

1. Admission and discharge criteria

Detailed discussions regarding admission and discharge to the PACU are addressed in Chapter 36. In general, most postoperative patients are expected to be admitted to the PACU for a period of time prior to final disposition to a general care unit or discharge from the institution (e.g., to a skilled nursing facility or to home). However, depending on institutional preference, certain patients, such as those having undergone a procedure under monitored anesthetic care or conscious sedation, may be transferred directly to a general care unit because expectations may suggest that the patient will have essentially returned to a preprocedural baseline at the completion of the procedure and requires no further specialized monitoring as available in a PACU. Clear guidelines must be established. Discharge of patients may be governed/guided by a set of criteria, such as the Aldrete scoring system (Table 37.2), and a protocol, or may require a more detailed review process.

2. Mandatory communications

With the evolution of communications systems, in addition to the phone system and overhead paging, alphanumeric pagers, walkie-talkies, body-worn communications devices, and so on may all be used for effective communication. However, there are several clinical scenarios that may mandate attending level communications and, as such, may be incorporated into a PACU Communications Guideline Document. Although to some degree institution specific, certain clinical issues have been incorporated into such a document at this institution.

TABLE 37.2	Modified Aldrete Score for Postanesthesia Recovery

Activity	Score
Able to move voluntary	
4 extremities:	2
2 extremities:	1
0 extremities:	0
Respiration	
Breathes deeply, coughs freely:	2
Dyspnea, shallow or limited:	1
Apneic:	0
Circulation	
BP $\pm$ 20% of preoperative:	2
BP $\pm$ 20%– 49% of preoperative:	1
BP $\pm$ 50% of preoperative:	0
Consciousness	
Fully awake:	2
Arousable with minimal stimulation:	1
Not responding:	0
O_2 saturation	
>92% on room air:	2
Needs O_2 to maintain >90%:	1
<90% even with O_2:	0

Patients are assessed on admission to the PACU, at 15, 30, and 60 minutes, as well as prior to discharge. A score of 8/10 is generally considered the minimal acceptable score for transfer.

Events, such as reintubation, arrest, death, and other scenarios may be considered for such a policy, which should be developed in such a manner as to facilitate communication by any member of the care team.

3. **Emergency support**

   Clearly urgent and emergent situations, such as a cardiac arrest or acute change in mental status, mandate that a predefined system be in place and understood by all clinicians working in the PACU. Response systems can range from calling the code or rapid response team to the PACU, to developing a program for resources already assigned to the perioperative area(s) for assistance. ACLS-related issues are discussed in detail in Chapter 35.

4. **Escalation of care**

   A small percentage of patients will be identified at some point during the transition through the PACU as requiring clinical care in excess of that typically associated with general care units. As such, there must be a definite plan addressing the issues associated with direct transfer to ICU or specialized step-down unit. Institutional policies may vary; however, a predetermined and efficient mechanism can serve the best needs of the patient and minimize impact on PACU and institutional resources.

5. **Infectious disease and immunocompromised/transplant patients**

   Management of infectious disease–related issues is paramount to every PACU, and basic planning must include coordination with infectious disease specialists. Determining critical requirements, such as positive pressure rooms and isolation factors, can markedly affect PACU operations. In addition, immunocompromised and/or immunosuppressed (i.e., transplant) patients will require close coordination in a multidisciplinary fashion and merit specific guidelines developed in a collaborative manner and readily available to all clinicians.

6. Recovered patients

The obvious goal of any PACU or recovery room is to closely monitor a postoperative patient until the effects of anesthesia have diminished to the point where the patient may safely receive care in a setting that provides a less robust suite of monitoring technology/capabilities and specialized personnel, typically a general care unit. However, on many occasions, most often because of institutional occupancy, appropriately recovered patients will remain in the PACU, awaiting a room on a general care unit. This can result in extended periods in the PACU, including remaining overnight, and may impact operating room schedules. As such, the PACU and the institution must specify the manner in which the patient is to be monitored and the clinician(s) who will be primarily responsible for directing patient management. Although urgent and emergent situations will always remain the domain of the personnel in the PACU, routine issues, such as dietary requirements, antibiotic plans, and so on, may be directed by the specialty that will assume direct care responsibilities, once the patient has transferred from the PACU.

7. Pediatric patients

Many institutions maintain separate PACUs for the management of the postoperative pediatric patient (see Chapter 30). Regardless of the physical site, a specially trained and certified team of clinicians must be available to care for the child recovering from anesthesia.

8. Special testing

Various tests, including the drawing of blood for laboratory testing, radiographic procedures, and/or the performance of an echocardiogram, are often performed in the PACU. Clear guidelines directing such procedures should be developed. In addition, as a function of geographic location, certain tests, such as a blood sample for HIV or hepatitis testing, require (by law) informed consent from the patient; surrogate consent is not or may not be appropriate. Given the likelihood that a patient in the PACU has received neuroactive agents (e.g., volatile anesthetics, opioids, benzodiazepines), the patient will not have the capacity to provide informed consent. Moreover, the PACU may be considered a "coercive site," similar to the manner in which the operating rooms are viewed. A policy should be established to direct personnel in the setting of situations often occurring in the perioperative areas (such as resulting from needle sticks, splashes, and other inadvertent exposure of personnel to bodily fluids). In addition, PACU personnel may observe the earliest observations of awareness under anesthesia. Consequently, a protocol establishing PACU guidelines for initial screening may be of use. The Brice protocol (Table 37.3), or a threshold modification, may be used by PACU clinicians as a screening device.

9. Visitation

Family members are often contacted by the proceduralist (surgeon) as the patient is being admitted to the PACU. Clearly anxious regarding a family member's condition, there is generally an immediate desire to visit with the patient in the PACU. Guidelines establishing criteria for visitations must be in place. This is in part because the patient's

TABLE 37.3	Modified Brice Protocol

What is the last thing you remember before going to sleep for the operation?
What is the first thing you remember on waking after the operation?
Do you remember anything between going to sleep and waking up?
Did you have any dreams?
What was the most unpleasant thing you remember from the operation and anesthesia?

condition may not permit visitors at certain times (drain management, wound inspection, etc.). Given the level of activity in a typical PACU, admitting multiple patients simultaneously, with specialists and support services coming through to perform various interventions, such as a chest x-ray or an echocardiogram, traffic management can become a challenge that visitation guidelines can help mitigate. Furthermore, the presence of family members may be disturbing to other patients. Institutions may also choose to specifically address visitation by children.

10. **PACU as a procedural area**

Institutions may choose to utilize the PACU for additional patient care activities. The PACU is often used as a short stay/overnight critical care unit. In this setting, patients having undergone procedures such as a carotid endarterectomy, requiring a short period of close hemodynamic control, may be maintained in the PACU, for planned discharge to a general care unit on the first postoperative day. Some institutions may utilize the PACU as a procedural area for the placement of PICC lines, or endoscopic procedures. In collaboration with psychiatry services, the PACU may be utilized as a site to provide a short duration of anesthetic and subsequent recovery for patients undergoing electroconvulsive therapy. Many institutions utilize the PACU as preoperative area, where patients are admitted for preparation in anticipation of undergoing a procedure placement of neuraxial anesthesia and regional blocks. Guidelines for any specialized use of the PACU should be clearly developed, documented, and disseminated collaboratively.

Suggested Readings

American Society of Anesthesiology. Standards for Postanesthesia Care Committee of Origin. Standards and Practice Parameters (Approved by the ASA House of Delegates on October 27, 2004, and last amended on October 15, 2014).

Brice DD, Hetherington RR, Utting JE. A simple study of awareness and dreaming during anaesthesia. *Br J Anaesth* 1970;42(6):535–542.

Levine WC, Dunn PF. Optimizing operating room scheduling. *Anesthesiol Clin* 2015;33(4):697–711.

Macario A, Glenn D, Dexter F. What can the post anesthesia care unit manager do to decrease costs in the post anesthesia care unit? *J Perianesth Nurs* 1999;14(5): 284–293.

Marcon E, Dexter F. Impact of surgical sequencing on post anesthesia care unit staffing. *Health Care Manag Sci* 2006;9(1):87–98.

Marcon E, Kharraja S, Smolski N, et al. Determining the number of beds in the post anesthesia care unit: a computer simulation flow approach. *Anesth Analg* 2003;96(5):1415–1423.

Infection Control

Erin J. Levering and Jean Kwo

I. INFECTION CONTROL

Infection control in the hospital setting encompasses the surveillance of epidemiologically important organisms and the prevention of transmission of healthcare-associated infections. Patients coming through the operating room can be colonized or infected with a variety of pathogens, which are often multidrug resistant and easily communicable. Infections caused by antibiotic-resistant pathogens lead to prolonged hospital stays and higher costs, as well as increased morbidity and mortality. Therefore, strict adherence to infection control practices is imperative throughout the perioperative course.

II. INFECTION CONTROL PROGRAMS

Infection control programs in the hospital became a requirement in the United States because of mandates from the Joint Commission for Accreditation of Hospitals (JCAHO) and guidelines set forth by the Centers for Disease Control (CDC). Infection control teams are responsible for ensuring proper adherence to standard and transmission-based precautions and for the surveillance of multidrug-resistant organisms (MDROs) and outbreaks. In addition, the hospital infection control team should provide education to both clinical and nonclinical staff regarding the harms of MDROs; the prevention of hospital-acquired infections; the proper cleaning, disinfection, sterilization of equipment; and the proper disposal of infectious wastes. Finally, it is the responsibility of the infection control committee to provide oversight from pharmacists and infectious disease specialists to promote appropriate antimicrobial use and encourage the preferred use of narrow-spectrum antibiotics to prevent the development of antimicrobial resistance. Antimicrobial stewardship teams should ensure the proper doses and durations of antibiotics are prescribed because an inadequate dose, duration, or both may make the evolution of a resistant organism more likely. An effective infection control program will be cost-effective while decreasing the incidence of hospital-acquired infections.

III. TRANSMISSION OF INFECTION

The transmission of infection requires three components: a source or reservoir of infection, a susceptible host, and a mode of transmission.

A. Sources of Infectious Agents

Pathogens transmitted during healthcare practices generally emanate from human sources (patients, healthcare workers [HCWs], family, and visitors), although inanimate objects and the environment can also be implicated. Source individuals may not show signs of active infection; they may be chronically colonized carriers or in the asymptomatic/ incubation phase.

B. Host

Most of the factors that influence the development of infection are related to the host. Some persons exposed to a potential pathogen never become infected, whereas others can become chronic carriers of the pathogen, and others develop clinically significant infections. Unique host factors that influence the development of infection once exposed include age, comorbidity, immunodeficiency, certain medications (immune modulators, drugs that interrupt the normal flora such as gastric acid inhibitors, other antimicrobial agents), surgical procedures and irradiation that can interrupt the skin's line of defense, indwelling catheters and lines, and permanently implanted devices.

C. **Mode of Transmission**

The three principal modes of transmission are by contact (direct or indirect), by droplet, or by the airborne route.

1. Contact transmission is the most common mode of transmission of pathogens. Direct contact occurs when microorganisms are transferred from one infected person to another, without an intermediate object or person. This generally requires blood or other bodily fluids from an infected patient directly entering the body of another person through mucous membranes or breaks in the skin. In addition, this includes infections or infestations that can occur from direct skin to skin contact (i.e., scabies infestations or herpes infection). Indirect contact involves transmission of an infectious agent through a contaminated intermediate object (i.e., electronic thermometers, glucose monitors) or person (i.e., HCW).

2. Droplet transmission from the source person occurs primarily during coughing, sneezing, talking and during certain procedures such as suctioning and bronchoscopy. Large-particle droplets, defined as those that are greater than 5 μm, must come into contact with the conjunctivae or mucous membranes of a susceptible person in order for the infection to be passed. Transmission of droplets generally requires close contact, because they cannot stay suspended in the air for more than about 3 feet. Given the inability for prolonged suspension, special air handling and ventilation are not necessary.

3. **Airborne transmission** occurs by dissemination of small particles in the respirable size range (less than 5 μm) containing the infectious agent, which can remain suspended in the air for long periods of time and distance. Pathogens carried in this manner can be easily dispersed by air currents in hospital ventilation systems and can be inhaled by a susceptible person in the same room. Special ventilation systems are required to prevent airborne transmission.

IV. **STANDARD PRECAUTIONS**

Standard precautions are the minimum practices of infection control to be followed when dealing with all patients, without knowledge of the patient's infection status, and in any healthcare environment. The components of standard precautions are listed below.

A. **Hand Hygiene**

Hand hygiene is the single most important measure for controlling the spread of MDROs and the most effective component of an infection prevention and control program. Wearing gloves does not replace the need for hand hygiene, because gloves may have small, not readily apparent defects or tears that may occur during wear, and contamination of hands may occur when gloves are removed. Diligent hand hygiene must occur prior to touching any patient and after contact with a patient or a patient's environment, even if gloves are worn. In addition, hand hygiene must be performed prior to donning sterile gloves to insert a catheter or device, before handling medications, and prior to manipulating respiratory devices, urinary catheters, and intravascular catheters.

1. Hand hygiene includes both hand washing with antimicrobial soap and water and the use of an alcohol-based hand rub (ABHR). In

2002, the CDC recommended that ABHR be the primary choice for hand hygiene (except in specific cases outlined later), because it has better in vivo and in vitro efficacy against drug-resistant bacteria. Additionally, the ABHRs have improved the ability for clinicians to easily and comfortably sanitize hands at frequent intervals, hence increasing compliance. Compared to soap and water, the ABHRs have superior microbiocidal activity against gram-positive and gram-negative organisms and viral pathogens, and have shown to decrease the incidence of nosocomially acquired methicillin-resistant *Staphylococcus aureus* (MRSA) and vancomycin-resistant enterococci (VRE). Frequent hand washing can cause drying of the hands, with potential skin damage and irritation, leading to changes in skin flora, increased skin shedding, and increased risk of transmission of microorganisms. However, in the case of certain pathogens such as *Clostridium difficile* and *norovirus*, hand washing with soap and water must be employed first, prior to using an ABHR. Furthermore, hands must be washed with soap and water prior to the use of an ABHR in the case of visibly soiled hands.

2. There has been a correlation between the use of artificial fingernails and more pathogenic organisms, especially bacilli and yeast. Artificial fingernails should not be worn by healthcare personnel in contact with high-risk patients (i.e., those in the ICU, OR, PACU). In addition, natural nails should be well maintained and kept less than 1/4 inch in length.

B. Personal Protective Equipment

Personal protective equipment (PPE) is used to protect the HCW from exposure to or contact with infectious materials. The choice of PPE depends on the pathogen and possible modes of transmission. Hand hygiene is always the first step prior to donning PPE and final step after the removal and disposal of PPE.

1. **Gloves:** should be used when there may be contact with blood or bodily fluid, mucous membranes, nonintact skin, or potentially infectious material. They should also be worn if there is any contact with a patient or patient's environment in the setting of pathogens transmitted via the contact route in the case of isolation precautions. Finally, gloves are necessary when having any contact with visibly contaminated patient equipment or environmental surfaces. When interacting with an individual patient, it is important to remember the practice of working from "clean" to "dirty," and it often may be necessary to change gloves when working with the same patient to reduce cross-contamination of body sites. When gloves are used with other PPE, they should be put on last.

2. **Gowns** are used as part of standard precautions if there is a chance of contamination of the HCW's arms or clothing with blood, bodily fluid, and other infectious material. In addition, gowns should be used as part of isolation precautions in the case of transmission via the contact route. Many studies have demonstrated the contamination of HCW's clothing with MDROs, and a decrease in transmission of MDROs when gowns are worn in addition to gloves compared to the use of gloves alone. Gowns should be donned first, prior to other PPE, and when patient care is complete, remove gowns before leaving a patient care area. The gown should be removed in such a way that the outer, contaminated side of the gown is turned inward and rolled into a bundle prior to discarding.

3. The use of **mouth, nose, and eye PPE** is considered standard precautions in situations where splash of blood or bodily fluid may occur and come in contact with the mucous membranes of the HCW.

Masks are required in the case of a sterile procedure, to protect the patient from pathogens carried in the HCW's mouth or nose. Lastly, masks and respirators are to be used in the case of droplet and airborne precautions, as detailed below.

C. Safe Injection and Sharps Practices

Safe injection and sharps practices aim to prevent transmission of infection between one patient and another and between patient and healthcare provider. Injuries due to sharps have been linked to the transmission of HIV, HBV, and HCV to HCWs. The principles of safe injection and sharps practices include:

1. Never recap used needles or manipulate them using more than one hand, instead using the one-handed "scoop" method to reapply the cap onto the needle;

2. Do not remove used needles from syringes by hand, and do not bend or break used needles by hand;

3. Place all used needles and sharps into the appropriate puncture-resistant containers; and

4. Whenever possible, use single-dose vials (SDVs) of medication, and if multidose vials (MDVs) are necessary, a new needle and syringe must be used for each patient.

    a. The American Society of Anesthesiologists (ASA) recommends using SDVs for parenteral medications whenever possible. SDVs should be used only once and for only one patient. Both the CDC and JCAHO warn against using SDVs in multiple patients because these vials typically lack antimicrobial preservatives and can serve as a source of infection when contaminated. Misuse of SDVs has been associated with outbreaks of blood-borne pathogen, bacterial bloodstream infections, meningitis, and epidural abscesses. If the SDV needs to be reaccessed for another dose in the same patient, a new needle/cannula/syringe must be used each time the vial is accessed. The SDV should be discarded at the end of the case.

    b. MDVs are approved by the Federal Food and Drug Administration for use on multiple persons. Prior to each entry, the vial's rubber septum should be disinfected by wiping with an antiseptic swab (e.g., sterile 70% isopropyl alcohol) and the septum should be allowed to dry before inserting a new needle and syringe. CDC guidelines require that MDVs be stored outside *immediate patient treatment areas* including surgery/procedure rooms where anesthesia is administered and any anesthesia medication carts used in or for those rooms. Thus the ASA recommends that if a medication (or other solution) is not available as a SDV and a MDV must be used (e.g., neostigmine, succinylcholine), discard the MDV after single-patient use.

    c. **Propofol** is formulated in a lipid emulsion that can support bacterial growth and has been associated with postoperative infections and sepsis. Though current propofol formulations contain a bacteriostatic agent (e.g., sodium metabisulfite or benzyl alcohol), these only slow the rate of growth of microorganisms. Propofol should be drawn up just prior to administration using strict aseptic technique including hand hygiene. The syringe containing propofol should be labeled with the date and time the vial was opened, and any unused propofol should be discarded at the end of the case or within 6 hours after the vial was opened. If propofol is administered as an infusion from a bottle (e.g., for ICU sedation), the tubing and any unused portion must be discarded within 12 hours after the vial has been entered.

D. Environmental Cleaning

The proper cleaning and disinfection of surfaces in the patient environment is part of standard precautions. Studies have shown that both MRSA and VRE can persist on dry environmental surfaces for weeks to months. Hospital infection control programs should provide rigorous policies and procedures for routine cleaning, disinfection, and sterilization of devices and environmental surfaces in between patient uses. These protocols should also address the prompt cleaning and removal of spills of blood, bodily fluid, and other infectious materials. Certain pathogens may be resistant to routinely used hospital disinfectants; it has been suggested that a 1:10 dilution of 5.25% household bleach be used in the case of *C. difficile*.

E. Medical Equipment

In order to prevent patient-to-patient transmission of infectious agents, reusable medical equipment and devices must be properly cleaned, disinfected, and sterilized. Whenever possible, patients on transmission-based precautions should be provided with dedicated noncritical equipment such as thermometers, stethoscopes, and blood pressure cuffs.

1. The **Spaulding classification** categorizes instruments and items for patient care according to the degree of risk for infection involved in use of the items.

   a. **Critical items** are objects that enter sterile tissues and, thus, confer a high risk of infection if they are contaminated with any microorganism. Critical items must be sterile at the time of use and include surgical instruments, vascular needles and catheters, regional needles and catheters, urinary catheters, syringes, stopcocks, etc. Most of these items are single-use items. Those that are not single use need to be sterilized.

   b. **Semicritical items** contact mucous membranes and nonintact skin and need high-level disinfection. Equipment such as laryngoscope blades, bronchoscopes, endotracheal tubes, transesophageal echocardiography probes, and the anesthesia circuit fall into this category. High-level disinfection using chemicals or heat will eliminate all organisms except bacterial spores. The rationale for this is that intact mucous membranes (e.g., lungs or gastrointestinal tract) are resistant to infection by common bacterial spores.

   c. **Noncritical items** come in contact with intact skin, which is an effective barrier against most microorganisms. Examples of noncritical items include the anesthesia machine and cart, blood pressure cuffs, pulse oximeters, bedside tables, etc. These items should be cleaned with an intermediate or low-level disinfectant when visibly soiled or after each use.

F. Respiratory Hygiene/Cough Etiquette

Hospital visitors have been implicated as the source of many different hospital-acquired infections, including influenza, pertussis, *Mycobacterium tuberculosis*, and other respiratory illnesses. The implementation of infection control measures directed at hospital visitors is recommended in triage and reception areas. This includes the dispensation of masks and tissues and signage that alerts visitors to the hospital to avoid entering clinical areas if they show any signs of communicable disease (cough, rhinorrhea, congestion, increased respiratory secretions). In addition, these notifications should include information about appropriate cough etiquette (i.e., coughing into tissue or arm rather than hand) and proper hand hygiene.

V. ISOLATION PRECAUTIONS
A. Contact Precautions

Contact precautions are designed to reduce the transmission of infection by either direct or indirect contact. A private room is preferred but cohorting between patients infected with the same microorganism is allowed if necessary. After hand hygiene, gloves are required prior to entering room, and a gown should be worn if there could be any contact with the patient, environmental surfaces, or other items in the patient's room because HCW's hands are the most common vector for transmission. Masks and eye protection should be worn when there is the risk of splash or droplet dispersal (tracheostomies, suctioning, intubation). Noncritical items (i.e., stethoscope) should be dedicated to use by a single patient if possible. The need for contact precautions should be reported during the transfer of care. The list below highlights some of the more epidemiologically important pathogens that require contact precautions. For a comprehensive list of organisms and diseases requiring contact precautions, consult with facility infection control programs.

1. Prevention and control of MRSA is a challenging, but essential aspect of infection control. The United States remains one of the nations with the highest MRSA prevalence worldwide. Important facets of decreasing the transmission of MRSA include surveillance cultures to identify those that are colonized and the subsequent isolation of these patients, and in certain cases decolonization with chlorhexidine and/or mupirocin. There are few published reports of a reduction in MRSA transmission through changes in antimicrobial use alone; therefore, the prevention of person-to-person spread of the bacteria using standard and transmission-based precautions is of utmost importance. In the past, MRSA has been found almost solely in healthcare facilities, but in recent years, there have been more and more reports of MRSA infection occurring in patients with little contact with healthcare facilities, making community-acquired MRSA of increasing concern.

2. The prevalence of VRE has also been steadily increasing, because this MDRO has become more difficult to treat. A minimum inhibitory concentration less than 4 μg/mL classifies the enterococci as susceptible, and greater than 32 qualifies resistance. Values in between are considered intermediate; however, vancomycin therapy is not recommended for these isolates. The vast majority of vancomycin resistance is found with *Enterococcus faecium*, with *E. faecalis* being only a small minority of VRE isolates. VRE colonize the gastrointestinal tract and can be found on the skin because of fecal shedding. Antimicrobial drug exposure has consistently been identified as a risk factor in VRE colonization, likely because the antimicrobial agent suppresses competing normal flora and provides selective advantage for VRE survival. As a result, the burden of VRE colonies in the stool is increased, increasing the probability of environmental or HCW contamination. However, as in the case of MRSA, the restriction of antimicrobial use alone is not sufficient in limiting the prevalence of VRE. This must be combined with rigorous hospital-wide interventions, aimed at stopping the transmission of the bacteria.

3. Extended-spectrum β-lactamases (ESBLs): β-Lactamases are enzymes that open the β-lactam ring, inactivating the antibiotic. Bacteria with ESBLs generally demonstrate resistance to penicillins and certain cephalosporins (cefotaxime, ceftazidime, ceftriaxone, or cefepime). In addition, β-lactamase inhibitors (i.e., clavulanate), which are used to overcome the bacteria's resistance to β-lactam

antibiotics, **are also rendered ineffective**. ESBLs have been found not only among gram-negative organisms, mainly *Klebsiella pneumoniae*, *K. oxytoca*, and *Escherichia coli*, but also in many others including *Acinetobacter*, *Pseudomonas*, *Enterobacter*, *Proteus*, and *Serratia*. The only current proven treatments of ESBLs are antibiotics in the carbapenem family.

4. Other MDROs of clinical concern that warrant the implementation of contact precautions include multidrug-resistant *Streptococcus pneumoniae* (resistant to penicillin, fluoroquinolones, and macrolides) and strains of *Staphylococcus aureus* that are intermediate or resistant to vancomycin (VISA or VRSA). There has been an increase in the prevalence of *Pseudomonas aeruginosa* resistant to imipenem or fluoroquinolones, *Acinetobacter baumannii* resistant to carbapenems, *Stenotrophomonas* species resistant to trimethoprim–sulfamethoxazole, and Enterobacteriaceae resistant to carbapenems. In order to prevent the further spread of resistant organisms, facilities should consider the implementation of contact precautions in patients colonized or infected with these MDROs. See Table 38.1 for risk factors in the development of colonization or infection with MDROs.

5. Herpes simplex: In the case of a severe primary outbreak, disseminated disease, or immunocompromised hosts, contact precautions should be maintained until lesions are crusted over.

6. Varicella zoster (chickenpox and shingles). Airborne and contact precautions should be instituted for chickenpox. Patients with disseminated shingles and immunocompromised patients with localized disease should be placed on airborne precautions. Patients with localized shingles and an intact immune system, and lesions that can be covered, need standard precautions only. Nonimmune HCWs should not provide direct care to patients with varicella zoster.

7. Gastroenteritis. Certain pathogens implicated in gastroenteritis, such as *E. coli* O157:H7 or *Giardia lamblia* do not typically require isolation precautions. However, contact precautions should be considered in the case of incontinent patients with severe symptoms.

8. Pediculosis (lice of the head, body, or anogenital area). The transmission of lice requires close physical contact with an infested patient or their clothes, hats, or combs. The incubation period for hatching of eggs is 6 to 10 days, and precautions should continue for 24 hours after effective treatment.

B. **Contact PLUS Precautions**

Certain microorganisms have been categorized into the requirement of Contact PLUS precautions. HCWs are required to wash hands with

TABLE 38.1	Risk Factors for the Development of MDROs	
Length of hospital/ICU stay	Central venous or arterial catheters	
Urinary catheters	Mechanical ventilation	
Prior antibiotic administration	Older age and lack of functional independence	
Presence of underlying comorbid conditions (diabetes, renal failure, immunosuppression, malignancy)	Emergency abdominal surgery, presence of gastrostomy tube and jejunostomy tube (in the case of ESBLs)	

soap and water, and then utilize the ABHR, because the ABHR alone may not remove all spores and other resistant infectious material. In addition, every attempt should be made to dedicate certain patient care devices, such as thermometers, stethoscopes, and blood pressure cuffs, to a single patient on Contact PLUS precautions.

1. *Clostridium difficile* infection (CDI) prolongs hospital length of stay by about 7 days, and the daily mortality rate of patients with CDI is nearly double that of noninfected patients. Rates of CDI more than doubled between 2000 and 2009, and levels now remain at an all-time high, especially among elderly patients. *C. difficile* now rivals MRSA as the most frequent cause of hospital-acquired infections in the United States. The severity of CDIs has increased, largely due to certain strains that produce more toxins and more spores. The clinical presentation of CDI can range from mild diarrhea to pseudomembranous colitis and even death. The virulence of CDI is attributable to environmental contamination, persistence of spores over long periods of time, the resistance of these spores to many traditional antiseptic and cleaning agents, and frequent use of antibiotics, predisposing patients to CDI. Antimicrobials most frequently associated with CDI are clindamycin, vancomycin, fluoroquinolones, and third-generation cephalosporins. Some studies have shown an association between gastric acid suppression and CDI.

   a. Duration of precautions for *C. difficile*. The CDC recommends continuing precautions for the duration of the illness, and many experts recommend continuing precautions for 48 hours after diarrhea resolves. Patients can continue to shed spores despite resolution of diarrhea, and these patients are at high risk for *C. difficile* recurrence. A common practice is to extend precautions until time of hospital discharge, although no data exist to support this approach. Patients with a history of CDI, who have completed a course of appropriate antibiotic therapy and are asymptomatic, do not need precautions when they are readmitted to a hospital.

2. Norovirus, formerly referred to as "Norwalk-like viruses," is a highly contagious virus that causes severe gastroenteritis with an incubation period of 12 to 48 hours and has a duration of 12 to 60 hours. The symptoms include nausea, vomiting, abdominal cramps, and diarrhea. The virus is transmitted via contaminated food or water, and by person to person contact. Transmission of the virus through contamination of the environment and fomites plays a role in outbreaks. On account of the fact that only a minimal dose of virus is needed to generate an infection and their frequent resistance to the usual cleaning solutions, patients infected with norovirus are maintained on Contact PLUS precautions.

3. Cutaneous anthrax (*Bacillus anthracis*)—Contact PLUS precautions is indicated for patients with suspected or laboratory-confirmed cutaneous anthrax because this is a spore-forming bacterium.

C. Droplet Precautions

Healthcare providers must wear a mask if within 3 feet of patient on droplet precautions, and the patient is required to wear a surgical mask for transport. A private room is preferred but cohorting patients who have active infection with the same microorganism is acceptable if necessary. For examples of pathogens that necessitate droplet precautions, see Table 38.2.

D. Airborne Precautions

Special ventilation systems are required to prevent airborne transmission. Patient should be placed in a room with a pressure that is negative

TABLE 38.2	Microorganisms That Necessitate Droplet Precautions

Neisseria meningitidis: meningitis, pneumonia, sepsis	*Haemophilus influenzae* type B in infants and children: meningitis or pneumonia or epiglottitis	*Mycoplasma pneumoniae*
Group A streptococcus: pneumonia in adults, pharyngitis and scarlet fever in children	Influenza virus	*Yersinia pestis*: pneumonic plague
Bordetella pertussis: whooping cough	Rubella (German measles)	Mumps virus
Corynebacterium diphtheria: pharyngeal diphtheria	Parvovirus B19	Respiratory syncytial virus (RSV) in infants, children, immunocompromised adults
Adenovirus: pneumonia	Rhinovirus	

relative to surrounding areas, with at least 6 to 12 exchanges per hour. Room exhaust must be discharged to the outdoors or be filtered through a high-efficiency particulate aerator (HEPA) filter before recirculation with the rest of the hospital. If the patient has confirmed or suspected tuberculosis (TB), caregivers must wear a certified respirator (i.e., a mask with N95 filtration). In the case of measles, varicella, or disseminated zoster, susceptible individuals should not enter the room if other immune healthcare personnel are available to provide care. Transport of the patient should be minimized. If transport is unavoidable, the patient must wear a surgical mask. See Table 38.3 for a list of pathogens that necessitate airborne precautions.

1. *M. tuberculosis*, the causative agent for TB, is spread by airborne transmission. Exposed individuals have a 10% lifetime risk for developing active disease, with the highest risk period in the first 1 to 2 years after exposure. Immunocompromised individuals (e.g., HIV patients) have a 10% risk per year of developing active TB. Antibiotic resistance is a growing problem in multidrug-resistant TB.

    a. Patients with active pulmonary or laryngeal TB should **postpone elective surgery** until the patient is no longer infectious.

    b. If patients with diagnosed or suspected TB require **urgent or emergent procedures**, measures must be taken to minimize the exposure of other patients and HCWs.

        1. HCWs should wear a fit-tested **N95 mask**.

        2. A **bacterial filter** with an efficiency rating of >95% for particle sizes of 0.3 μm should be placed in the anesthesia circuit. This should be routine practice as we often learn in retrospect that a patient has a respiratory infectious disease.

        3. Keep in mind that the operating room is kept positive pressure in relation to the surrounding corridors to minimize the risk of surgical site infections. Select an OR room in the presence of the fewest patients and personnel and an OR with highest number of air exchanges per hour (preferably >12). Commercially

TABLE 38.3	Microorganisms That Necessitate Airborne Precautions

Mycobacterium tuberculosis: in any patient with pulmonary symptoms; in HIV+ patient with extrapulmonary symptoms	Varicella virus: in any patient with chickenpox; in immunocompromised patients with herpes zoster; or if disseminated
Measles virus (rubeola)	Variola (smallpox)
SARS virus (severe acute respiratory syndrome)	Influenza A/subtype H5N1 (avian influenza)
Ebola, Lassa, Marburg viruses (hemorrhagic fevers)	

available portable negative pressure containment units with HEPA air filtration can be used to transform an OR into an airborne isolation room.

4. The patients should be recovered in a negative pressure room. If no such room is available in the postanesthesia care unit, consideration should be given to recovering the patient in the OR.

5. The OR should be kept vacant until a 99.9% turnover of air has occurred. This time will vary depending on the number of air exchanges per hour.

E. Immunocompromised Patients

Immunocompromised patients are frequently seen in the perioperative setting and are at increased risk of developing infection. Immunocompromise has many etiologies, including immunosuppressive therapy (i.e., bone marrow transplant and solid organ transplant patients), burns, corticosteroids, malnutrition, HIV infection, and critical illness. The specific defects in the immune system determine what type of infection is likely to develop. For example, patients with a deficiency in T-cell production are more likely to succumb to viral infections, whereas those who are neutropenic are more likely to develop bacterial infections.

1. Neutropenic precautions—Neutropenia is defined as an absolute neutrophil count (ANC) <500 cells/mm^3 or the anticipation that the ANC will reach that level within 48 hours. Neutropenia most commonly occurs in the setting of leukemia, chemotherapy, or bone marrow transplantation. Patients on neutropenic precautions should be placed in a positive pressure room (room pressure positive relative to surrounding areas) with HEPA filtration. The room door should be closed at all times. Patient should wear a N95 mask or powered air purifying respirator (PAPR) when being transported from the room.

2. Hematopoietic stem cell transplantation patients require additional precautions in order to prevent invasive environmental fungal infections such as aspergillosis. Caregivers should wear gloves and mask when caring for these patients. Patients should be placed in rooms with HEPA filtration of air incoming into patient's room, positive room air pressure relative to corridors, seals to prevent flow of air from the outside, ventilation systems that provide at least 12 air exchanges per hour, and anterooms to promote the appropriate air balance relative to the corridor. There should be dust control measures, and flowers and plants should be prohibited in patient rooms. Patients should wear a N95 mask or PAPR when being transported from the room.

3. Lung transplant patients in their first year posttransplant or who are receiving T-cell-depleting therapies should be placed in a HEPA-filtered, positive pressure room with the door closed. HCWs should wear gloves, gown, and surgical mask when entering the room. Patients should wear an N95 mask or PAPR when being transported from the room.

VI. DURATION OF ISOLATION PRECAUTIONS

For most infectious diseases, the natural history of the infection, including patterns of persistence and shedding of infectious materials, is well known. However, viral shedding can continue for a prolonged period of time (weeks to months) in immunocompromised patients. Therefore, the duration of precautions in these patients may be prolonged. For certain diseases, such as diphtheria and respiratory syncytial virus, precautions should remain in effect until testing results document eradication of the pathogen. On the other hand, certain MDROs, such as MRSA and VRE, may persist and become part of the patient's normal flora even after adequate treatment of an infection. Thus, patients infected or colonized with MRSA, VRE, and multidrug-resistant gram-negative bacilli are assumed to be colonized permanently and should be placed on contact precautions on every hospitalization. See earlier for information about the duration of isolation precautions in the case of *C. difficile*. Consult with facility infection control personnel regarding the duration of precautions for other transmission-based organisms.

VII. DISCONTINUATION OF ISOLATION PRECAUTIONS

Patients on contact precautions experience decreased patient–provider interaction leading to possible delays in care and decreased quality of care, increased symptoms of depression and anxiety, and decreased patient satisfaction with care. From an institutional perspective, the need of contact precautions can lead to decreased bed availability and delays in bed assignment because of cohorting requirements. It is known that MRSA and VRE colonization can clear spontaneously. There are no national guidelines regarding when or how contact precautions for MRSA/VRE may be discontinued, though most institutions have local guidelines. Active screening for clearance of colonization of MRSA results in a higher frequency of discontinuation of MRSA contact precautions.

VIII. SURVEILLANCE

Surveillance of nosocomial infections allows for the identification of particular nosocomial and non-nosocomial pathogens, and the detection of epidemics and outbreaks. In addition, surveillance cultures are important tools for detecting patients who are colonized with organisms that require isolation precautions to prevent transmission, for the early identification and control of outbreaks, and for identifying increases in the rates of resistant bacteria. Routine surveillance practices have been found to be essential in the reduction of multidrug-resistant pathogens such as MRSA and VRE and certain strains of *A. baumannii* and *Enterobacter aerogenes*. Routine surveillance also decreases hospital-acquired infections such as urinary tract infections, ventilator-associated pneumonia, surgical site infections, and central line–associated bloodstream infections. Surveillance methods can be targeted to areas with high-risk patients (e.g., the intensive care unit), but for certain epidemiologically important organisms (MRSA and VRE), it may be preferable to perform surveillance facility-wide. At our institution, a nasal swab for MRSA and a rectal swab for VRE are performed at the time of admission in all ICUs, hospital wards with immunosuppressed patients, and on other selected wards that have had two or more positive healthcare-associated infections within 2 weeks. Depending on results of surveillance cultures, patients can be placed on the proper type of isolation precautions, and the data can be used to track clusters or outbreaks of certain microorganisms. Weekly surveillance cultures should be considered for hospitalized patients at high risk for MRSA or VRE carriage because of ward location, antibiotic usage, underlying disease, or duration of stay.

Suggested Readings

Ellingson K, Haas JP, Aiello AE, et al. Strategies to prevent healthcare-associated infections through hand hygiene. *Infect Control Hosp Epidemiol* 2014;35:937–960.

Gaspard P, Eschbach E, Gunther D, et al. Methicillin-resistant *Staphylococcus aureus* contamination of healthcare workers' uniforms in long-term care facilities. *J Hosp Infect* 2009;71:170–175.

Gordin FM, Schultz ME, Huber R, et al. Reduction in nosocomial transmission of drug-resistant bacteria after introduction of an alcohol-based handrub. *Infect Control Hosp Epidemiol* 2005;26:650–653.

Huang GKL, Stewardson AJ, Grayson ML. Back to basics: hand hygiene and isolation. *Curr Opin Infect Dis* 2014;27:379–389.

Mathai E, Allegranzi B, Kilpatrick C, et al. Prevention and control of healthcare-associated infections through improved hand hygiene. *Indian J Med Microbiol* 2010;28:100–106.

Morgan DJ, Diekema DJ, Sepkowitz K, et al. Adverse outcomes associated with contact precautions: a review of the literature. *Am J Infect Control* 2009;37:85–93.

Muto CA, Jernigan JA, Ostrowsky BE, et al. SHEA guideline for preventing nosocomial transmission of multidrug-resistant strains of *Staphylococcus aureus* and *Enterococcus*. *Infect Control Hosp Epidemiol* 2003;24:362–386.

Rutala WA, Weber DJ. Disinfection and sterilization in healthcare facilities: what clinicians need to know. *Clin Infect Dis* 2004;39:702–709.

Shenoy ES, Kim J, Rosenberg ES, et al. Discontinuation of contact precautions for methicillin-resistant *Staphylococcus aureus*: a randomized controlled trial comparing passive and active screening with culture and polymerase chain reaction. *Clin Infect Dis* 2013;57:176–184.

Siegel JD, Rhinehart E, Jackson M, et al. 2007 Guideline for Isolation Precautions: Preventing Transmission of Infectious Agents in Healthcare Settings. Healthcare Infection Control Practices Advisory Committee, Centers for Disease Control; 2007. Available at: http://www.cdc.gov/hicpac/pdf/isolation/Isolation2007.pdf. Accessed January 20, 2015.

Stackhouse RA, Beers R, Brown D, et al; the ASA committee on Occupational Health Task Force on Infection Control. *Recommendations for Infection Control for the Practice of Anesthesiology*. 3rd ed. Available at: http://www.asahq.org/For-Members/Standards-Guidelines-and-Statements.aspx. Accessed February 28, 2015.

The Hospital Infection Control Practices Advisory Committee, Centers for Disease Control and Prevention, Public Health Service, U.S. Department of Health and Human Services. Guideline for isolation precautions in hospitals: Part II. Recommendations for isolation precautions in hospitals. *Am J Infect Control* 1996;24:32–52.

Van Kleef E, Green N, Goldenberg SD, et al. Excess length of stay and mortality due to *Clostridium difficile* infection: a multi-state modelling approach. *J Hosp Infect* 2014;88:213–217.

39 Healthcare-Associated Infections

Erin J. Levering and Jean Kwo

I. INTRODUCTION

Healthcare-associated infections (HAIs) are a major source of morbidity and mortality in the United States. In acute care hospitals in the United States, on any given day, about 1 patient out of 25 carries some form of HAI, and more than half of HAIs occur outside of the intensive care unit. These HAIs include surgical site infections (SSIs), catheter-associated urinary tract infections (CAUTIs), central line–associated bloodstream infections (CLABSIs), and ventilator-associated pneumonia (VAP). The most frequent organisms causing HAIs are coagulase-negative staphylococci, *Staphylococcus aureus*, *Enterococcus* species, *Candida* species, *Escherichia coli*, *Pseudomonas aeruginosa*, *Klebsiella pneumoniae*, *Enterobacter species*, *Acinetobacter baumannii*, and *Klebsiella oxytoca*. Of concern, up to 16% of HAIs are caused by antimicrobial-resistant pathogens, the most common being methicillin-resistant *S. aureus* (MRSA), vancomycin-resistant *Enterococcus faecium* (VRE), extended-spectrum β-lactamases and carbapenem-resistant pathogens. The detection, prevention, and reduction of HAIs are a top priority of hospital infection control programs and governmental agencies such as the Centers for Disease Control and Prevention (CDC).

II. SURGICAL SITE INFECTIONS

Careful attention to sterile surgical technique and the appropriate timing and dosing of perioperative antibiotics remain the most important measures in preventing SSIs, which is the most common nosocomial infection among postoperative patients.

A. Definition

The CDC defines SSI as an infection that occurs at or near a surgical site within 30 days of the surgical procedure, or within 90 days if hardware was implanted. The site can be incisional (superficial or deep) or related to the organ/space and involve any part of the anatomy that may have been incised, shifted, or manipulated during the procedure.

B. Diagnosis of SSI

The diagnosis of SSI can be made from any of the following criteria: purulent drainage from operative site, positive culture obtained from surgical site that was closed primarily, the surgeon's diagnosis of infection, or a surgical site that requires reopening.

C. Classification of Wounds

Classification of wounds based on the definition from the CDC National Healthcare Safety Network and Healthcare Infection Control Practice Advisory Committee:

1. Clean wounds arise from operations done electively and atraumatically, neither with no inflammation or break in sterile technique. In addition, the respiratory, biliary, gastrointestinal (GI), nor genitourinary (GU) tracts were entered during the procedure. These wounds are associated with a less than 2% risk of infection.

2. **Clean-contaminated** wounds are from urgent or emergent cases in which the respiratory, biliary, GI or GU tracts were entered electively with minimal spillage of contents, and without encountering urine or bile. There is a less than 4% risk of infection.

3. **Contaminated** wounds are from procedures in which there was gross spillage from the GI tract, infected bile or urine was encountered, there was a major break in sterile technique, penetrating trauma <4 hours old, or chronic, open wounds that are to be grafted or covered. There is an approximately 20% risk of infection.

4. **Dirty** wounds arise from operations in which there was purulent inflammation (i.e., an abscess). In addition, this encompasses pre-operative perforation of the respiratory, biliary, GI or GU tract, or penetrating trauma >4 hours old. These wounds carry an approximately 40% risk of infection.

D. **Risk Factors for the Development of SSI**

1. **Systemic factors:** diabetes, steroid use, age, obesity, malnutrition, recent surgery, massive transfusion, and American Society of Anesthesiologists physical status class 3 or 4.

   a. **Local factors:** foreign body, electrocautery, epinephrine injection, prior irradiation, wound drains, and hair removal with razor (preferable to remove hair using depilatory or clippers).

E. **Prevention of SSI**

1. **Perioperative considerations**

   Hair should be removed only if necessary and done immediately before the operation, preferably with electric clippers. Serum blood glucose should be controlled perioperatively. Hyperglycemia (>200 mg/dL) has been associated with increased SSI risk. Normothermia should be maintained intraoperatively and postoperatively, because a core temperature of <36° Celsius is associated with increased SSI risk.

2. **Operating rooms** should be maintained with a positive pressure relative to corridors and adjacent areas to prevent airflow from the "less clean" areas. There should be a minimum of 15 air changes per hour, of which at least 3 should be fresh air. Operating room doors should be kept closed, except as needed for passage of equipment, personnel, and the patient.

3. Selection of the appropriate **perioperative antibiotic** requires consideration of the most likely involved pathogen and ability for adequate tissue penetration at the site of surgery.

   a. Antibiotics should be **dosed within 60 minutes** prior to incision in order to achieve the appropriate tissue concentration. In the case of antibiotics with longer infusion times, such as vancomycin or fluoroquinolones, doses should be given within 60 to 120 minutes prior to the incision.

      1. **Organisms by wound type.** The predominant organisms seen in clean cases are skin flora, including streptococcal species, *Staphylococcus aureus*, and coagulase-negative staphylococci. The predominant organisms seen in clean-contaminated cases: gram-negative rods, enterococci, and skin flora, as above. Finally, in the case of procedures that involve entering a viscus, organisms reflect the flora of that viscus or nearby mucosal surfaces, and infections are usually polymicrobial.

      2. For a list of common types of **organisms by surgical site**, see Table 39.1.

      3. **Cefazolin** is the most widely used perioperative antibiotic with proven efficacy for antimicrobial prophylaxis. It is safe, carries a low cost, possesses a desirable duration of action, and is effective

| TABLE 39.1 | Most Likely Pathogen in Surgical Site Infections by Operative Site |

Operative Site	Likely Pathogen(s)
Placement of graft, prosthesis, or implant	*Staphylococcus aureus*, coagulase-negative staphylococci
Cardiac surgery	*S. aureus*, coagulase-negative staphylococci
Neurosurgery	*S. aureus*, coagulase-negative staphylococci
Breast	*S. aureus*, coagulase-negative staphylococci
Ophthalmic	*S. aureus*, coagulase-negative staphylococci, streptococci, gram-negative bacilli
Orthopedic	*S. aureus*, coagulase-negative staphylococci, gram-negative bacilli
Thoracic	*S. aureus*, coagulase-negative staphylococci, *Streptococcus pneumoniae*, gram-negative bacilli
Vascular	*S. aureus*, coagulase-negative staphylococci
Appendectomy	Gram-negative bacilli, anaerobes
Biliary	Gram-negative bacilli, anaerobes
Colorectal	Gram-negative bacilli, anaerobes
Gastroduodenal	Gram-negative bacilli, streptococci, oropharyngeal anaerobes
Head and neck	*S. aureus*, streptococci, oropharyngeal anaerobes
Obstetric and gynecologic	Gram-negative bacilli, enterococci, group B streptococci, anaerobes
Urological	Gram-negative bacilli

against streptococci, methicillin-sensitive staphylococci, and some gram-negative organisms. Alternatives to penicillins include vancomycin and clindamycin. However, in these cases, antimicrobials with activity against gram-negative organisms must sometimes be added (i.e., gentamicin, fluoroquinolones, or aztreonam).

b. An **additional dose** should be considered if the procedure lasts for greater than 3 hours, for longer than two half-lives of the drug, or there is more than 1,500 mL of blood loss. Special consideration should be taken in situations where the half-life may be shortened (i.e., extensive burns) or prolonged (i.e., renal insufficiency). Further dose adjustments and weight-based dosing must be employed in obese patients.

c. The use of perioperative antibiotics is considered prophylaxis for clean and clean-contaminated cases. The use of antimicrobial agents is considered therapeutic treatment of the presumed infection in contaminated and dirty cases.

d. **Duration** of antimicrobial prophylaxis should be less than 24 hours.

4. ***Staphylococcus aureus* decolonization**

Patients colonized with MRSA have an increased risk for SSI with MRSA compared with noncarriers. There lacks a consensus regarding decolonization of patients with known MRSA, because some studies have shown it to be neither beneficial nor cost-effective. However, certain high-risk surgical subgroups (e.g., cardiac surgery, joint replacements, or spinal procedures involving implants) may benefit from decolonization. Decolonization methods in past clinical trials have varied and include intranasal mupirocin with or without the addition of chlorhexidine bathing.

III. CATHETER-ASSOCIATED URINARY TRACT INFECTIONS (CAUTI)

Urinary tract infections (UTIs) are the most frequent nosocomial infections, and 70% to 80% of these are associated with an indwelling catheter. Although most individual UTIs do not cause severe morbidity and mortality, the cumulative burden of UTIs on the medical system is large. CAUTIs can lead to urosepsis, which is the second most frequent type of nosocomial bloodstream infection. Finally, asymptomatic bacteriuria often leads to inappropriate and costly laboratory testing, as well as treatment with antibiotics, which can increase the prevalence of antimicrobial prevalence, resistance, and *Clostridium difficile* in the hospital setting.

A. **Risk factors** for the development of CAUTIs: The duration of the indwelling catheter is the most important risk in the development of infection. In addition, risks include female sex, advanced age, and the failure to maintain a closed catheter to drainage bag system.

B. **Detection of CAUTI.** The typical signs and symptoms used to recognize UTIs may not be present in the patient with a catheter. In addition, many postoperative patients may not be able to accurately report symptoms of UTI because of factors such as sedation, delirium, location of surgical incisions, and confounding pain or other symptoms. The most common presentation is fever with a positive urine culture result; however, this definition lacks specificity because of the high number of patients with bacteriuria, which is usually asymptomatic. Diagnosis usually requires a growth of at least 10^6 CFU/mL of an organism from a urine specimen that was collected aseptically. Although lower quantitative counts can occasionally represent true infection in symptomatic individuals, this usually represents colonization of the drainage system.

C. **Methods of prevention.** For a list of strategies to prevent CAUTI, both those shown to be effective and ineffective, see Table 39.2. The implementation of a facility-wide CAUTI prevention program has been shown to decrease the frequency of unnecessary catheterization and CAUTIs. Further, a facility-established list (Table 39.3) of criteria for the acceptable uses of indwelling catheters should be readily available and adhered to.

D. In the case of **neurogenic bladder**, avoidance of catheterization, if possible, is preferred. If bladder drainage must be assisted, clean-intermittent catheterization is preferable to leaving an indwelling catheter.

IV. CENTRAL LINE-ASSOCIATED BLOOD STREAM INFECTION (CLABSI)

Central line–associated bloodstream infection has historically been associated with ICU patients because of the fact that they are often placed in emergency situations, they are accessed very frequently, and they are needed for extended periods of time. However, the majority of CLABSIs actually occur in patients outside of the ICU setting, such as in the perioperative setting, hemodialysis areas, and oncology units. CLABSI has been associated with increased length of hospital stay and significant increases in cost.

A. **Risk factors** for the development of CLABSIs, see Table 39.4.

B. Prevention of CLABSIs depends largely on the education of clinicians inserting the catheters and on those caring for catheters on a daily basis. Standardized protocols and checklists to ensure the appropriateness of catheter insertion, the daily reassessment of catheter need, the maintenance of aseptic technique on insertion, and the proper daily care of the catheter and catheter site have been demonstrated to decrease CLABSI rates and should be made available at all acute care facilities. Other measures recommended for the prevention of CLABSIs include:

1. Have a central line cart and kits with all supplies needed for inserting a central line available.

| TABLE 39.2 | Strategies for the Prevention of CAUTI |

Effective	Not Effective
Avoidance of the placement of indwelling catheter unless deemed absolutely necessary by facility-established criteria	Systemic antibiotic prophylaxis
Aseptic technique at insertion and the avoidance of trauma at insertion by using appropriate lubricant	Irrigation of bladder and collecting system with an antiseptic solution
Properly secure the indwelling catheter after insertion to prevent movement and urethral traction/trauma	Antimicrobial coated catheters
Keep a closed system at all times	Daily antiseptic perineal cleaning
Replace the catheter and collecting system when breaks in aseptic technique, disconnection, or leakage occur	Antiseptic solution added to drainage bag
Maintain unobstructed drainage of urine from the bladder to the collection bag, with the bag positioned below the level of the bladder at all times	
Use the needleless collection port for collecting samples of fresh urine, taking care to disinfect the port prior to attaching a sterile syringe	
Limit duration of indwelling catheter and reassess catheter need on a daily basis by medical and nursing teams	
Implementation of a facility-wide CAUTI prevention program	

| TABLE 39.3 | Examples of Appropriate Uses of Indwelling Urinary Catheters |

In the perioperative setting for certain surgical procedures, i.e., urologic or gynecologic surgeries, diuretics given during procedure, cases with large volume of blood/bodily fluid loss and resuscitation, procedures during which the monitoring of urine output is necessary

A patient who is in shock and/or requiring vasopressor agents

A patient who is sedated with a score on the Richmond Agitation Sedation Scale of 2 or less

To assist in the management of chronic pressure wounds or ulcers that may be affected by urinary incontinence

In the management of acute urinary retention or obstruction

For comfort in the care of end-of-life patients

TABLE 39.4	Risk Factors in the Development of CLABSIs
Prolonged hospitalization prior to central line placement	Prolonged duration of indwelling central line and excessive manipulation of the catheter
Microbial colonization at the insertion site or at the catheter port	Catheter selection site: subclavian lines have the lowest risk of infection, followed by internal jugular. Femoral lines carry the highest risk
Neutropenia	Total parenteral nutrition

2. Strict adherence to aseptic techniques including hand hygiene before insertion and full barrier precaution (cap, mask, gown, sterile gloves, and a sterile full-body drape).

3. A clinician designated as an "observer" should monitor the procedure for breaks in sterile technique.

4. Choose a catheter with the minimum number of ports needed, because multilumen catheters are associated with a higher risk of infection than single-lumen catheters.

5. Use ultrasound guidance for the placement of internal jugular lines.

6. Use chlorhexidine–alcohol solution (containing more than 0.5% chlorhexidine) for topical antisepsis of skin prior to the line placement. The solution must be allowed to dry completely prior to skin puncture.

7. Use either sterile gauze or a sterile, transparent, semipermeable dressing to cover the catheter site. Transparent dressings permit moisture to escape and are associated with lower rates of skin colonization and catheter-related infection.

8. Scrub the catheter ports with antiseptic solution to reduce microbial contamination prior to accessing. Use mechanical friction lasting no less than 5 seconds.

9. Change tubing and needleless access devices every 96 hours.

10. Antimicrobial- and antiseptic-impregnated catheters can be considered in special circumstances. Both minocycline/rifampin– and chlorhexidine/silver sulfadiazine–impregnated catheters lead to a reduction in CLABSIs. Other products that may decrease infection rates include chlorhexidine-containing dressings and antiseptic-containing caps and covers.

11. Do not use peripherally inserted central catheters (PICCs) as a way to reduce CLABSIs, because PICCs hold similar infection rates to central lines in the internal jugular and the subclavian veins.

12. Prophylactic systemic antibiotics are not recommended to reduce CLABSI risk.

13. Routine changing of central lines, either by a new insertion or guidewire exchange, is not recommended. Rather, daily evaluation for the necessity of the central line and assessment of the patient for catheter infection is warranted.

14. Guidewire exchange technique can be utilized to replace a malfunctioning nontunneled catheter if there is no evidence of infection. Catheter replacement over a guidewire is associated with less discomfort and a significantly lower rate of mechanical complications as compared to another catheter insertion.

V. VENTILATOR-ASSOCIATE PNEUMONIA

Ventilator-associated pneumonia is defined as an infection in the lungs that occurs 48 or more hours after tracheal intubation in mechanically ventilated patients. Data have shown that anywhere between 5% and 20% of ventilated patients develop nosocomial pneumonia. A VAP is defined by clinical, radiographic, and microbiology data. However, these criteria can often be subjective, causing the rates of VAP diagnosis and treatment to vary among clinicians.

A. **Prevention of VAP.** See Table 39.5 for a list of practices that are widely recommended in the prevention of VAP, in that they have been shown to decrease number of ventilator days, length of hospital stay, mortality, and/or costs with little risk of harm.

B. Other interventions that may be beneficial in the reduction of VAP:

1. Oral care with chlorhexidine can reduce pneumonia rate by 10% to 30%, but has no clear impact on duration of mechanical ventilator, length of hospital stay, or mortality.

2. Use of prophylactic probiotics has been associated with lower VAP rates. However, they should not be used in immunosuppressed patients and those with a risk of gut translocation. Data on probiotic use are equivocal on length of hospital stay and mortality.

3. Silver-coated endotracheal tubes (ETTs) have been shown to decrease the incidence of VAP by as much as 30%, but have not shown to have any impact on duration of mechanical ventilation, hospital length of stay, and mortality.

4. Use of a **mucus shaver**, an inflatable catheter for the removal of mucus and secretions from the interior surface of the ETT, has been shown to decrease bacterial colonization and biofilm formation on the ETT.

5. **Subglottic secretion drainage** is associated with decreased VAP rate, decreased ICU length of stay, decreased duration of mechanical ventilation, and increased time to first episode of VAP.

6. **Kinetic beds and prone positioning** have not been shown to reduce duration of mechanical ventilation and mortality.

TABLE 39.5	Recommendations for the Prevention of Ventilator-Associated Pneumonia	
Intervention		**Quality of Evidence**
• Avoidance of intubation and the use of noninvasive ventilation in the appropriate circumstances		High
• Minimize sedation, perform daily spontaneous awakening trials once daily for patients without contraindications		Moderate
• Perform spontaneous breathing trials once daily		High
• Early physical therapy and mobilization		Moderate
• Minimize pooling of secretions above the cuff, use endotracheal tubes with subglottic secretion drainage devices as intubation is expected to last more than 48 h		Moderate
• Elevate head of the bed to 30–45 degrees		Low
• Ventilator circuit: change only if soiled or malfunctioning, and follow CDC guidelines for sterilization and disinfection of equipment		Moderate

7. **Early tracheostomy** had no impact on VAP rates, length of hospital stay, or mortality in several meta-analyses.

8. **Monitoring gastric residual volumes** was not more effective than simply monitoring for vomiting and oral regurgitation in terms of VAP rates, length of mechanical ventilation, and mortality.

VI. CHLORHEXIDINE

Chlorhexidine is a topical antiseptic with a wide range of activity against gram-positive bacteria (including *S. aureus* and *Enterococcus* species), gram-negative bacteria, some viruses, and molds, but has no sporicidal activity. Chlorhexidine has residual antimicrobial activity on patients' skin for up to 24 hours and may also help prevent secondary environmental contamination.

A. **Preoperative use.** Chlorhexidine bathing, showering, and scrubs in the preoperative settings have been shown to significantly decrease the burden of microbes found on the skin. However, there is no clear evidence demonstrating a reduction in SSIs with the use of chlorhexidine bathing versus placebo or regular soap. The local application of chlorhexidine to the surgical site immediately prior to surgery achieves a greater reduction in skin flora and has a longer duration of action than povidone–iodine, but no clear data demonstrating a reduction in SSI. Although topical antiseptics are effective in reducing skin microorganisms, they are not effective in eliminating bacteria from hair follicles or sebaceous glands.

B. **Daily use.** Chlorhexidine bathing on a daily basis has been associated with a decrease in the transmission of multidrug-resistant organisms (especially MRSA and VRE) and a decrease in the number of hospital-acquired bloodstream infections in intensive care units and bone marrow transplantation units. Specifically, daily bathing with chlorhexidine was associated with fewer catheter-related fungal bloodstream infections and gram-positive bacteremias. However, concern regarding the development of nosocomial pathogens resistant to disinfectants like chlorhexidine has limited the wider use of these agents for daily bathing, and more studies are needed to evaluate this possibility. The use of chlorhexidine plus mupirocin has been effective in reducing colonization of MRSA in patients and, thus, the incidence of nosocomial MRSA infection.

Suggested Readings

Bratzler DW, Dellinger EP, Olsen KM, et al. Clinical practice guidelines for antimicrobial prophylaxis in surgery. *Am J Health Syst Pharm* 2013;70:195–283.

Chlebicki MP, Safdar N, O'Horo JC, et al. Preoperative chlorhexidine shower or bath for prevention of surgical site infection: a meta-analysis. *Am J Infect Control* 2013;41(2):167–173.

Climo MW, Yokoe DS, Warren DK, et al. The effect of daily chlorhexidine bathing on hospital-acquired infection. *N Engl J Med* 2013;368:533–542.

Ducel G, Fabry J, Nicolle L, eds. *Prevention of Hospital Acquired Infections: A Practical Guide*. 2nd ed. World Health Organization, Department of Communicable Disease, Surveillance and Response; 2002. Retrieved from http://www.who.int/csr/resources/publications/whocdscsreph200212.pdf. Accessed March 10, 2015.

Hidron AI, Edwards JR, Patel J, et al. Antimicrobial-resistant pathogens associated with healthcare-associated infections: annual summary data reported to the National Healthcare Safety Network at the Centers for Disease Control and Prevention, 2006–2007. *Infect Control Hosp Epidemiol* 2008;29:996–1011.

Holzheimer RG, Mannick JA, eds. *Surgical Treatment: Evidence-Based and Problem-Oriented*. Munich, Germany: Zuckschwerdt; 2001.

Klompas M, Branson R, Eichenwald EC. Strategies to prevent ventilator-associated pneumonia in acute care hospitals: 2014 update. *Infect Control Hosp Epidemiol* 2014;35(8):915–936.

Lo E, Nicolle LE, Coffin SE, et al. Strategies to prevent catheter-associated urinary tract infections in acute care hospitals: 2014 update. *Infect Control Hosp Epidemiol* 2014;35:464–479.

Mangram AJ, Horan TC, Pearson ML, et al. Guideline for the prevention of surgical site infection. Hospital Infections Program National Center for Infectious Diseases Centers for Disease Control and Prevention Public Health Service US Department of Health and Human Services. *Infect Control Hosp Epidemiol* 1999;20:247–278.

Marshall J, Mermel L, Fakih M, et al. Strategies to prevent central line–associated bloodstream infections in acute care hospitals: 2014 update. *Infect Control Hosp Epidemiol* 2014;35:S89–107.

Martinez-Resendez MF, Garza-Gonzalez E, Mendoza-Olazaran S, et al. Impact of daily chlorhexidine baths and hand hygiene compliance on nosocomial infection rates in critically ill patients. *Am J Infect Control* 2014;42:713–717.

Milstone AM, Passaretti CL, Perl TM. Chlorhexidine: expanding the armamentarium for infection control and prevention. *Clin Infect Dis* 2008;46:274–281.

Pronovost P, Needham D, Berenholtz S, et al. An intervention to decrease catheter-related bloodstream infections in the ICU. *N Engl J Med* 2006;355:2725–2732.

Note: Page numbers followed by "*f*" indicate figure; those followed by "*t*" indicate table.